Pediatric Tumors: Immunological and Molecular Markers

Editor

John T. Kemshead, B.Sc., Ph.D.
Head, ICRF Oncology Laboratory
Imperial Cancer Research Fund
London, England

CRC Press, Inc.
Boca Raton, Florida

Library of Congress Cataloging-in-Publication Data

Pediatric tumors : immunological and molecular markers / editor, John
T. Kemshead.
p. cm.
Includes bibliographies and index.
ISBN 0-8493-6752-2
1. Tumors in children. 2. Tumor markers--Diagnostic use.
3. Immunodiagnosis. [1. Genetic Marker. 2. Neoplasms--diagnosis.
3. Neoplasms--in infancy and childhood.] I. Kemshead, John T.
[DNLM: QZ 241 P3713]
RC281.C4P46 1989
618.92'9940758--dc19
DNLM/DLC
for Library of Congress 88-7362
CIP

This book represents information obtained from authentic and highly regarded sources. Reprinted material is quoted with permission, and sources are indicated. A wide variety of references are listed. Every reasonable effort has been made to give reliable data and information, but the author and the publisher cannot assume responsibility for the validity of all materials or for the consequences of their use.

Direct all inquiries to CRC Press, Inc., 2000 Corporate Blvd., N.W., Boca Raton, Florida, 33431.

International Standard Book Number 0-8493-6752-2

Library of Congress Card Number 88-7362
Printed in the United States

PREFACE

Review of the field of pediatric oncology shows that major advances in the treatment of some childhood malignancies have been made over the last twenty years. This change has been brought about by the introduction of more effective combination chemotherapy and radiotherapy. Treatment protocols have also become more effective as they have become tailored to particular tumor types. Our understanding of these malignancies has become considerably more sophisticated, particularly with the application of immunological and molecular approaches to tumor diagnosis. This volume documents some of these innovative approaches to tumor diagnosis and also reviews how these are being applied to the *in vivo* diagnosis and therapy of childhood tumors.

Monoclonal antibodies have made a major impact in aiding in the diagnosis of relatively anaplastic tumors, difficult to classify by conventional histopathological criteria. Lymphoid tumors can be accurately subclassified and antibodies used to assist in the differential diagnosis of the small round cell tumors of childhood: namely, lymphoblastic leukemia/lymphoma, neuroblastoma, rhabdomyosarcoma, and Ewing's sarcoma. These studies have been extended to radioimmunoscintigraphy and targeted radiation therapy for neuroblastoma; both topics are reviewed in this volume.

Cytogenetics, molecular cytogenetics, and molecular biology are also playing an important role in our understanding of pediatric malignancies. It is these tumors that are often responsible for demonstrating important relationships between oncogene amplification and malignancy, and further work in this area will almost certainly reveal valuable information regarding the histogenesis of childhood tumors.

The contributors to this volume represent research workers actively studying different aspects of childhood malignancy. They are all experts in their fields, and have attempted to clearly review the current state of our knowledge in their particular areas. In addition, they have speculated as to where the work may lead in the future in furthering our understanding of childhood malignancies.

THE EDITOR

John T. Kemshead, Ph.D., is head of the Imperial Cancer Research Fund Oncology Laboratory at the Institute of Child Health in London. In addition, he holds an Honorary Senior Lectureship in the Department of Haematology/Oncology in the Institute, a Post graduate center of the University of London.

Dr. Kemshead graduated with a B.Sc. in Biochemistry from King's College, London in 1979, after completing his 2MB examination at Westminster Medical School. He went on to complete a Ph.D. in Natural Sciences at King's College undertaking studies on the degradation of abnormal proteins in *Escherichia coli.* After undertaking a Post Doctoral Fellowship in Immunology at the National Institute for Medical Research in Mill Hill, Dr. Kemshead joined the Imperial Cancer Research Fund in 1978. He was given his current position in 1982 specializing in innovative approaches to the diagnosis and therapy of pediatric tumors.

Dr. Kemshead has been involved in establishing a collaborative European group to study neuroblastoma, namely, the European Neuroblastoma Study Group. In addition, he is a trustee to the Neuroblastoma Society in the UK and a Scientific advisor to the Forbeck Foundation in the U.S. In 1987 he was elected to the Royal Society of Science in Norway, following his work with Professor J. Ugelstad on the immunomagnetic separation of tumor cells from bone marrow.

Dr. Kemshead has been invited to lecture extensively on his field and has published over 100 papers on topics relating to pediatric oncology. His current interests remain in the area of pediatric oncology, where his laboratory is extending its work to cover molecular aspects of this field as well as nuero-oncology.

CONTRIBUTORS

Stephen Paul Bourne, B.Sc.
Research Assistant
Brain Tumour Research Laboratory
Frenchay Hospital
Bristol, Avon, England

Nai-Kong V. Cheung, Ph.D.
Associate Member
Department of Pediatrics
Memorial Sloan Kettering Cancer Center
New York, New York

J. P. Clayton, Ph.D.
Doctor
Department of Microbiology
University of California
Los Angeles, California

Hugh B. Coakham, M.R.C.P.
Consultant Neurological Surgeon
Department of Neurosurgery
Frenchay Hospital
Bristol, Avon, England

John K. Cowell, Ph.D.
Honorary Lecturer
Department of Hematology and Oncology
Institute of Child Health
London, England

J. A. Garson
Oncology Laboratory
Institute of Child Health
London, England

Adrian Gee, Ph.D.
Research Scientist
Fenwal Scientific Affairs
Baxter Healthcare Corporation
Santa Ana, California

J. T. Kemshead, Ph.D.
Doctor and Head
Oncology Laboratory
Imperial Cancer Research Foundation
London, England

L. S. Lashford
Oncology Laboratory
Institute of Child Health
London, England

Floro Miraldi, Sc.D.
Professor
Department of Radiology
University Hospitals of Cleveland
Case Western Reserve University
Cleveland, Ohio

K. Patel, Ph.D.
Doctor
Oncology Laboratory
Imperial Cancer Research Foundation
London, England

John R. Pincott, M.D.
Group Director
Department of Pathology & Toxicology
Smith Kline & French Research Limited
Welwyn, Hertfordshire, England

W. Smith, Ph.D.
Postdoctoral Scientist
Department of Histopathology
University College Hospital Medical School
London, England

Paul M. Zeltzer, M. P.
Associate Professor
Brain Tumor Program
University of Southern California
Los Angeles, California

TABLE OF CONTENTS

Chapter 1

PATHOLOGY AND EPIDEMIOLOGY

John R. Pincott

TABLE OF CONTENTS

I. INTRODUCTION

The management of many adult and childhood tumors has been transformed in recent years. Part of this change has derived from improved accuracy of diagnosis which has allowed the more appropriate tailoring of therapeutic regimens. Consequently, the effectiveness of radiotherapy and combinations of potent chemotherapeutic agents has been enhanced while their concomitant toxicity has been minimized. As a result, the prognosis of many tumors has been improved and the quality of life of the patients bearing them enhanced.

An integral part of this diagnostic improvement has been a change in the approach to the histopathological assessment of the tumors. Refinements of classification with recognition of new tumor types and subtypes and the employment of more sensitive methods of diagnosis have all contributed to improved diagnostic precision, on which more effective treatment can be based.

Some of the methodological advances introduced in recent years have been the result of direct study of childhood tumors. Others, however, have stemmed from related fields such as adult oncology, from which techniques have been adapted, often with great effect.

One of the more subtle changes in the area of childhood tumor assessment which has, however, contributed significantly to these improvements is the pooling of knowledge and resources for a concerted effort to examine specific aspects of particular oncological problems. It has been recognized that for most pathologists, a childhood tumor is an uncommon occurrence, so that even a lifetime of experience will be an insufficient database to make a significant impact on clinical management. In addition, limitations on manpower and financial constraints have also encouraged a collaborative approach to this numerically relatively small, but clinically very important area. Hence, scientific and financial considerations have, exceptionally, tended to work towards the same logical end.

This pooling of knowledge and experience has particularly manifested itself in the creation of specialist centers for the treatment of tumors of childhood, and the establishment of multicenter collaborative studies between these groups, each designed to address a particular oncological issue or gather data on a specific tumor. An early consequence of this approach has been the classification of some of the more common tumors histopathologically in a manner which has proved to have demonstrably more clinical relevance. A particular advantage of this approach has been the recognition of classes of tumor which bear a particularly poor prognosis, and for which an especially intensive therapeutic regimen can therefore be justified. Just as important as these are the tumors which, despite past opinions to the contrary, systematic study has demonstrated to have an especially good prognosis. In these cases therapy can be minimized, thus improving the trauma to the child and reducing the risk of early and late sequelae of treatment.

Occurring independently of developments in approaches and organization of scientific investigation have been improvements and exciting innovations in the scientific techniques themselves. Many of these are based on existing methods, well proven over many years of use, but which utilize the techniques in a different way, or with added refinements to tailor them to specific diagnostic needs. In this regard, for example, the increasing use of fine needle aspiration cytology has, from the patient's viewpoint, made some histological diagnoses considerably less troublesome than an open biopsy, while for the physician it has provided a far speedier tissue diagnosis.

The method is, however, largely based on many years' experience in the established techniques of morphological assessment in the field of exfoliative cytology. Elsewhere, investigative techniques such as electron microscopy, long valued for the insight they have provided into the subcellular basis of pathological appearances, have developed through the stage of supporting diagnoses made primarily by traditional histological methods to a vital component of the pathologist's armamentarium in the laboratory investigation of tumors, requiring great skill, experience, and patience.

Within the science of histochemistry, progress has been made in recent years beyond the level of the use of "special stains" to characterize cells merely by cataloguing their staining characteristics. More advanced techniques are now utilized to identify individual cytoplasmic components and contents, such as enzymes, which permit not only observations on the functions of the cells, but also some deduction as to the histogenesis of the tumor.

Among the many techniques available for the investigation of tumors, immunohistology has probably made the greatest impact. Methods have been developed to identify both surface and cytoplasmic antigens which have considerably enhanced the identification and elucidation of histogenesis of tumor cells. In addition, the use of particular forms of fixation and proteolytic enzymes to "unmask" cytoplasmic antigens has allowed the application of some of these techniques to paraffin wax-embedded tissues. In turn, this has permitted immunohistology to be applied in diagnostic pathology laboratories with minimal disturbance of routine, and has also released much archive material for more detailed assessment. Unfortunately, surface antigens are, on the whole, less amenable to demonstration under these conditions, and tissues under investigation require to be processed separately, usually by frozen section or cytology from impressions of fresh tumor. Monoclonal antibodies to surface antigens are most effectively applied in this manner. They are highly specific, which makes them a very useful tool in the differential diagnosis of morphologically similar tumors. However, as antigen expression can vary considerably between tumors of the same type, and even between individual cells in the same tumor, it is a necessary precaution to employ monoclonal antibodies in panels, rather than individually for diagnostic purposes.

Other less widely used techniques may also be appropriate in the investigation of individual cases, and in some instances have been developed or differently applied in recent times to considerable effect. For example, observation of the differentiation and behavior of tumor cells in tissue culture can be time consuming and resource intensive, but in combination with other techniques (such as catecholamine fluorescence for the diagnosis of neuroblastoma or monoclonal antibodies for the differential diagnosis of small round cell tumors of childhood) can be very effective and specific. Cytogenetic examination can be of interest in particular areas, such as specific types of Wilms' tumors or retinoblastomas, though more for etiological and clinical genetic purposes than diagnostic. In the related areas of oncogene expression and amplification, however, there has been a recent upsurge in interest, though the diagnostic application and specificity of such techniques remain to be validated.

In conclusion, it should be said that a broad spectrum of histopathological methods is available for the diagnosis and classification of childhood tumors. Many of these are relatively recent innovations, and new developments are continually being applied to this field of study. For convenience, this variety of investigative techniques is presented as a sequence of separate fields of study, though in practice matters work out very differently.

It is usual in the process of diagnosis of a specific tumor for the techniques considered most appropriate to that case to be selected from each of the groups of investigations and applied in the order dictated by clinical circumstances, likely diagnosis and its differential diagnosis, as well as the availability of manpower and other resources. It is clear that for intelligent planning of these various studies and the setting of priorities, there must be close liaison between physician and pathologist.

It is also worth recording that many of the techniques described require preparation and planning to perform. Many investigations, particularly histochemical and immunohistological, can only be carried out on fresh, snap-frozen material, which require the advance preparation of a freezing mixture. Cytology on tumor imprints cannot be carried out if the specimen is plunged directly into formalin directly after resection or biopsy, and this act also considerably increases the difficulty of rapid diagnostic or specialist frozen section work. Good ultrastructural examination is best done on fresh, refrigerated glutaraldehyde which clearly requires to be prepared in advance.

Further, few laboratories have the resources to carry out all the investigations listed. In addition to the establishment of specialist centers for particular investigations, the need for close collaboration between physician and pathologist is also valuable in permitting advance arrangements to be made for transfer of the material in question to the laboratory where the required investigations will be undertaken.

The same considerations apply to the establishment of a central diagnostic registry where material may be sent for review, collation, or comparison. Collaboration between specialist centers of pediatric oncology in this manner considerably benefits the individual patient while speeding the accumulation of knowledge of particular tumors, especially those which occur infrequently.

II. COLLABORATIVE INVESTIGATIONS AND CLASSIFICATIONS

Despite the establishment of specialist centers dedicated to the diagnosis and treatment of childhood malignancies, the number of tumors of any particular type seen in an individual center is still small. This has been one of the main stimuli to the setting up of collaborative investigations between specialist centers and others, on a national and international basis.

One of the more successful collaborative ventures of this nature to have developed in recent years has been the National Wilms' Tumor Study in the U.S., where the pathology review mechanism has both catered for the cases entered into the study and functioned as a referral center for pathologists outside the group.[1] Pathology review of cases as part of this study led to the proposal of a classification of renal tumors in childhood[2] which has subsequently been the mainstay of not only the National Wilms' Tumor Study, but investigations of childhood renal tumors in many other countries.

One of the major achievements of this study was to draw attention to two distinct histological types of tumor, termed "favorable" and "unfavorable" according to their ultimate clinical prognosis (Figure 1). Although only 12% of the renal tumors were placed in the "unfavorable" category, they accounted for 52% of the deaths due to tumor.[2] The clinical relevance of this histopathological classification is emphasized by the fact that 98% of the children with "favorable histology" tumors survived two years, while only 39% of those with "unfavorable histology" tumors survived the same length of time.[3] The histological group classified as "unfavorable" included tumors demonstrating several different histological patterns, grouped into anaplastic and sarcomatous. The anaplastic, which Beckwith and Palmer observed tended to occur in older children, could contain the usual Wilms' tumor components of tubular differentiation, blastema and stroma, but in addition showed areas of marked pleomorphism. This anaplasia was described as focal when it occupied less than 10% of the tumor and diffuse if it was seen in an area greater than 10%. Anaplasia was found to be important in increasing both the relapse and the mortality rate, and the effect of its presence was greater in the diffuse than the focal form. It is interesting to note, however, in the context of a discussion of the value of multicenter collaborative studies, that the number of anaplastic tumors was still so small that there were insufficient cases to separate statistically the focal anaplastic from the diffuse. Consequently, only the presence or absence of anaplasia was noted in the final proposed classification, and this was regarded as sufficient to label the tumor as "unfavorable" histological type.

The sarcomatous renal tumors were subclassified into rhabdomyosarcomatoid, clear cell, and hyaline types. Patients with all three types of tumor had a poor prognosis, but unlike the anaplastic Wilms' tumors, more of the sarcomatous variety were found in younger children — approximately one in three of these tumors were found in children under 2 years old.

More recently however, the view has developed that these sarcomatous tumors are not likely to be variants of Wilms' tumors per se, even though they are primary tumors of renal

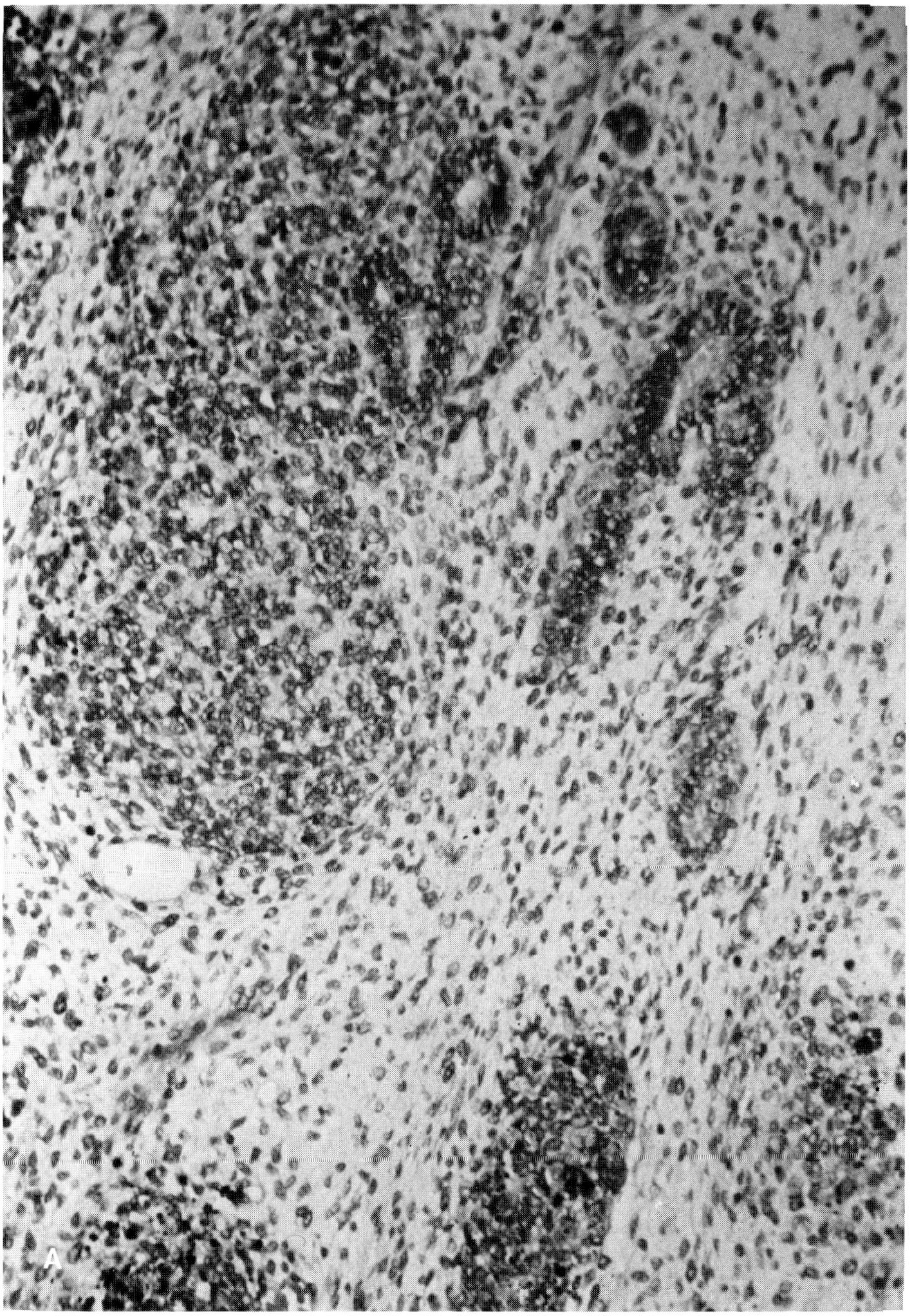

FIGURE 1. Wilms' tumor, (A) ''Favorable'' histological type comprises a trimorphic mixture of tubules, condensations of blastema, and more sparsely-cellular stroma. (H.E.; magnification × 200.) (B) A rhabdoid tumor which is an example of an ''unfavorable'' histological tumor type of the sarcomatous category. Tumor cells are monomorphic, of uniform size and have indented nuclei. Eosinophilic inclusions are often seen adjacent to the nucleus. (H.E.; magnification × 500.)

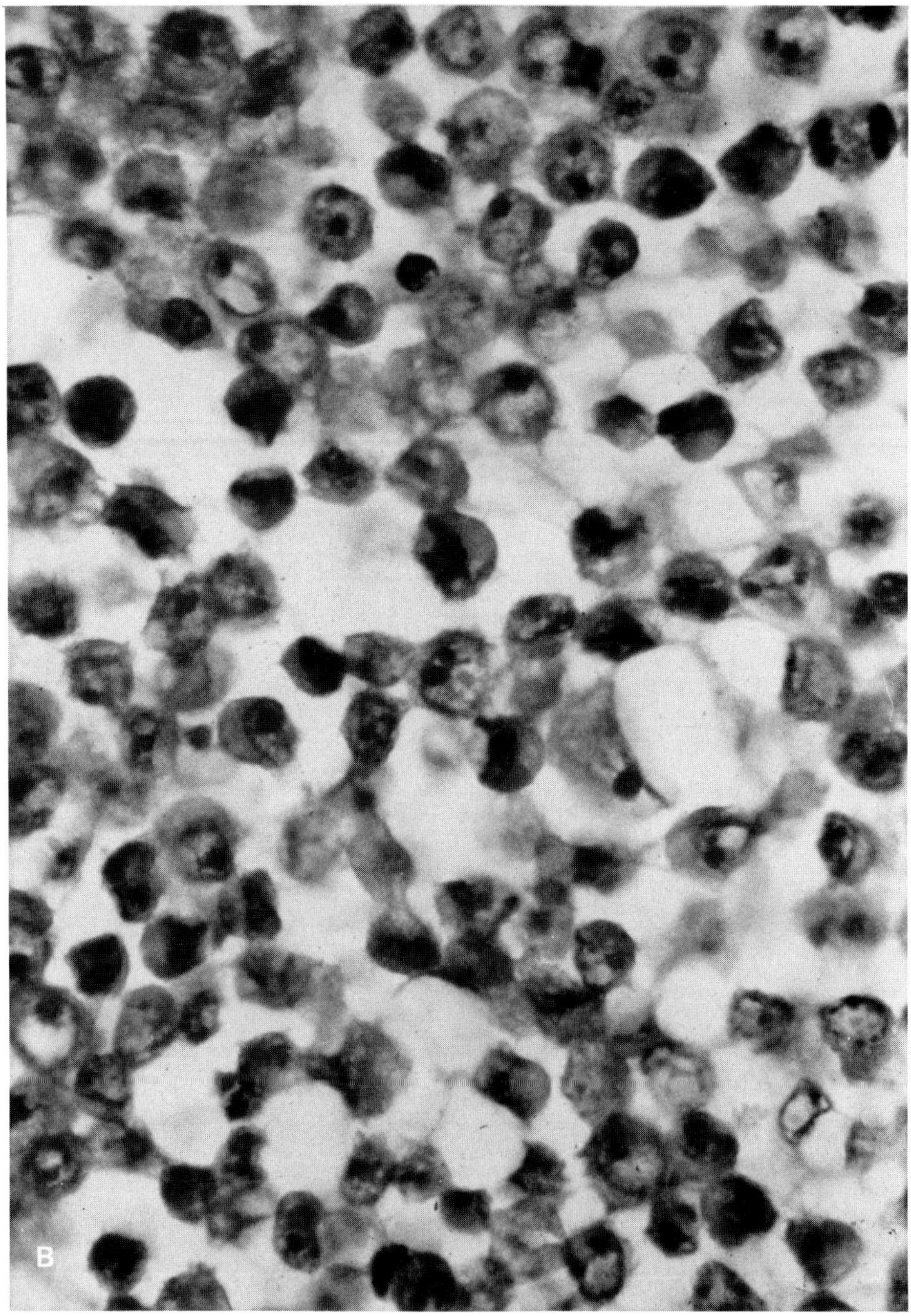

FIGURE 1B.

origin. This change in attitude would seem to endorse the view of Marsden and Lawler[4] who, when they originally described the clear-cell tumors, emphasized their separate identity by describing them as "bone-metastasizing renal tumors of childhood" — a title which also drew attention to their distinctive clinical behavior. In addition, attitudes to the hyaline tumor have also changed, and it is now seen by some as a variant of either the rhabdoid or clear-cell tumor.[5]

As implied above, the title of *rhabdomyosarcomatoid tumors* has since been shorted to rhabdoid tumors, partly for brevity and partly in recognition of their morphological separation from true rhabdomyosarcomas. Despite early suggestions[2] of a striated muscle lineage for rhabdoid tumors, subsequent investigations have not supported this contention. In particular, electron microscopy has failed to demonstrate Z-bands or myofibrils,[6] though it has highlighted an apparently characteristic whorling of intermediate filaments. Additionally, myoglobin, a characteristic cytoplasmic component of rhabdomyosarcomas, is conspicuously absent in rhabdoid tumors.[7] These tumors have also been found in the posterior fossa of the brain, in the liver, and elsewhere, and have also been associated with hypercalcemia in the absence of bony metastases.[8]

The renal tumors of unfavorable histological type have thus been clearly defined as demonstrating one of several specific histological patterns. Those of favorable designation are broadly regarded as all which remain after these specific types have been identified — albeit the majority of childhood renal tumors. They comprise a mixture in varying proportions of blastematous, tubular, and stromal tissues which lack any evidence of anaplasia.

The group also includes a tumor subtype which previously had been otherwise — and inappropriately — classified. This subtype is composed entirely of uniform blastema; this group had been considered to be "undifferentiated" and by analogy with some other tumors to have a poor prognosis. Assessment in a large, collaborative study[2] with a sufficient number of cases, however, has shown that the prognosis of these cases is no worse than the more common histologically "mixed" tumors in the favorable histology group.

Another renal tumor of childhood which reclassification has separated from Wilms' tumors has been the congenital mesoblastic nephroma, which in the great majority of instances behaves in an entirely benign fashion. The benefit to the patient of this diagnostic separation has been considerable, as previously such tumors were treated aggressively, as though malignant, whereas since the recognition by Bolande[9] of their relatively benign nature, it has been found that adequate nephrectomy alone usually achieves a cure. This finding alone has led to the removal of much of the morbidity and even mortality associated with the treatment of these tumors in the past.

As always however, these classifications develop and modify. More recently, a subtype of the mesoblastic nephroma has been described[10] which does not follow this benign course. This subtype does not demonstrate the usual fascicular pattern, and may even appear frankly sarcomatous; it usually presents in the latter part of the first year of life. Although it tends not to metastasize, its propensity for aggressive local infiltration qualifies it for a malignant classification.

The tendency to classify childhood tumors into the broad groups of "favorable" and "unfavorable" histological types has been extended to collaborative investigations of other tumors, particularly rhabdomyosarcoma.[11] Another multicenter organization established for the purpose of investigating a particular tumor type is the Inter-Group Rhabdomyosarcoma Study, and as a part of their collaborative enquiry this broad histological categorization of tumor types has been developed. In this instance, the unfavorable histological features have been identified as anaplasia and a monomorphous round cell pattern of tumor; as with Wilms' tumors, the histologically favorable tumors are those which remain after exclusion of the specific unfavorable types. Time and repeated application of this potentially very valuable classification by other groups will be the surest test of its validity.

In the study of childhood liver tumors, identification of prognostically favorable and unfavorable histological patterns has also occurred, though they have not formally received these appellations. It has been observed[12] that hepatoblastomas comprising mainly tumor which resembles embryonic liver, and therefore classified as embryonal, carry a poor prognosis, with only 2 of 19 such patients in this particular study surviving 5 years. In contrast, those hepatoblastomas containing tumor tissue similar in appearance to the more mature fetal liver, and thus categorized as fetal hepatoblastoma, had a much better prognosis. These tumors were found to be more susceptible to complete resection, and subsequently it was seen that all the children in whom this was accomplished survived 5 years. This study also served to allay fears as to the prognostic significance of mesenchymal tissues such as osteoid, sometimes seen in hepatoblastomas. It was found that the presence or absence of such tissues as such had no significant influence on the progress or ultimate outcome of the tumor.

The identification of tumor subtypes with a better prognosis than the rest of their class has also been seen with another form of liver tumor, namely hepatocellular carcinoma. A morphologically clearly distinguishable form of hepatocellular carcinoma, the fibrolamellar carcinoma,[13] has been identified as being particularly prone to develop in older children and young adults. Unlike other forms of hepatocellular carcinoma, this tumor occurs in livers not predisposed to tumor formation by factors such as cirrhosis. Fibrolamellar carcinomas are also, on the whole, more amenable to complete surgical resection and are commonly associated with considerably longer patient survival times.

One of the most difficult childhood tumors to treat, and which also carries one of the worst prognoses overall, is neuroblastoma. Yet over the years, even collaborative attempts between specialist oncology centers to produce a clinically relevant classification have met with only limited success. In recent years however, there have been developments which have tended to reverse this trend.

The first of these was the recognition of an important variant of neuroblastoma,[14] known as stage IVs. Despite its being apparently widely disseminated at the time of presentation, children with this tumor have a good prognosis. The definition of this tumor includes the following features: a small adrenal neuroblastoma sometimes regarded as the primary tumor (Figure 2), with distant disease in the liver, skin, and bone marrow, though with no radiological evidence of bone disease. The liver tumor is often very large and may cause clinical problems by its compressive effects on the thorax and abdomen, though these can be relieved temporarily by the insertion of a silastic patch in the abdominal wall until the child grows and the tumor shrinks and matures. The skin tumors tend to be multiple and also mature spontaneously with time.

The importance of the identification of this subtype of neuroblastoma, which has been frequently confirmed by workers internationally, is that it regresses spontaneously, and thus care should be taken to avoid over-treatment by chemotherapy and radiotherapy with their attendant morbidity.

More recently,[15] favorable and unfavorable tumor types have been identified in neuroblastoma and related tumors. In summary, the tumors in this study were divided into the majority stroma-poor cases and minority stroma-rich group. The stroma-poor cases were divided into favorable and unfavorable types according to the patient's age at diagnosis, degree of tumor maturation, and the number of mitoses or karyorrhectic nuclei (termed mitosis-karyorrhexis index or MKI) of tumor cells. The stroma-rich cases were divided into well-differentiated, intermixed and nodular types on the basis of the least well-differentiated elements in the tumor; the age of the patient and relative proportions of well- and poorly differentiated tumor tissue were disregarded at this stage.

Favorable stroma-poor and well-differentiated stroma-rich types constituted good-prognosis groups, with 87% survival for at least 2 years; within these groups a greater degree of maturation was seen in the older patients. Conversely, a poor prognosis, with a survival of only 7% at 2 years, was seen in the unfavorable stroma-poor and nodular stroma-rich groups. These groups also showed cytological features generally associated with more malignant tumors, had poor maturity for the age of the patient, a high MKI, the formation of nodules of poorly differentiated neuroblasts, and manifested a more aggressive clinical behavior.

Although this classification is not totally independent of the age of the patient, it represents

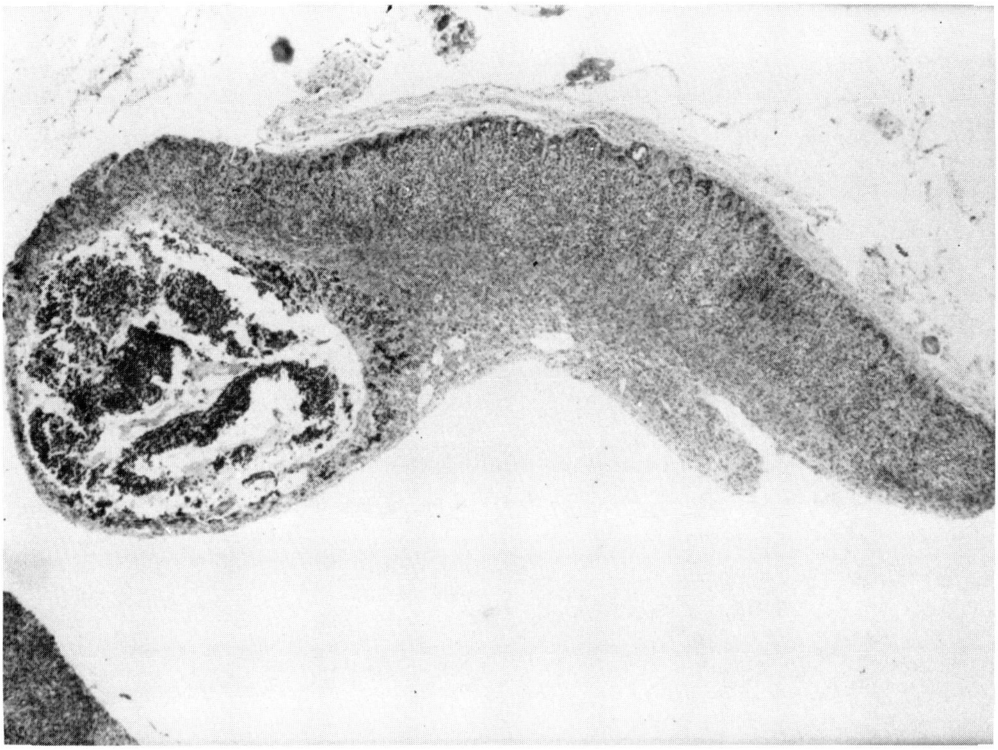

FIGURE 2. Neuroblastoma, Stage IVs. A small adrenal medullary tumor is barely large enough to distort the profile of the adrenal gland on section. (H.E.; magnification × 20.)

a considerable advance on previous classifications of neuroblastoma. Again, time and testing of the hypotheses contained in the classification by other investigators will be the ultimate tests of its validity.

III. LIGHT MICROSCOPIC METHODS OF DIAGNOSIS

Traditionally, the biopsy diagnosis of tumors has relied heavily on the use of formalin-fixed, paraffin wax-embedded tissues, sections of which are usually stained by the tried and tested techniques of hematoxylin and eosin. With the development in recent years of progressively more powerful chemotherapeutic agents and radiotherapeutic techniques, the use of the modalities in various combinations has enabled treatment regimens to be tailored to suit different tumor types and even individual tumors. These refinements in treatment have exposed the inadequacies of formerly perfectly acceptable histological diagnostic techniques and promoted the development of technical advances and innovations to allow the accuracy of tissue diagnosis to remain a step ahead of subsequent therapy.

Rapid diagnosis has usually required the use of frozen tissue sections, formerly using the freezing microtome and latterly the cryostat. It has been recognized that the artifactual tissue distortions caused by these techniques compromise to some extent the level of detail to which a section can be examined, but this was accepted and pathologists worked within these limitations. With the establishment of a reliable, speedy, diagnostic service, however, the need for improved demonstration of cellular features and their more detailed assessment have come to the fore, and new techniques have had to be developed to cater for these requirements.

It has long been recognized that the morphological assessment of tumor tissue of paraffin

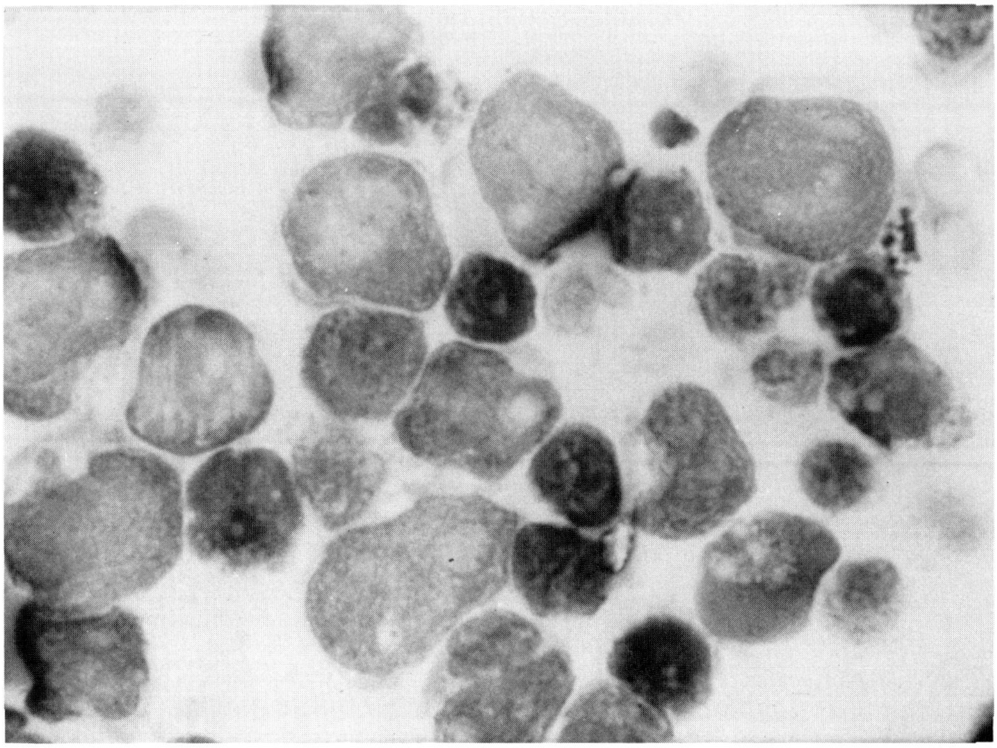

FIGURE 3. Acute lymphoblastic leukemia. A cytological impression demonstrates cells with large nuclei containing several paler-staining nucleoli and with little cytoplasm. (May-Grunwald-Giemsa; magnification × 2,000.)

wax-embedded tissues can be difficult or even completely inadequate for the finer cytological assessment necessary to differentiate tumor subtypes. One of the stimuli to the appreciation of this fact was the development in the 1970s of several classifications of non-Hodgkin's lymphomas which require microscopic scrutiny of material to a level of detail which was simply not possible on paraffin wax sections alone. For this reason, it was suggested[16] that these sections be supplemented by the use of Giemsa-stained impressions from the cut surface of fresh lymph nodes. The use of these impressions had the additional advantages of speed, and the fact that cytochemical and immunocytological methods could be applied to them if necessary to improve diagnostic accuracy.

As might be expected, the earliest beneficiaries of these diagnostic techniques among childhood tumors were the lymphomas and leukemias, a useful benefit for malignancies which are the commonest in this age group (Figure 3). It was soon appreciated however, that these methods could be utilized for other solid pediatric tumors, particularly that perennial thorny problem, the differentiation of the "small round cell" tumors of childhood (Figure 4). Techniques utilized for the preparation of specimens and their use for cytological diagnosis were naturally developed from the established methods used for many years in exfoliative cytology, though traditional exfoliative cytology itself found little direct application in the diagnosis of childhood tumors.

These same principles of preparation and examination of tumor imprints and exfoliative cytology have also been extrapolated into the development of fine-needle aspiration cytology. The technique has been in use for some years in the field of adult oncology,[17] but unaccountably pediatric pathologists have been reluctant to follow this early lead.[18]

Several advantages might accrue from the use of fine-needle aspiration cytology for pediatric tumor diagnosis. On occasion, under the right circumstances, the patient might

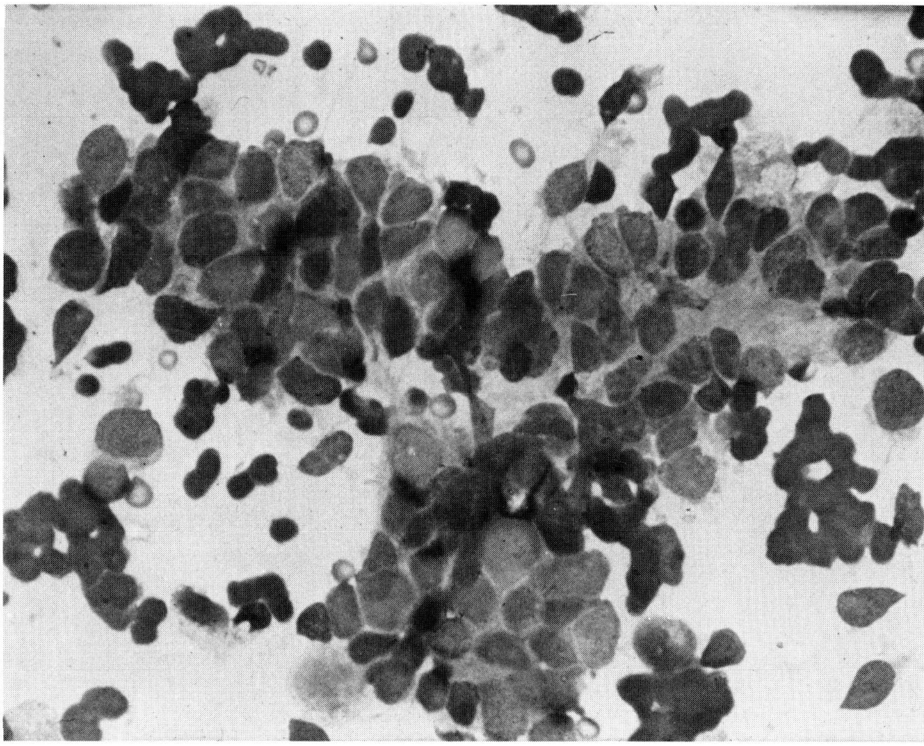

FIGURE 4. Neuroblastoma. A cytological preparation demonstrates groups of rather elongated tumor cells with a little fibrillary stroma and the suggestion (right) of a rudimentary rosette. (May-Grunwald-Giemsa; magnification × 800.)

even be spared the necessity of an open biopsy, at a time of possible great physical debility and distress. At the very least, the use of general anesthesia — not without its own dangers — can be minimized at a time when the child is least fit for such a procedure. Certain tumors, such as intrathoracic masses, may be so sited that they are inaccessible to open biopsy without recourse to major surgery, for which the patient may not be fit or the facilities not readily available, whereas a fine-needle biopsy with appropriate precautions with regard to site would be a relatively minor procedure.

The speed of processing of aspiration specimens and hence the rapidity of diagnosis and accurate treatment are of course a great advantage of this technique, and in experienced hands these objectives can be attained without loss of diagnostic accuracy (Figure 5). It should also be stressed that the method shares with tumor imprints the facility for the application of immunocytological and cytochemical aids to diagnosis and tumor classification. Finally, the financial saving entailed in the use of this technique as a substitute for surgical biopsy cannot be overlooked in times of financial constraint, and to a large extent accounts for its rapidly increasing popularity, especially in Third World countries.

Despite these obvious advantages, the technique is unlikely to supplant the use of open biopsy completely, nor the use of resection biopsy for simultaneous tissue diagnosis and treatment. Obvious applications of the technique however, would be the investigation of possible metastatic disease localized clinically, radiologically, or ultrasonically where a primary tumor has already been characterized, or its contribution to the monitoring of the effects of treatment on an established tumor.

The degree of definition seen on a biopsy viewed microscopically is closely related to the thinness of the section. For this reason, techniques orientated towards the production of

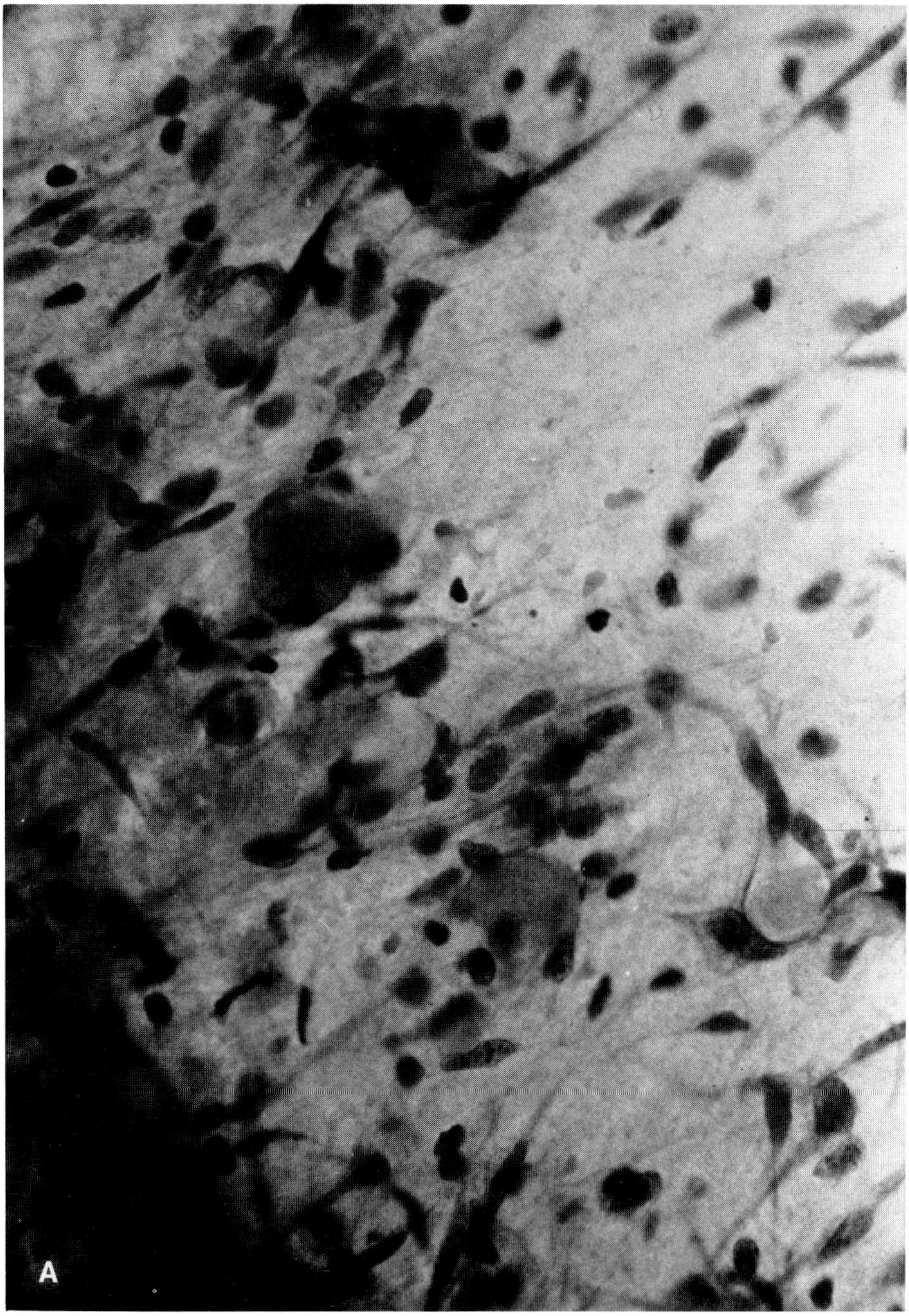

FIGURE 5. Low grade astrocytoma. (A) A speedy diagnosis is provided by the use of a smear preparation in which astrocytes are identified, together with large spheroidal structures. (Toluidine blue; magnification × 500.) (B) The accuracy of the rapid diagnosis is confirmed in the same biopsy on paraffin wax sections where astrocytes and eosinophilic spheroids are demonstrated, albeit having a different appearance with this different technique of preparation. (H.E.; magnification × 500.)

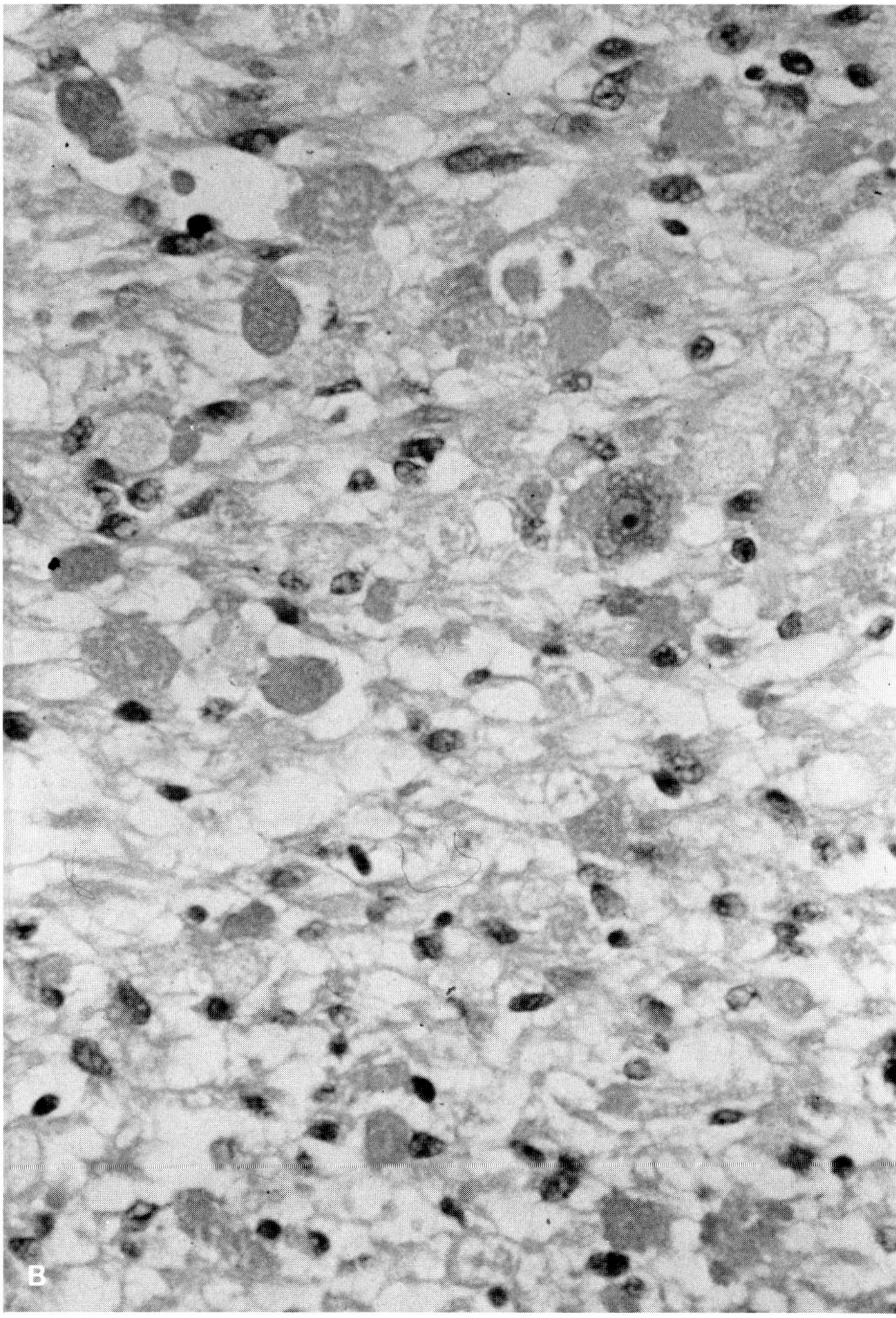

FIGURE 5B.

thinner sections have become popular as an inexpensive means of achieving this end. Higher melting-point paraffin wax and ester wax have been used to an extent effectively, but by far the greatest advance towards achieving this objective has been the routine use of epoxy resin-embedded semithin sections to supplement paraffin wax histology.

The thickness of these resin-embedded sections can be varied considerably, using specially designed microtomes or ultramicrotomes to range from the thickness of paraffin wax sections down to the ultrathin sections used for electron microscopy; it was indeed the use of these semithin sections as survey sections for electron microscopy which to a large extent drew attention to their value as an end in themselves. Some embedding resins such as Araldite or Epon are very restrictive in the stains which they will permit, as the resin is not removed prior to staining. This allows only the use of a few regular staining techniques such as toluidine blue or certain silver impregnation methods. If a range of stains is required for diagnostic purposes, however, other resins such as methacrylates can be utilized very effectively.

The use of resin-embedded material for light microscopic examination carries the obvious advantage that if the tissue has been appropriately fixed in glutaraldehyde, it is usually easy to progress to electron microscopic examination of the same block of tissue. The use of semithin sections has, however, been specifically recommended[19] for the purpose of substituting for electron microscopy, especially in the very demanding area of the differential diagnosis of the malignant lymphomas. Whether or not one wholly accepts this point of view, their use can certainly defer the use of the very expensive and time-consuming modality of electron microscopy until time and facilities permit.

Because of the greatly reduced level of processing artifact associated with this technique, its popularity in aiding histological diagnosis and fine classifying of tumors is likely to continue to increase. Where a wide range of histological methods needs to be applied, however, it will still need to be supplemented by the use of other techniques; but even now, the method in one or other of its forms is widely recognized as standing in its own right as a means of improving the quality of morphology on microscopic sections.[20]

IV. ULTRASTRUCTURAL EXAMINATION

Transmission electron microscopy, long regarded as an interesting research tool, is now firmly established as an indispensable diagnostic method in the identification of and differentiation between the tumors of childhood. Scanning electron microscopy, though it appears promising in certain well-defined areas, has yet to make a significant contribution to routine diagnostic function in this area.

One of the major diagnostic problems in the histological diagnosis of childhood tumors is the differentiation between that group of morphologically similar malignancies known as the small round cell tumors of childhood, which bedevil pediatric oncology. It is to the answering of this particular diagnostic conundrum that electron microscopy makes its greatest contribution.

Ultrastructurally, the identification of neuroblastoma and related tumors is greatly aided by the location of neurosecretory or "dense core" granules measuring 90-240 μm in their cytoplasm (Figure 6).[21] Fine cytoplasmic filaments are also identifiable by electron microscopy, which correspond to the fibrillary stroma frequently seen in the tumor on light microscopic examination. This observation is of particular value, as it is in these filaments and the peripheral part of the tumor-cell cytoplasm that the neurosecretory granules are most frequently seen. Even in the most histological undifferentiated of neuroblastomas, diagnosis can be facilitated by the use of electron microscopy, so frequently are the dense core granules seen in this type of tumor. In certain tumors of otherwise obscure origin, such as that described in the chest wall of children by Askin et al.,[22] an indication of possible neuroepithelial origin may be given by the presence, albeit in small numbers, of cytoplasmic neurosecretory granules.

There have been many proponents of the value of electron microscopy in the identification and differentiation of malignant lymphomas,[19,23] though in recent years this facet of the investigation of their histopathological characteristics has been to a large extent reduced by the use of semithin epoxy resin-embedded sections and of late almost eclipsed by the advent of immunohistological methods.

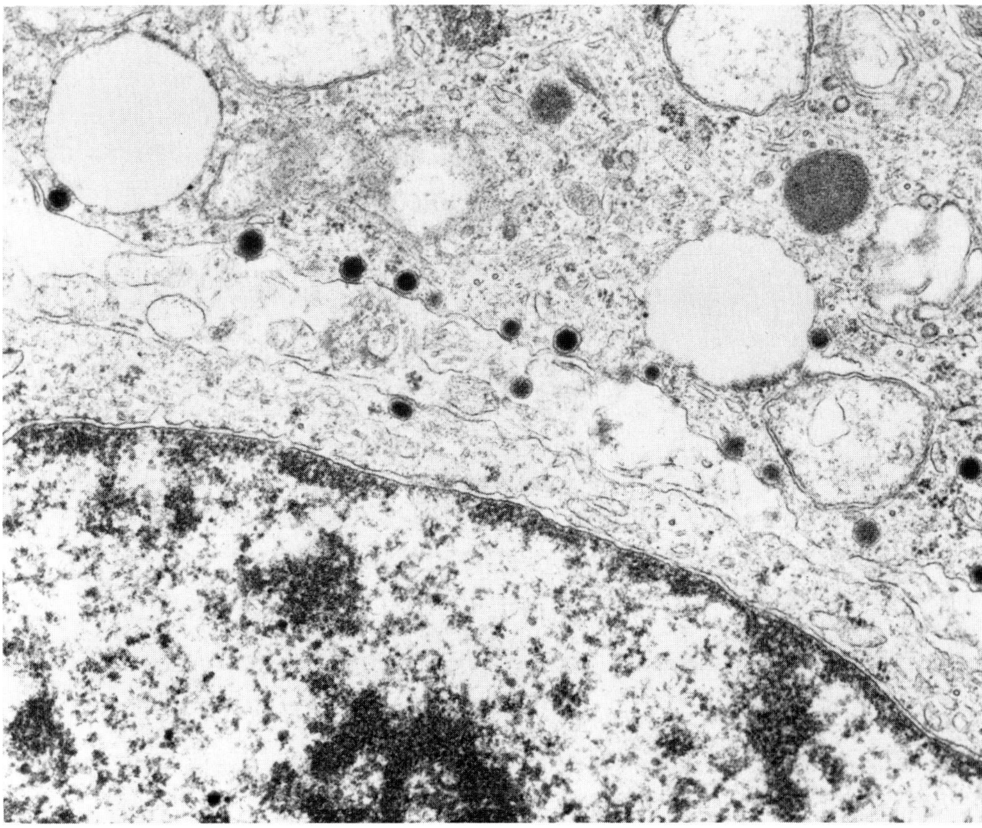

FIGURE 6. Neuroblastoma. Ultrastructurally, "dense core" granules with a pale halo and fine limiting membrane are seen to be concentrated peripherally in the cytoplasm of the tumor cells and in the neurofibrils. (Magnification × 40,000.)

A diagnostic finding of great value in histiocytosis X however are the trilaminar and racquet-shaped Birbeck granules; indeed most would agree that the ultrastructural presence of these granules is pathognomonic of this group of disorders. Attempts have been made[24] to correlate the presence of these structures with a histological subtype of the disease bearing a particularly good prognosis, and characterized by a mixed population of cells in the tumor infiltrate, including a high proportion of multinucleate giant cells. It is also probable that the identification of Birbeck granules ultrastructurally is at least as reliable, and probably more so, than the use of such immunohistological techniques as S-100 protein or histochemical methods as α-1 mannosidase.

In the diagnosis of Ewing's sarcoma, ultrastructural support for the diagnosis may be obtained by the identification of cytoplasmic glycogen, even when this is not visible histochemically at the light microscopic level. Care should be taken in the interpretation of this finding, however, as its presence and quantity can be extremely variable in Ewing's sarcomas and glycogen may also be present in the cytoplasm of a variety of other tumor cells. Another interesting ultrastructural observation in Ewing's sarcoma is the presence of two apparently distinct cell types: the larger, primary cells are the predominant cell type and have more abundant, paler cytoplasm, while the secondary cells are smaller and darker, having less cytoplasm.[25] In all probability, however, these are merely variants of the same cell type.

The use of electron microscopy in the examination of rhabdomyosarcomas does, however,

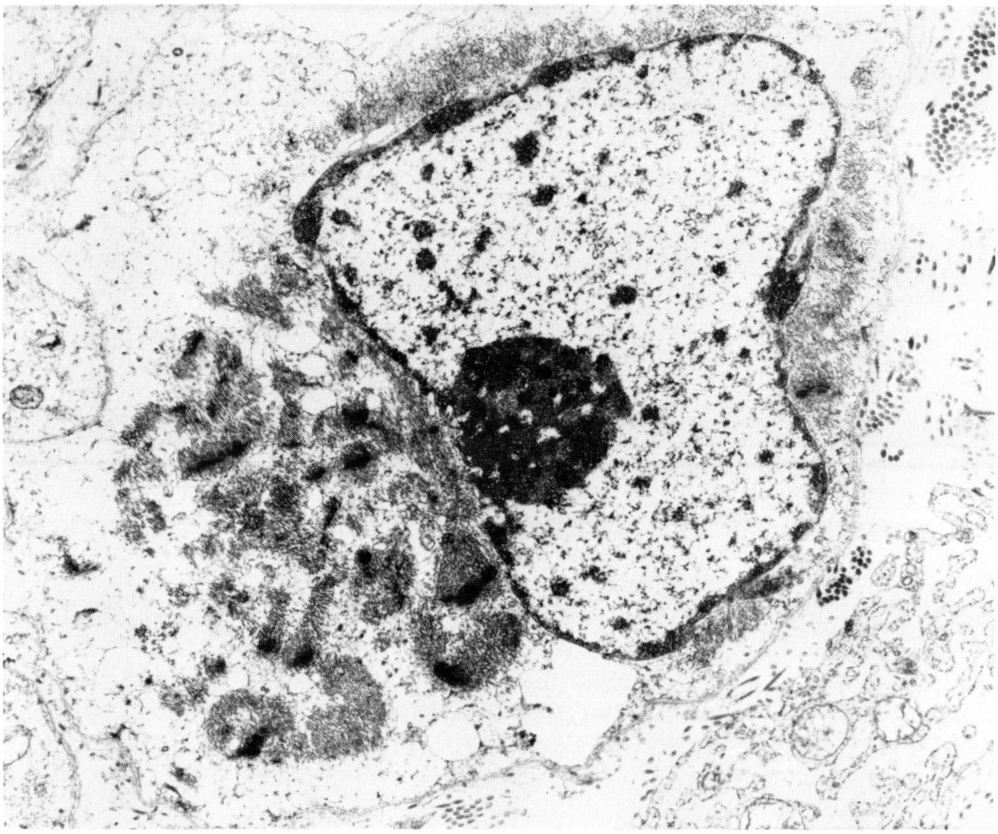

FIGURE 7. Rhabdomyosarcoma. Disorganized myofibrils with irregular, densely staining Z-band material are seen by electron microscopy (left). (Magnification × 10,000.)

seem to have little more than confirmatory value. If seen, the presence of thick and thin myofibrils, and especially Z-bands, is pathognomonic (Figure 7).[26] They are, however, infrequently seen in childhood rhabdomyosarcomas as these are most frequently embryonal in type, a class of rhabdomyosarcoma in which these structures are seldom seen.[27] This is another tumor in which glycogen may be readily identifiable ultrastructurally even when it is scanty or absent at the light microscopic level.

The electron microscopic examination of tumors of childhood may provide information essential to the characterization of the tumors and their differentiation from others with similar morphology by light microscopy. An obvious application of this technique is in the often extremely difficult area of the differential diagnosis of the small round cell tumors of childhood. There are occasions when use of ultrastructural examination alone may be diagnostic, or where this method may, in a particular tumor, be the only one by which a specific diagnosis is capable of formulation. On the whole, however, it is widely recognized that electron microscopy achieves its greatest potential as a diagnostic tool when used in conjunction with other methods. This may be accomplished by applying the different techniques to separate portions of the same tumor, such as fixing a piece in buffered formalin for light microscopy, a piece in glutaraldehyde for electron microscopy and freezing some for immunohistology or histochemistry. Alternatively, different techniques may be applied to the same sections, as with the application of colloidal gold methods using suitably small particle size to the ultrathin sections for electron microscopy to utilize the hybrid technique of immunoelectron microscopy.

V. IMMUNOHISTOLOGY

One of the most significant advances seen in recent years in the field of tumor histopathology has been the development of immunohistopathological methods for diagnostic purposes. In many instances, the needs of adult oncology have provided the stimulus for these innovations, though on occasion the study of childhood tumors has been the motive force; in either instance the advantages provided by these methods in the identification and classification of childhood tumors has been considerable. In many areas, the specificity of diagnosis has improved beyond recognition with the advent of these methods, and on occasion an empirical morphological diagnosis has been transformed almost overnight into a highly specific classification based on antigen expression or cellular function of the cells.

Diagnostic antibodies are now available to cover a wide range of tumor classes, and many of them are produced commercially. Polyclonal and monoclonal antibodies are widely used for diagnostic purposes, each class having its own advantages and disadvantages, specificities, and "cross-reactions." Polyclonal antibodies are produced by the immunization of animals with purified antigen and harvesting the antibody subsequently produced by the animal. Though this simplistic description is subject to certain refinements, the fact remains that the production of polyclonal antibodies is highly dependent on the availability of antigen of adequate purity in sufficient quantity for immunization. There is also the risk of a degree of variability of the antibody between batches.

Monoclonal antibodies, however, are produced by the immunization of animals with antigen and subsequently rendering their immunoglobulin-producing lymphoid cells "immortal" by fusion with cultured mouse myeloma cells.

The hybrid cells so formed are screened individually for their antigenic specificities, and the selected antibody-producing clones are subsequently grown continuously in tissue-culture, and their antibody harvested. Such techniques can be very labor-intensive in their early stages, when the specificity of the antibody produced by a particular cell line is a rather hit-or-miss procedure, but once these specificities are fully characterized against a range of normal and tumorous tissues, the value of this technique comes into its own.

The diagnostic application of immunohistological methods received a considerable stimulus in the routine histopathology laboratory when it was found that they were ideally suited to the diagnosis and detailed characterization of malignant and pseudomalignant disease of the reticuloendothelial system (Figure 8). Indeed, the application of immunohistological methods to the diagnosis of and differentiation between malignant lymphomas has been the subject of several detailed reviews.[28,29]

Polyclonal antibodies have been raised and are widely available to individual cytoplasmic immunoglobulins, light chains, and J-chains. Initially the application of these antibodies was restricted to their use on frozen sections, but use of the cryostat for this purpose was rendered to a large extent superfluous by the discovery that protease digestion of formalin-fixed paraffin wax-embedded tissues can unmask tissue antigens previously disguised by alteration during fixation (Figure 9). The position of this technique has been further enhanced by the use of fixatives other than formalin prior to processing. Polyclonal antibodies are also widely available to other reticuloendothelial-associated antigens such as α1-antitrypsin contained in histiocytes and myeloid cells.

Pretreatment by protease digestion, however, does little to help the demonstration of surface antigens, as these do not appear to survive formalin fixation and paraffin wax-embedding. Monoclonal antibodies to such surface antigens as HLA-DR (found on most B-cell lymphomas), T-cells and their subsets, and leukocyte common antigen cannot therefore benefit from these unmasking techniques and need to be applied to cryostat sections and tumor imprints.

In the earlier days of the application of immunohistological methods to tumor diagnosis,

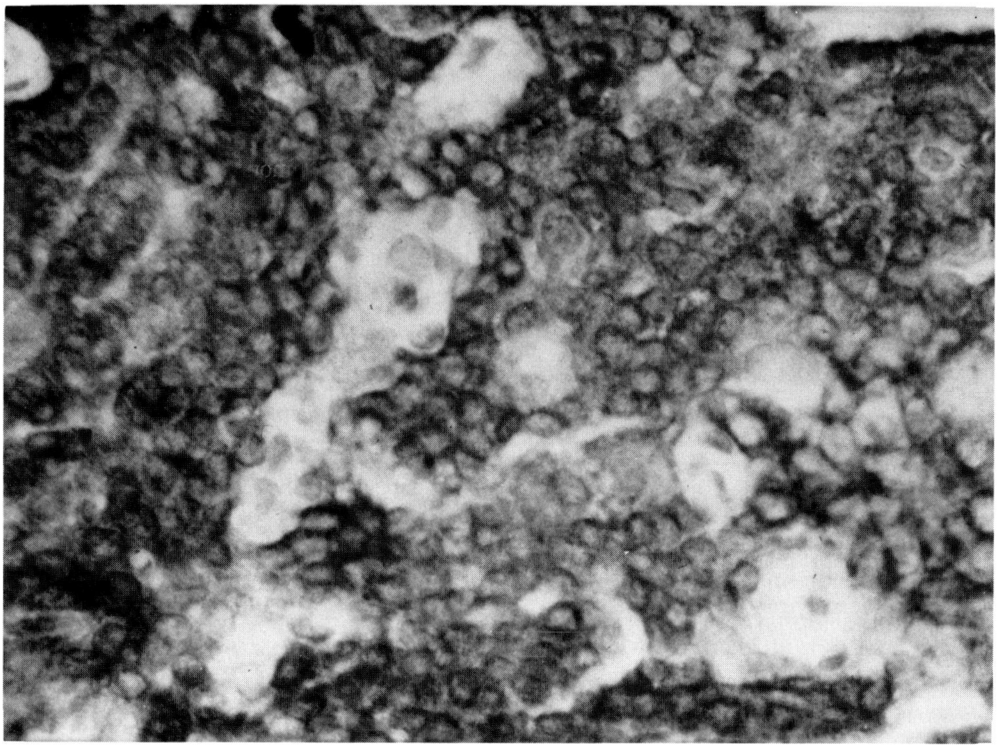

FIGURE 8. Thyroid, malignant lymphoma. Immuno-peroxidase preparation utilizing a polyclonal T-cell marker demonstrates the precise character of the infiltrating tumor, enabling the employment of appropriately tailored therapy. (Magnification × 800.)

the method used to demonstrate the site of antigen localization was immunofluorescence using the action of ultraviolet light on antibodies conjugated with fluorescein or other fluorogen. Indeed, immunofluorescence is still the method of choice in some areas of study because of its high degree of sensitivity and ability to locate small quantities of antigen. It does suffer from disadvantages in the short storage life of the sections and the inconvenience of requiring a separate facility for ultraviolet light microscopy in addition to the white light microscopy available in most laboratories.

These criticisms led to the development of alternative methods of immunohistological demonstration, particularly using horseradish peroxidase and alkaline phosphatase. These have the dual advantages of prolonged storage life and availability for examination by white light. A major disadvantage of the peroxidase technique is that diamino-benzidine used in the terminal color reaction, is carcinogenic. Utilizing the immuno-peroxidase technique, several methods are available for use, as indeed is the case with the other immunohistological techniques. The direct immuno-peroxidase method utilizes the peroxidase directly conjugated to the antibody, and is simple, but not very sensitive, and limited in its range of applications. Sensitivity is greatly increased by the use of indirect techniques where the antibody is applied to the tissue and a further peroxidase-labeled antibody is applied to the first layer antibody, or alternatively where a peroxidase-antiperoxidase bridge is utilized.

A further development in recent years has been the use of colloidal gold as the indicator in immunohistological methods. This has the additional advantage of routine applicability to electron microscopic as well as light microscopic preparations, and reagents of different particle size have been developed for this purpose.

Also available for diagnostic purposes are monoclonal antibodies to individual constituents

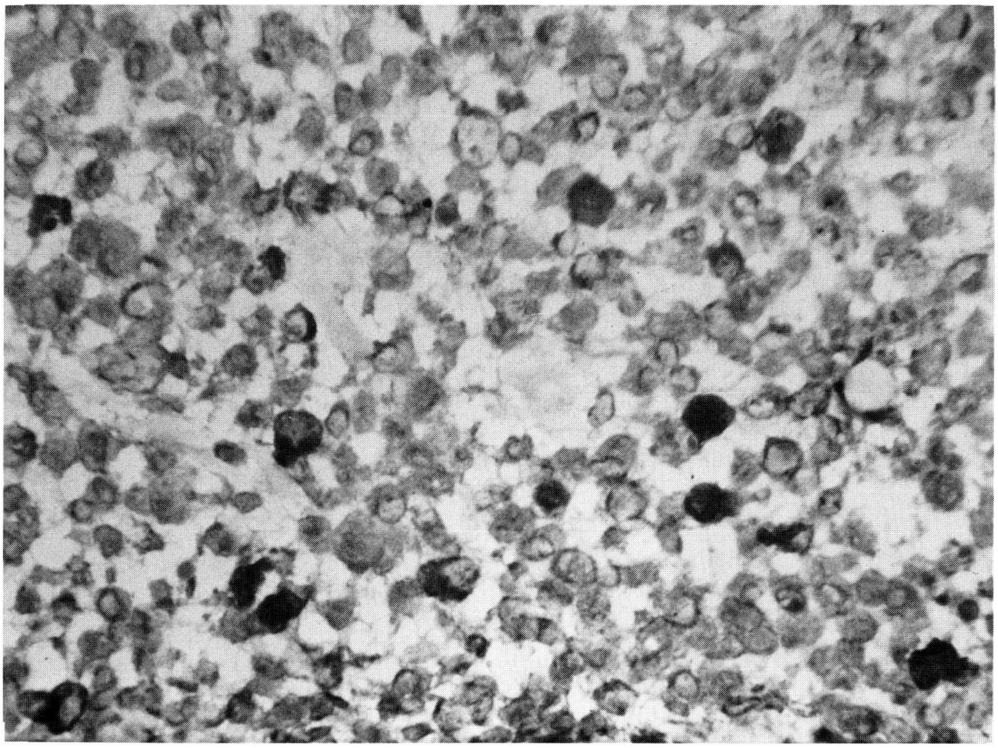

FIGURE 9. Embryonal rhabdomyosarcoma. Protease digestion of a paraffin wax-embedded section, followed by immuno-peroxidase demonstration of cytoplasmic desmin utilizes a polyclonal reagent. The intensity of demonstration of the antigen in different cells varies considerably. (Magnification × 800.)

in the cytoplasm of nonlymphoid cells. A particularly valuable group of antibodies in this category are those which have been raised to intermediate filaments, which are so described because of the fact that their size is intermediate between actin (6 nm) and the larger myosin (15 nm) and microtubules (22 nm). Several types of intermediate filament are recognized using monoclonal antibodies, and their presence in particular tumors can be most helpful in formulating a precise histopathological diagnosis.

Cytokeratins are a characteristic component of epithelial cells, and as such are also seen in many carcinomas.[30,31] Vimentin (see Figure 16) is seen in sarcomas, particularly rhabdomyosarcomas, though its diagnostic value is considerably reduced by its relative nonspecificity; it is also seen for example in lymphomas and melanomas. Desmin (see Figure 9) is another intermediate filament found in many rhabdomyosarcomas, but in this case its diagnostic value is enhanced by its rather greater specificity than vimentin. In the field of neuropathology, the accurate diagnosis of astrocytomas has been greatly enhanced by the development of polyclonal and monoclonal antibodies to the intermediate filament glial fibrillary acidic protein (Figure 10). Additional valuable monoclonal antibodies have also been raised against neurofilaments,[32] and these have been used to identify cells of neural origin in the central and peripheral nervous systems.

The identification of other cytoplasmic components in cells of childhood tumors has also attained diagnostic importance with the advent of reliable immunohistological reagents for their demonstration. In particular, α-fetoprotein is present in the cells of both hepatoblastomas and hepatocellular carcinomas, as well as certain forms of malignant teratoma (Figure 11); fortunately, the morphological appearances of these tumors are quite distinctive, so the use of this immunohistological reagent can be regarded as a valuable confirmatory investigation.

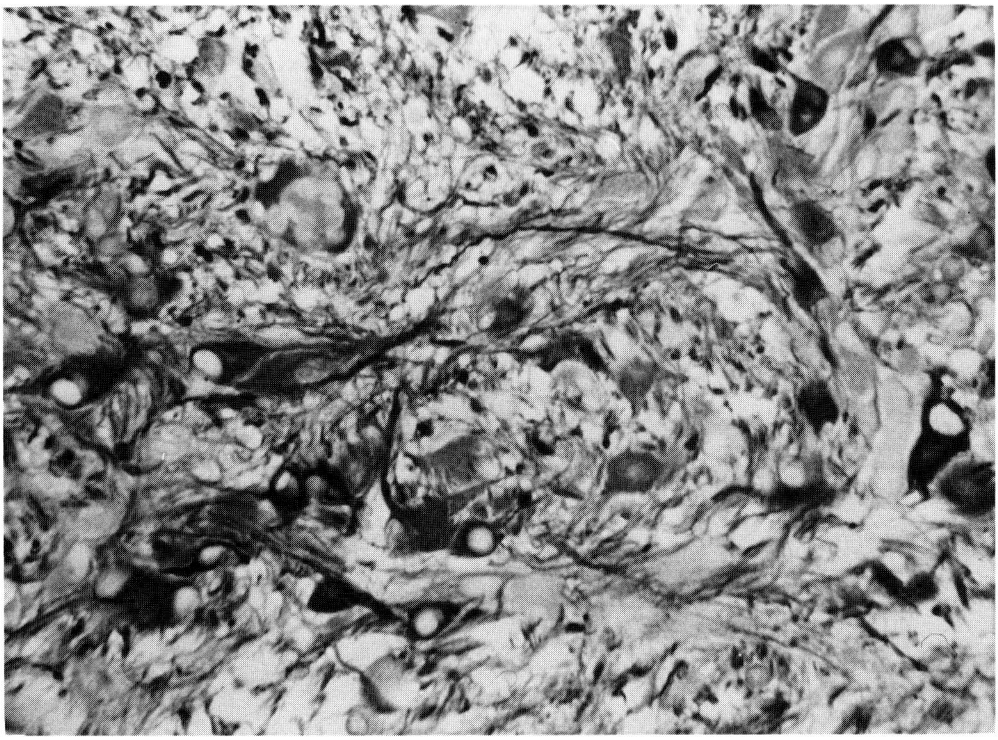

FIGURE 10. Low-grade astrocytoma. A polyclonal antibody locates glial fibrillary acidic protein in the cytoplasm and fibrils of astrocytes; the absence of staining in nuclei has resulted in pale circular areas appearing in the cells. Paraffin wax-embedded section, protease digested, indirect immuno-peroxidase preparation. (Magnification × 500.)

The presence of myoglobin in rhabdomyosarcomas and specific hormones in some endocrine tumors are specific, and the use of these antibodies can be of major diagnostic importance.

Neuron-specific enolase can also be identified immunohistologically in the cytoplasm of cells of the neuroblastoma lineage. Many investigators find that this antigen is expressed poorly, if at all, in those morphologically undifferentiated tumors where diagnostic assistance is most needed. Tsokos et al.,[33] found that this cytoplasmic component was demonstrable in every one of a group of neuroblastomas which they investigated, while it was found in one rhabdomyosarcoma among a large, heterogeneous group of other tumors. A similar criticism can be leveled at S-100 protein in neuroblastoma, in that it is only expressed in the better differentiated tumors, but in this latter group it has proved to be of some diagnostic value. Epithelial-membrane antigen is another marker of considerable value demonstrable immunohistologically on the surface of epithelial-derived tumors such as primary or secondary carcinomas.

The diagnostic value of monoclonal antibodies has been proved with respect to a number of tumors. Among several such tumors in the pediatric age group, neuroblastoma has received particular attention in recent years, in large part because of the difficulty in managing these tumors. Antibodies applied against a particular tumor, however, may not always be specific to that tumor, and in this instance may for example bind to other neuroectodetermally derived tissues or other tumors. Conversely, any individual antigen identified by a monoclonal antibody need not necessarily be expressed in every tumor of a particular class, nor even on every cell in a particular tumor. This implicit heterogeneity which is a characteristic in so many ways of any group of tumors dictates that for effective use and significant, reliable results, monoclonal antibodies should be applied in panels rather than individually.[34,35]

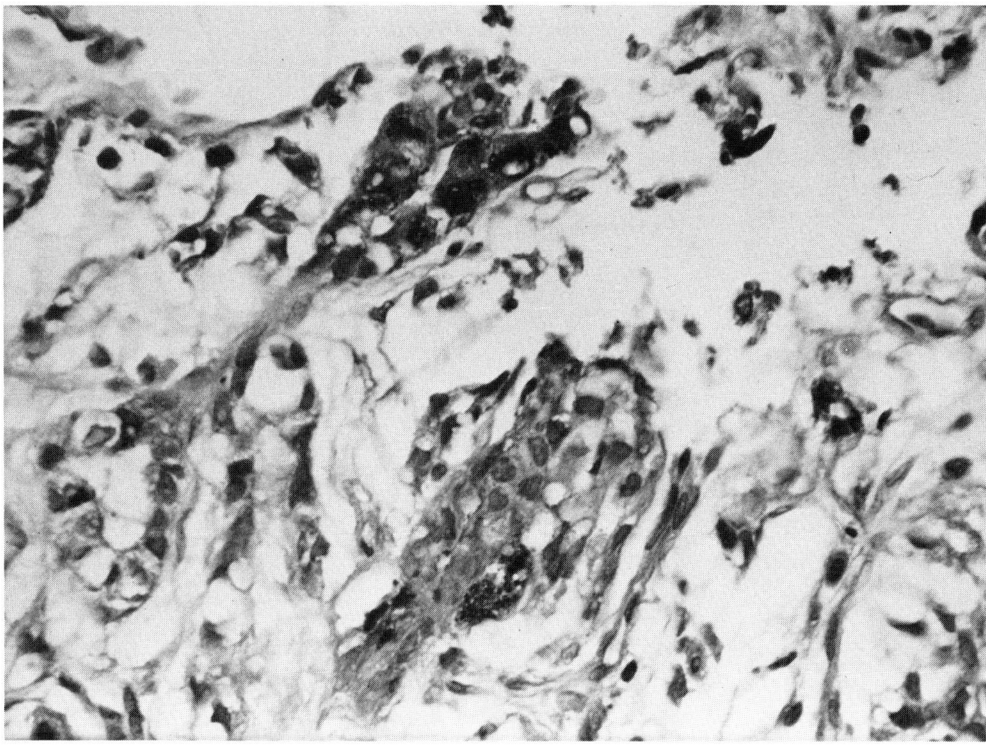

FIGURE 11. Malignant teratoma. Yolk sac tissue is identified (top center) by the presence of α-feto protein staining darkly in the cytoplasm. Indirect immuno-peroxidase, utilizing a polyclonal antibody. (Magnification × 500.)

VI. HISTOCHEMISTRY AND CYTOCHEMISTRY

The modification of qualitative and quantitative biochemical assay techniques to tissue sections and tumor impressions has provided histochemical and cytochemical methods of considerable variety and great diagnostic value in the field of childhood tumors.

Some of these techniques are undertaken merely to amplify the morphological description of the tumor in a purely empirical fashion, without necessarily indicating an understanding of the physiological reason for the presence of the identified component. A good example of this situation is diagnostic reliance on the demonstration of glycogen in the cytoplasm of tumor cells in Ewing's sarcoma (Figure 12). This is achieved by staining with the Periodic Acid-Schiff (PAS) technique in duplicate, once with, and once without diastase digestion; the reaction is enhanced by prior fixation in an alcohol-based fixative, which reduces loss of glycogen. The cell of derivation of the Ewing's sarcoma remains speculative, so the presence of glycogen is of unknown significance and furthermore does little itself to elucidate that question. The observation, however, remains of considerable diagnostic value.

Other histochemical and cytochemical techniques are employed which are much more specific, whose significance is better understood and which give some clue as to the histogenesis of a tumor by virtue of deduction of cellular function from its cytoplasmic constituents. Cellular enzymes are particularly amenable to this approach, and especially prominent in this respect is the identification of cytoplasmic alkaline phosphatase in the diagnosis of osteosarcomas (Figure 13). This is a useful diagnostic technique for this tumor under any circumstances, but where differentiation towards fibroblastic or chondroblastic types predominates, the osteoblastic origin of the tumor is still revealed by the presence of alkaline phosphatase activity.

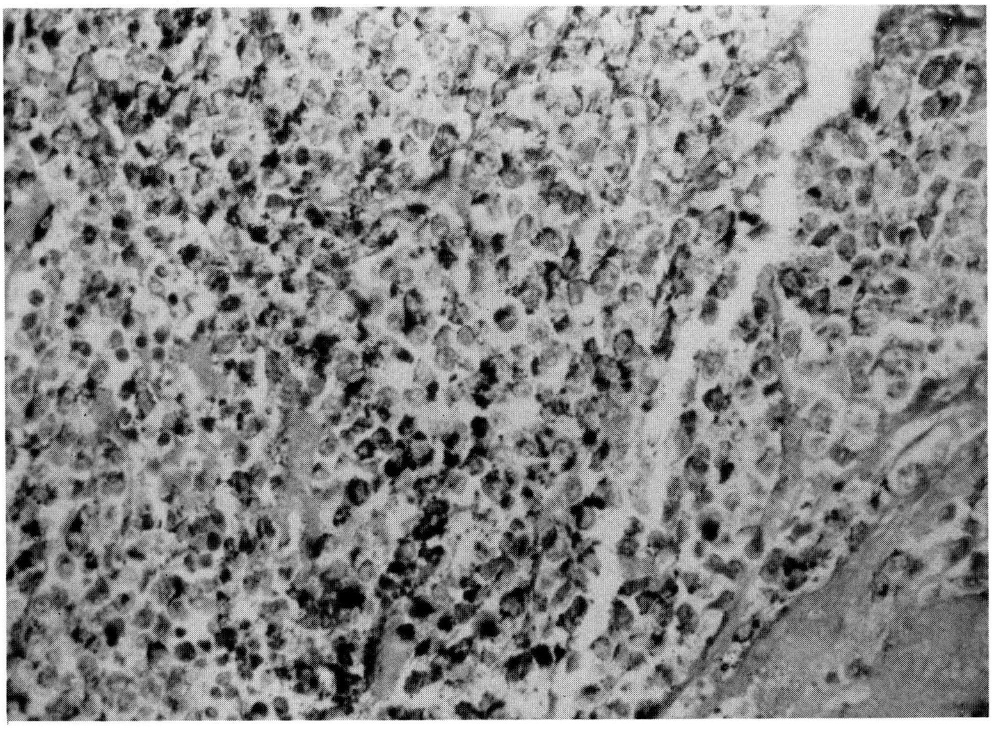

FIGURE 12. Ewing's sarcoma. The uniform tumor cells contain much cytoplasmic glycogen and little intercellular stroma is seen. Periodic Acid-Schiff stain on a celloidinized section. (Magnification × 200.)

In the identification of and differentiation between forms of childhood leukemia and lymphoma, cytochemical techniques again assume great importance. When considering the lymphoblastic leukemias, those of T-cell origin demonstrate strong staining for acid phosphatase and β-glucuronidase in coarse granules. In contrast, B-cell lymphomas are negative to both of these investigations, and the non-B, non-T cell tumors show only weak positivity.[36] Coarse PAS-positive granules are found in the cytoplasm of both T-cell and non-B, non-T cell leukemias, while none are seen in B-cell leukemias. The different types of non-Hodgkin's lymphoma tend to show similar cytochemical reactions to their leukemic counterparts.

Acute myeloid leukemia can be identified by the presence of cytoplasmic myeloperoxidase and a positive Sudan black stain. Chloro-acetate esterase is also positive in this situation and is a particularly important histochemical technique as it is available for use even on formalin-fixed, paraffin wax-embedded tissues. Acid phosphatase and β-glucuronidase activities are variable, but are usually weakly positive in the cytoplasm of acute myeloid leukemic cells.

Particularly valuable in the differential diagnosis of soft tissue tumors is the fact that rhabdomyosarcoma cells tend to demonstrate myophosphorylase and adenosine triphosphatase activity. Positive staining for fat in adipose tissue tumors is an obvious diagnostic technique, but is not always reliable as not all such tumors necessarily contain fat, and furthermore, fat deposition may be found in association with areas of degeneration in other types of soft tissue tumors.

Acid phosphatase activity in the cytoplasm of histiocytes is a useful technique in identifying cells of this type. It is of particular value in demonstrating the histiocytic origin of malignant histiocytosis when used in conjunction with the immunohistological demonstration of lysozyme and α1-anti-chymotrypsin. In osteosarcomas with many tumor giant cells the tech-

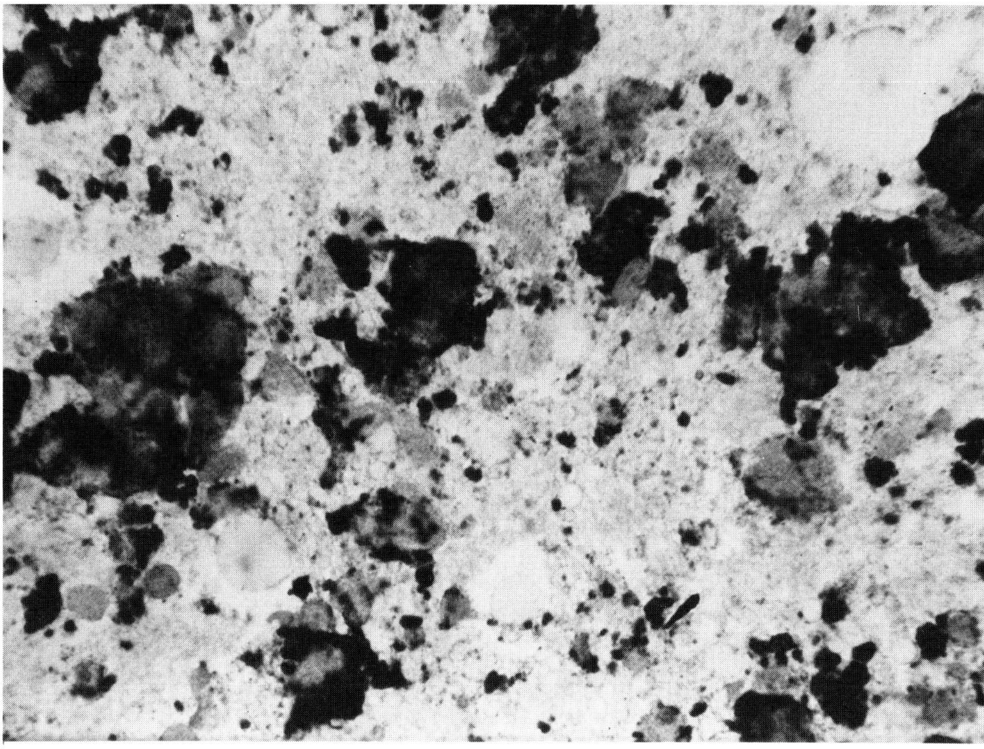

FIGURE 13. Osteosarcoma. A fresh imprint of tumor tissue shows the presence of alkaline phosphatase in the tumor cells, though cells not of tumor origin are negative. (Magnification × 800.)

nique can be usefully employed to distinguish between the acid phosphatase-positive osteoclasts and the alkaline phosphatase-positive malignant giant cells of osteoblastic derivation.

Many would contest the suggestion that histiocytosis X is a malignant tumor, though there is no denying that some forms of this curious entity certainly behave in a malignant fashion. Identification of histiocytosis X cells, particularly in the diagnostically more difficult monomorphic cellular form, has been aided by the observation[37] that the cytoplasm of the infiltrating cells in histiocytosis X shows α-mannosidase activity. The observation is of particular value as, though the reaction is short-lasting and must be applied to frozen sections, it can be used on small biopsies with minimal trauma to the patient.

Histochemical methods are also available for the identification of neuroblastoma and related tumors. In particular, the presence of cytoplasmic catecholamines renders them susceptible to formaldehyde[38] or glyoxylic acid[39] induced fluorescence (Figure 14). Acetyl cholinesterase can also be identified in the cytoplasm of neuroblastoma cells at all degrees of maturation.

VII. *IN VITRO* CULTURE

Over a long period of time, *in vitro* tissue culture was advocated as a useful adjunct to traditional histological methods in tumor diagnosis. Stout and Lattes[40] particularly applied this technique in their investigations of soft tissue tumors, and enhanced the accuracy of their diagnoses by the observation of cytological features on explant which they considered diagnostic. They demonstrated that nine days' culture of a rhabdomyosarcoma *in vitro* resulted in the development of cells having some of the cytological characteristics of mature striated muscle.[40] In another area of endeavor,[41] they were able to confirm the histiocytic

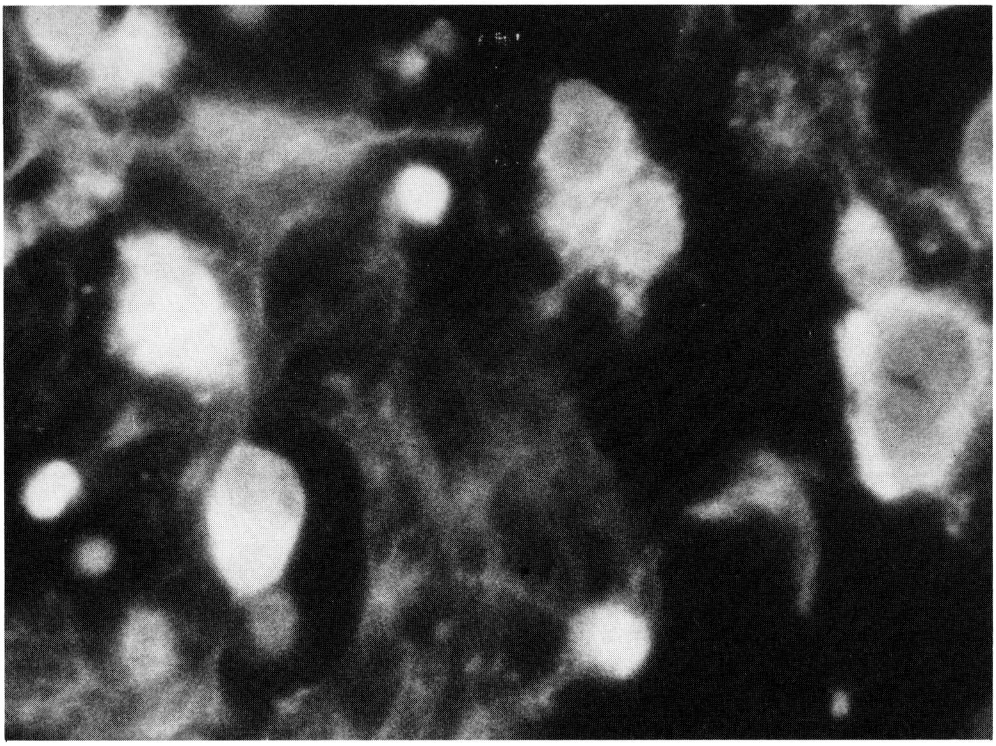

FIGURE 14. Neuroblastoma. Formalin-induced fluorescence when sections are viewed under ultra-violet light reveals the presence of catecholamines in the cytoplasm of tumor cells. (Magnification × 2,000.)

derivation of both malignant histiocytosis and fibrous xanthoma by cytological observations on *in vitro* cultures. These techniques were, and remain, very slow and for this reason alone can have very limited application in isolation for diagnostic purposes.

Certain aspects of this technique have been further developed in recent years with some enhancement of their diagnostic potential (Figures 15, 16). Although Murray and Stout[42] first called attention to the morphological features of cytological differentiation shown by neuroblastoma when cultured *in vitro* many years ago, the technique remained largely unused. In more recent times, however, it has been taken up again[39] in conjunction with the more recently applied glyoxylic acid-induced catecholamine fluorescence. In combination, these techniques demonstrate within 48 h the development of reliably identifiable neurites which are characteristic of this tumor. The combined technique is said to be as reliable as electron microscopy in the diagnosis of this class of tumor and appreciably quicker. Only a little less reliable, but speedier again in application was the use of catecholamine fluorescence alone.

VIII. CYTOGENETICS

Several tumors of childhood are recognized to occur, in certain forms, in association with chromosomal anomalies. Despite this observation, the knowledge is of limited diagnostic value, and is considered to be more relevant to epidemiological studies. The relationship between chromosomal abnormalities and human malignancies has been reviewed.[43]

Certain associations between chromosomal abnormalities and the occurrence of solid tumors are well known. One of these is the deletion in a small proportion of retinoblastoma patients of the q14 region of chromosome 13.[43] Another is the 11p deletion in those cases of Wilms' tumor associated with aniridia and gonadal dysgenesis.

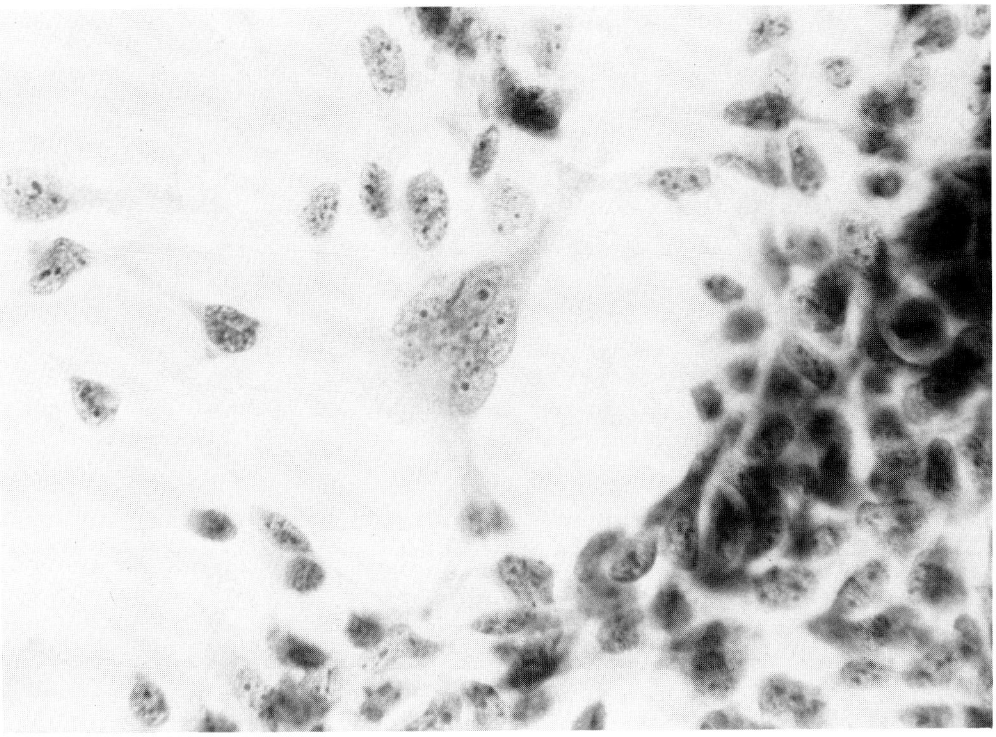

FIGURE 15. Rhabdomyosarcoma, embryonal type. In tissue culture, cells with the characteristic morphology of rhabdomyosarcoma can sometimes be identified, such as this multinucleate cell with elongated cytoplasmic processes. (H.E.; magnification × 800.)

With regard to the tumors themselves, cytogenetic studies on tumor cells have yielded variable results. Sometimes double minute chromatin bodies or other structural anomalies may be recognized as in neuroblastoma,[44] but little prognostic reliance can be attached to these observations. Still within the field of neuroblastoma study, however, the estimation of total cellular DNA content by flow cytometry[45] has provided evidence that neuroblastomas may be divided by this technique into two groups of differing clinical outlook. Those neuroblastomas with a hyperdiploid DNA content seem to be associated with a better response to chemotherapy than those with a diploid DNA content.

In a related area, the investigation of oncogene expression and amplification has recently caused much interest. These studies are likely to add much to knowledge of the etiology and pathogenesis of tumor development in childhood, and possibly also to the accuracy of diagnosis. Although this latter point shows every sign of being a long way off in development, its significance should not be overlooked, and many will observe this field with interest.

IX. EPIDEMIOLOGY

The epidemiology of childhood tumors is a broad and fascinating field, touching on many areas of investigation, and meriting a volume in its own right. Detailed reviews of the present situation are available[46] and for the present purpose a summary of the salient features will be made as relevant to succeeding chapters.

The epidemiological factors of significance in the development of childhood tumors may be broadly categorized as intrinsic, i.e., originating from the patient's internal environment and extrinsic, i.e., deriving from the external environment.

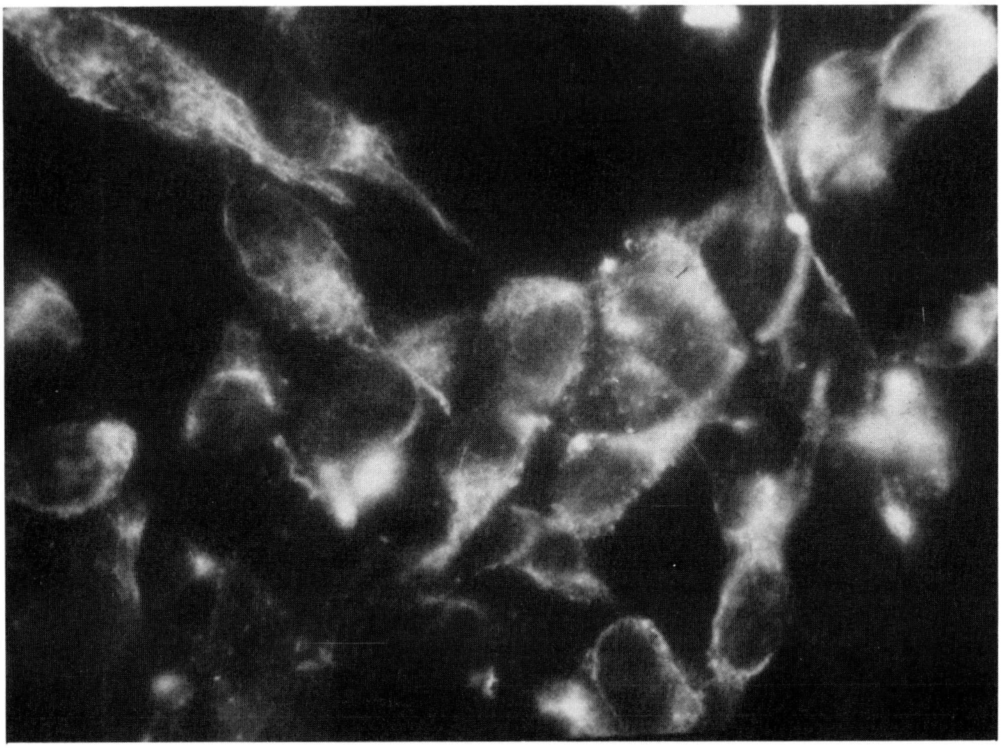

FIGURE 16. Embryonal rhabdomyosarcoma. A monoclonal antibody to vimentin (courtesy of Dr. J. P. Clayton) demonstrates cytoplasmic positivity utilizing an indirect immunofluorescence technique. (Magnification × 2,000.)

The intrinsic factors are largely genetic in origin, but are varied in their nature and presentation. Very many hereditary disorders exist which are associated with an increased risk of malignancy, and it is of considerable importance to recognize these clinically so as to predict the development of any malignancy, and hence diagnose and treat it promptly as and when it arises.

A well-recognized example of an inherited disorder with malignant connotations is neurofibromatosis. This is inherited in an autosomal dominant fashion, and in addition to sarcomatous transformation of the neurofibromata may be associated with sarcoma formation elsewhere, leukemia and other malignancies. In the Beckwith-Wiedemann syndrome, also inherited as an autosomal dominant condition, embryonic tumors may occur in kidney, liver, pancreas, or elsewhere in association with macroglossia and organomegaly.

Among the autosomal recessively inherited conditions associated with malignant tumor development are several, such as some cases of glycogen storage disorders, which predispose to hepatic cirrhosis, and which in turn lead to hepatocellular carcinoma formation. Other metabolic disorders which tend to cause major liver abnormalities, such as galactosemia or α-1 anti-trypsin deficiency may also follow this pathway through hepatic cirrhosis to hepatocellular carcinoma.

Prominent among the childhood disorders in which malignant tumors may develop are several where immune deficiency of one form or another is involved. Many of these are inherited in an X-linked recessive manner, as is the case with X-linked lymphoproliferative syndrome and severe combined immunodeficiency, in both of which conditions non-Hodgkin's lymphoma has the potential to develop.

Ataxia-telangiectasia also incorporates an important element of immunodeficiency, but is, however, more properly classified with such other conditions as Bloom's and Fanconi's syndromes as disorders of DNA repair. All three are inherited in an autosomal dominant fashion and may be associated with one of a number of different malignancies, notably leukemia, Hodgkin's disease or non-Hodgkin's lymphomas. Ataxia-telangiectasia is also exquisitely sensitive to even small doses of radiotherapy.

In patients with chromosomal deletions or trisomies, there is also an increased tendency to malignant tumor formation. The association between Down's syndrome and myeloid leukemia is well known, though the tendency is for this to develop predominantly in the early years. Down's syndrome, like several other of these genetically based disorders, is also associated with other abnormalities, in this instance severe congenital cardiac malformations, most commonly atrioventricular canal defect. These are often fatal at an early age, a fact which tends to distort statistics away from the recognition of late-developing tumors. Conditions associated with deletion or duplication of sex chromosomes such as Turner's or Klinefelter's syndromes may also be prone to malignant tumor formation, especially leukemias and germ-cell tumors.

Certain tumors may be associated with more specific deletions of parts of chromosomes. For example there is a constant association between chromosome 13q14 deletion and the development of retinoblastoma. Bilateral tumors occur in about half the cases, which is rather fewer than those occurring bilaterally in the autosomal dominant-inherited form of the disorder, but the similarity is striking. In certain Wilms' tumors also, there is an association between the tumor occurring in conjunction with aniridia and gonadal dysgenesis, and chromosal 11p deletion.

The situation with regard to the relationship between extrinsic environmental factors and the development of childhood tumors is much less clear, and where studies have been performed these tend to be conflicting in their conclusions.[47,48]

One widely-studied area is the effect of pre- and postnatal irradiation. There seems little doubt[49] that exposure of fetuses to diagnostic X-irradiation while *in utero* causes an increase in malignant tumors in the child at a later date. Some doubt does however surround the role of environmental radiation in the causation of childhood malignancies, especially leukemia.[47,48] It is also known that therapeutic irradiation in childhood can cause a subsequent malignancy; this was the case when thymic irradiation was considered necessary for the treatment of enlargement of that organ and this therapeutic maneuver was followed by the occurrence of an increased number of thyroid carcinomas some years later.[50]

Drug therapy, before and after birth, has also been implicated in the causation of tumors in children. Much evidence has accumulated to support the contention that treatment of pregnant women with di-ethyl stilbestrol can lead to the occurrence of clear-cell carcinoma of the vagina in the offspring many years later.[51] It is also known that children treated with antitumor chemotherapy, or immunosuppressant therapy as for organ transplantation run a considerably increased risk of developing a malignancy, or in the former situation a second, separate, malignant tumor. The development of malignant lymphoma is particularly prone to occur under the latter circumstances.

A further environmental factor, at least in certain parts of the world, which can be implicated in tumor causation in childhood is viral infection. In particular, the Epstein-Barr virus has been incriminated in at least aiding the development of certain non-Hodgkin's lymphomas, notably the African form of Burkitt's lymphoma. It has been postulated that infection with the Epstein-Barr virus causes B-cell proliferation, at first polyclonal and later monoclonal when malignant lymphoma of B-cell type develops.

For the future, developments in molecular biology can be expected to add much to our knowledge of specific genetic abnormalities or defects associated with malignant tumors. In particular the use of DNA restriction enzymes to identify the affected fragments of chromosomes, and the location and demonstration of oncogenes in specific tumors can be expected to be fruitful areas of inquiry.

REFERENCES

1. **Beckwith, J. B.,** personal communication.
2. **Beckwith, J. B. and Palmer, N. F.,** Histopathology and prognosis of Wilms' tumour: results from the First National Wilms' Tumour Study, *Cancer,* 41, 1937, 1978.
3. **D'Angio, G. J., Beckwith, J. B., Breslow, N. E., Bishop, H. C., Evans, A. E., Farewell, V., Fernbach, D., Goodwin, W. E., Jones, B., Leape, L. L., Palmer, N. F., Tefft, M., and Wolff, J. A.,** Wilms' tumor: an update, *Cancer,* 45, 1791, 1980.
4. **Marsden, H. B. and Lawler, W.,** Bone metastasising renal tumour of childhood, *Br. J. Cancer,* 38, 437, 1978.
5. **Beckwith, J. B.,** Wilms' tumour and other renal tumours of childhood: a selective review from the National Wilms' Tumor Study Pathology Center, *Hum. Pathol.,* 14, 481, 1983.
6. **Haas, J. E., Palmer, N. F., Weinberg, A. G., and Beckwith, J. B.,** Ultrastructure of the malignant rhabdoid tumour of the kidney: a distinctive renal tumour of childhood, *Hum. Pathol.,* 12, 646, 1981.
7. **Rutledge, J., Beckwith, J. B., Benjamin, D., and Haas, J. E.,** Absence of immunoperoxidase staining for myoglobin in the malignant rhabdoid tumor of the kidney, *Pediatr. Pathol.,* 1, 93, 1983.
8. **Rousseau-Merck, M. F., Boccon-Gibod, L., Nogues, C., Lesec, G., Lenoir, G., Chatelet, F., Avril, S., and Nezelof, C.,** An original hypercalcaemic infantile renal tumor without bone metastasis: heterotransplantation to nude mice, *Cancer,* 50, 85, 1982.
9. **Bolande, R. P., Brough, A. J., and Izant, J. R.,** Congenital mesoblastic nephroma of infancy, *Pediatrics,* 40, 272, 1967.
10. **Gonzales-Crussi, F.,** Variants and miscellaneous, in, *Wilms' Tumor (Nephroblastoma) and Related Renal Neoplasms of Childhood,* CRC Press, Boca Raton, FL, 1984, 77.
11. **Palmer, N. and Foulkes, M.,** Histopathology and prognosis in the second Intergroup Rhabdomyosarcoma Study (IRS-II). Proc. American Society of Clinical Oncology, 1984.
12. **Weinberg, A. G. and Finegold, M. J.,** Primary hepatic tumours of childhood, *Hum. Pathol.,* 14, 512, 1983.
13. **Craig, J. R., Peters, R. L., Edmondson, H. A., and Omata, M.,** Fibrolamellar carcinoma of the liver: a tumor of adolescents and young adults with distinctive clinico-pathologic features, *Cancer,* 46, 272, 1980.
14. **Evans, A. E., Chatten, J., D'Angio, G. J., Gerson, J. M., Robinson, J., and Schnaufer, L.,** A review of 17 IV-s neuroblastoma patients at the Children's Hospital of Philadelphia, *Cancer,* 45, 833, 1980.
15. **Shimada, H., Chatten, J., Newton, W. A., Jr., Sachs, N., Hamoudi, A. B., Chiba, T., Marsden, H. B., and Misugi, K.,** Histopathologic prognostic factors in neuroblastic tumours: definition of subtypes of ganglioneuroblastoma and an age-linked classification of neuroblastomas, *J. Natl. Cancer Inst.,* 73, 405, 1984.
16. **Lennert, K., Stein, H., and Kaiserling, E.,** Cytological and functional criteria for the classification of malignant lymphomata, *Br. J. Cancer,* 31 (Suppl. 2), 29, 1975.
17. **Jereb, M. and Us-Krasovec, M.,** Trans-thoracic needle biopsy of mediastinal and hilar lesions, *Cancer,* 40, 1354, 1977.
18. **Schaller, R. T., Schaller, J. F., Buschmann, C., and Kiviat, N.,** The usefulness of percutaneous fine needle aspiration biopsy in infants and children, *J. Pediatr. Surg.,* 18, 398, 1983.
19. **Henry, K., Bennett, M. H., and Farrer-Brown, G.,** Classification of the non-Hodgkin's lymphomas, in *Recent Advances in Histopathology,* Vol. 10, Anthony, P. P., and MacSween, R. N. M., Eds., Churchill Livingstone, Edinburgh, 1978, 275.
20. **Beckwith, J. B.,** (1984) Pathology, in *Clinical Pediatric Oncology,* Sutow, W. W., Fernbach, D. J., and Vietti, T. J., Eds., C. V. Mosby, St. Louis, 1984, 55.
21. **Misugi, K., Misugi, N., and Newton, W. A., Jr.,** Fine structural study of neuroblastoma, ganglioneuroblastoma and phaeochromocytoma, *Arch. Pathol.,* 86, 160, 1968.
22. **Askin, F. B., Rosai, J., Sibley, R. K., Dehner, L. P., and McAlister, W. H.,** Malignant small cell tumor of the thoracopulmonary region in childhood: a distinctive clinico-pathologic entity of uncertain histogenesis, *Cancer,* 43, 2438, 1979.
23. **Mori, Y. and Lennert, K.,** *Electron Microscopic Atlas of Lymph Node Cytology and Pathology,* Springer, Berlin, 1969.
24. **Newton, W. A., Jr. and Hamoudi, A. B.,** Histiocytosis: a histological classification with clinical correlation, *Perspect. Paediatr. Pathol.,* 1, 251, 1973.
25. **Llombart-Bosch, A., Blache, R., and Peydro-Olaya, A.,** Ultrastructural study of 28 cases of Ewing's sarcoma: typical and atypical forms, *Cancer,* 41, 1362, 1978.
26. **Henderson, D. W., Raven, J. L., Pollard, J. A., and Walters, M. N.-I.,** Bone marrow metastases in disseminated alveolar rhabdomyosarcoma: case report with ultrastructural study and review, *Pathology,* 8, 329, 1976.
27. **Henderson, D. W. and Papadimitriou, J. M.,** *Ultrastructural Appearances of Tumours: a Diagnostic Atlas,* Churchill Livingstone, Edinburgh, 1982.

28. **Isaacson, P. and Wright, D. H.,** (1983) Immunocytochemistry of lymphoreticular tumours, in *Immunocytochemistry: Practical Applications in Pathology and Biology,* Polak, J. M. and Van Noorden, S., Eds., Wright, Bristol, 1983, 249.
29. **Mason, D. Y.,** Immunohistology of lymphoid tissue, in *Histochemistry in Pathology,* Filipe, M. I. and Lake, B. D., Eds., Churchill Livingstone, Edinburgh, 1983, 215.
30. **Pinkus, G. S.,** Diagnostic immunocytochemistry of paraffin-embedded tissues, *Hum. Pathol.,* 13, 411, 1982.
31. **Gabbiani, G. and Krocher, O.,** Cytocontractile and cytoskeletal elements in pathologic processes: pathogenetic role and diagnostic value, *Arch. Pathol. Lab. Med.,* 107, 622, 1983.
32. **Trojanowski, J. Q., Lee, V. M.-Y., and Schlaepfer, W. W.,** An immunohistochemical study of human central and peripheral nervous system tumours, using monoclonal antibodies against neurofilaments and glial filaments, *Hum. Pathol.,* 15, 248, 1984.
33. **Tsokos, M., Linnoila, R. I., Chandra, R. S., and Triche, T. J.,** Neuron-specific enolase in the diagnosis of neuroblastoma and other small round cell tumours in children, *Hum. Pathol.,* 15, 575, 1984.
34. **Kemshead, J. T. and Coakham, H.,** The use of monoclonal antibodies for the diagnosis of intracerebral malignancies and small round cell tumours of childhood, *J. Pathol.,* 141, 249, 1983.
35. **Kemshead, J. T., Goldman, A., Fritschy, J., Malpas, J. S., and Pritchard, J.,** The use of panels of monoclonal antibodies in the differential diagnosis of neuroblastoma and lymphoblastic disorders, *Lancet,* 1, 12, 1983.
36. **Smith, H.,** The leukaemias, in *Histochemistry in Pathology,* Filipe, M. I. and Lake, B. D., Eds., Churchill Livingstone, Edinburgh, 1983, 206.
37. **Elleder, M., Povysil, C., Rozkovcova, J., and Cihula, J.,** Alpha-D-mannosidase activity in histiocytosis X, Virchows Archiv Abteilung B, *Cell. Pathol.,* (Berlin) 26, 139, 1977.
39. **Pearse, A. G. E.,** Neuroendocrine tumours and hyperplasia, in *Histochemistry in Pathology,* Filipe, M. I. and Lake, B. D., Eds., Churchill Livingstone, Edinburgh, 1983, 274.
39. **Reynolds, C. P., German, D. C., Weinberg, A. G., and Smith, R. G.,** Catecholamine fluorescence and tissue culture morphology. Technics in the diagnosis of neuroblastoma, *Am. J. Clin. Pathol.,* 75, 275, 1981.
40. **Stout, A. P. and Lattes, R.,** Tumors of the soft tissues, in *Atlas of Tumor Pathology,* Fascicle 1, Second Series, Armed Forces Institute of Pathology, Washington, D.C., 1967.
41. **Ozello, L., Stout, A. P., and Murray, M. R.,** Cultural characteristics of malignant histiocytomas and fibrous xanthomas, *Cancer,* 16, 331, 1963.
42. **Murray, M. R. and Stout, A. P.,** Distinctive characteristics of the sympathicoblastoma cultivated *in vitro, Am. J. Pathol.,* 23, 429, 1947.
43. **Yunis, J. J. and Ramsey, N.,** Retinoblastoma and sub-band deletion of chromosome 13, *Am. J. Dis. Child.,* 132, 161, 1978.
44. **Brodeur, G. M., Green, A. A., Hayes, F. A., Williams, K. J., Williams, D. L., and Isiatis, A. A.,** Cytogenetic features of human neuroblastomas and cell lines, *Cancer Res.,* 41, 4678, 1981.
45. **Look, A. T., Hayes, F. A., Nitschke, R., McWilliams, N. B., and Green, A. A.,** Cellular DNA content as a predictor of response to chemotherapy in infants with unresectable neuroblastoma, *N. Engl. J. Med.,* 311, 231, 1984.
46. **Strong, L. C.,** Genetics, etiology, and epidemiology of childhood cancer, in *Clinical Pediatric Oncology,* Sutow, W. W., Fernbach, D. J., Vietti, T. J., Eds., C. V. Mosby, St. Louis, 1984, 14.
47. **Romas, E., Beral, V., Carpenter, L., Watson, A., Barton, C., Ryder, H., and Aston, D. L.,** Childhood leukaemia in the West Berkshire and Basingstoke and North Hampshire District Health Authorities in relation to nuclear establishments in the vicinity, *Br. Med. J.,* 294, 597, 1987.
48. **Darby, S. C. and Doll, R.,** Fallout, radiation doses near Dounreay, and childhood leukaemia, *Br. Med. J.,* 294, 603, 1987.
49. **Bithell, J. F. and Stewart, A. M.,** Prenatal irradiation and childhood malignancy: a review of British data from the Oxford survey, *Br. J. Cancer,* 31, 271, 1975.
50. **Boice, J. D.,** Cancer following medical irradiation, *Cancer,* 47, 1081, 1981.
51. **Herbst, A. L.,** Clear cell adenocarcinoma and the current status of DES-exposed females, *Cancer,* 48, 484, 1981.
52. **Purtilo, D. T.,** Malignant lymphoproliferative diseases induced by Epstein-Barr virus in immuno-deficient patients, including X-linked cytogenetic and familial syndromes, *Cancer Gen. Cytogen.,* 4, 251, 1981.

Chapter 2

MONOCLONAL ANTIBODIES USED FOR THE DIAGNOSIS OF THE SMALL ROUND CELL TUMORS OF CHILDHOOD

J. T. Kemshead, J. Clayton, and K. Patel

TABLE OF CONTENTS

I. INTRODUCTION

Neuroblastoma, rhabdomyosarcoma, Ewing's sarcoma, acute lymphoblastic leukemia/lymphoma, and the blastematous component of Wilms' tumor can be grouped together as the small round blue cell tumors of childhood.[1] While it is often relatively straightforward to arrive at a diagnosis on clinical and conventional pathological information, in a small proportion of cases this is not the case. The pathologist can be left in doubt about the origin of a tumor when presented with biopsies consisting of small uncharacteristic cells with hyperchromatin nuclei and scanty cytoplasm. The accurate classification and subclassification of these tumors is far from academic, particularly as combination chemotherapy has become more specialized.

Immunohistochemistry has proved to be a valuable tool in the identification and characterization of tumor cells.[2] Monoclonal antibodies are playing an ever-increasing role in this area of diagnostic pathology. A great deal of effort has been placed into identifying antigens that are tumor specific. This, however, has not been achieved as no antibody has been obtained that recognizes an antigen uniquely expressed on tumor cells. The closest approximation of a tumor specific antibody one can arrive at is one that reacts with tumor tissue, fetal tissue, and not normal pediatric or adult tissue (i.e., oncofetal specificity). In spite of this, once the specificity of an antibody has been fully established, reagents cross-reacting with normal tissues may be diagnostically useful. This review discusses the various approaches to producing heteroantisera and monoclonal antibodies. The pitfalls associated with the use of monoclonal antibodies are reviewed along with the various types of antigens that are being studied. A panel of antibodies currently available for the differential diagnosis of the small round cell tumors of childhood is also discussed in detail.

II. PRACTICAL CONSIDERATIONS IN THE USE OF MONOCLONAL ANTIBODIES

A. Antigenic Expression

1. Heterogeneity

It is now well accepted that there is a considerable degree of antigenic heterogeneity found in any tumor cell population.[3] This means that when exquisitely specific reagents such as monoclonal antibodies are used, panels of reagents are needed to maximize the detection of the malignant population.

The underlying cause of tumor cell heterogeneity is under debate. While it is generally accepted that tumors are monoclonal in origin, a degree of tumor progression is observed. This is shown by variability in antigen expression as well as instability of the malignant karyotype. It is not possible to generalize about whether the heterogeneity in antigen density is due to qualitative and/or quantitative changes in expression. In the majority of cases it is probable that quantitative changes in antigen levels will occur due to a fine disturbance of the normal homeostatic processes involved in transcription and translation of any particular gene/gene complex.

2. Aberrant Expression

Many antigens identified by monoclonal antibodies appear to have a very restricted distribution, e.g., only being expressed on hemopoietic cells. However, occasionally the antigen may be found on what appears to be a totally unrelated cell type. Such an example is the C-ALLA antigen found on acute lymphoblastic leukemia cells.[4] Studies of many cell lines and tissues have also identified this antigen on a small number of neuroblastomas.[5]

The reasons underlying the apparent aberrant expression of a particular antigen on a cell type are not easy to explain. When this is observed it is generally noted in very anaplastic tumors. The differential antigen expression occurring in cells very early during embryonic development remains ill understood. It is tempting to speculate that if tumors arise from cells becoming frozen at a particular step in their normal differentiation pathway, then what is being observed is the sharing of antigens early in development.[6] These differentiation antigens became "switched off" in one cell type early in their maturation pathway, while they are maintained in other cells. If tumors arise at a sufficiently early developmental stage coexpression of antigens on apparently unrelated cell types will, therefore, be observed.

Alternatively, as it is known that the karyotype of many tumor cells is abnormal, it is possible that during complex translocations/deletions/amplifications, genes may become activated in cells where they are normally quiescent.

B. Identification of Shared Antigens

The assumption is often made that one monoclonal antibody binds to a single antigen. It is forgotten that binding of antibody to antigen is a dynamic event. Antibodies can bind to different epitopes with different affinities. It has been calculated that seven amino acids form a structure that allows the maximal possible three-dimensional fit of a high affinity antibody. Obviously, part of the sequence forming a three-dimensional structure may be shared between antigens, allowing a reagent to bind to different molecules with different affinities.[7]

C. Tissue Preparation

It has been found that many of the monoclonal antibodies currently available to us do not work on conventionally prepared formalin fixed, paraffin wax-embedded sections. This means that frozen sections have to be used which make morphological studies often difficult to interpret.

Formaldehyde fixation is achieved by chemically cross-linking proteins via amino acid residues. This may bring about denaturation which in turn can lead to the destruction or masking of certain antigenic sites.[7] As an alternative, dehydrating fixatives may be used to preserve specimen morphology (e.g., acetone/methanol). These function by disrupting hydrogen bonds and have a hardening effect on tissues. In general, brief exposure to this type of fixative does not damage antigenic structure, and most monoclonal antibodies will function on such tissue. As an alternative, protease digestion of formalin fixed tissue has been attempted with limited success. This breaks formaldehyde induced cross-links, allowing greater penetration of an antibody into tissues. Unfortunately, the precise enzyme and conditions for digestion vary for any particular antigen, making the technique extremely labor intensive.

Paraffin wax with its high melting point may also have a deleterious effect on antigens that are heat labile. This problem can now be overcome using low melting point waxes that can be used at 37°C.

III. APPROACHES TO OBTAINING IMMUNOLOGICAL REAGENTS

A. Heteroantisera

1. Cell Lines and Tissues as Immunogens

A variety of human neuroectodermally derived tissues and/or cell lines have been used to raise antisera specific to human neuroblastoma cells. Using human fetal brain, Casper et al.[8] raised an antiserum that detects antigens shared between neuroblastoma and other normal neural tissues. Following extensive absorption, indirect immunofluorescence and radiobinding studies indicated the reagent bound to fetal brain, adult brain, neuroblastoma, and embryonal rhabdomyosarcoma. No reactivity to glial cells or hemopoietic cells was reported, suggesting that the cross-reactivity between neuroectodermal and mesenchymal tumors (neuroblastoma, rhabdomyosarcoma) was not artifactual.

Seeger et al.[9] have also described a heteroantiserum, raised against the human neuroblastoma cell line LAN 1. Following absorption, the antiserum bound to a relatively large group of tumors, namely: neuroblastoma, Oat cell carcinoma, Wilms' tumor, and sarcomas. In addition, the reagent bound to normal fetal and adult brain as well as adrenal gland. Antisera of the type described above always cross-react with tissue/tumors other than neuroblastoma and related normal tissues. Whether this is due to lack of sufficient absorption has always been questioned, as no biochemical studies on the antigens detected by these reagents have been reported.

2. Purified Antigens as Immunogens

Until recently some of the best high titer and well characterized heteroantisera to neural tissue have been those reacting with the Thy-1 molecule in rodents.[10-11] These have been produced using highly purified Thy-1 as an antigen and require little or no absorption to confirm their specificity. Originally using one of these reagents and more recently monoclonal antibodies to the antigen, we have identified the human homologue of Thy-1 on several human neuroblastoma cell lines. Using a Skatchard analysis, the neuroblastoma cell line TR14 has been shown to express 2—2.25 $\times$ 10^6 molecules of antigen/cell.[10] The specificity of rabbit anti-rat Thy-1 antisera to the human homologue of this molecule was demonstrated by blocking all reactivity of the reagent by prior incubation with an excess of highly purified human Thy-1. It was estimated that approximately 25% of the total anti-rat Thy-1 antibodies in the heteroantisera bind to the human homologue of Thy-1. This suggests that the primary sequence of the Thy-1 antigen is at least partially conserved between species.

Despite structural homology, the distribution of Thy-1 differs markedly in different species. There is considerable variation among the cells expressing the Thy-1 antigen within the nervous system. In addition rat thymocytes express the Thy-1 antigen, but this is not the case in the human. Analysis of bone marrow cells in humans shows Thy-1 to be expressed on less than 0.1% of the nucleated cell population. This is important as a monoclonal antibody to Thy-1 has been used as one of a panel of reagents in studying the metastatic spread of neuroblastoma cells to bone marrow.[10]

3. Synthetic Peptides as Immunogens

Using DNA sequencing techniques, it is possible to predict the amino acid sequence of a particular gene. Based on this sequence it is possible to produce synthetic peptides that can be used as immunogens. To determine the amino acid sequence of peptides to be synthesized, a hydrophobicity plot (Figure 1) is often produced to determine sequences that lie in either particular hydrophilic or hydrophobic regions of the molecule.[12] Synthetic peptides are then usually linked to a carrier molecule such as Keyhole Limpet Hemocyanin to render them more immunogenic. Antisera and/or monoclonal antibodies produced in this way can be purified by affinity chromatography, as it is possible to obtain the synthetic peptide/immunogen in relatively large amounts. Examples of antisera prepared by this approach are reagents recognizing oncogene products such as the C-myc[13] and N-myc proteins. While the expression of the C-myc gene occurs in a relatively wide variety of tumors/tissues, the N-myc gene product is far more restricted. (See Garson et al., Chapter 10.)

B. Monoclonal Antibodies

A very large number of monoclonal antibodies have been either produced against or shown to cross-react with the "small round cell tumors of childhood". It is inappropriate to list all of these reagents, as many have been made against tumors such as melanoma[14] and small lung cell carcinoma.[15] Instead of this, examples of antibodies recognizing different cell structures will be reviewed and those most useful as diagnostic aids will be discussed in detail.

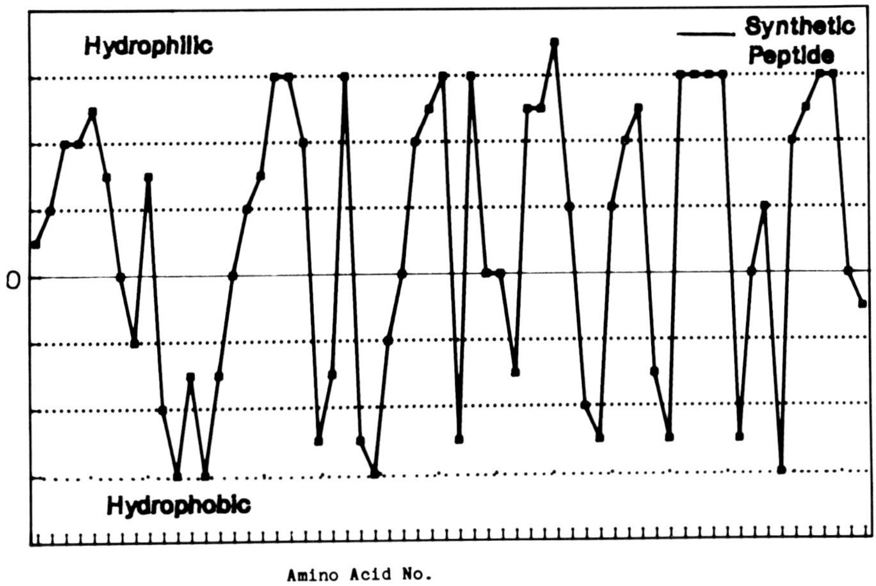

FIGURE 1. Hydrophobicity plot of a selected protein, based on predicted amino acid sequence. The amino acid sequence of a protein can be arrived at by either direct sequencing or determined from the DNA sequence of the particular gene. The hydrophobicity plot represents a plot of amino acid number V charge to demonstrate areas that lie in particular hydrophobic or hydrophillic areas.

Antibodies can be broken down into those recognizing cell membrane, cytoplasmic, and nuclear associated antigens.

1. Cell Membrane/ECM

Monoclonal antibodies recognizing cell membrane components bind to either glycoprotein or glycolipid antigens within the bilayer. Included in this section are also reagents that react with extracellular matrix material, as it is often difficult to distinguish these antibodies from those directly binding to the outer membrane of the cell.

The first published monoclonal antibody to neuroblastoma was PI 153/3 a reagent that binds to human neuroblastoma, retinoblastoma, and glioblastoma.[16] This antibody, of the IgM isotype, also binds to pre-B and common acute lymphoblastic leukemia cells (C-ALL). The antigen recognized by this monoclonal has been demonstrated to be a 20 kDa protein/glycoprotein expressed on the membranes of both neuroblasts and leukemic cells.[17] Conversely, several antibodies raised against hemopoietic cells have also been shown to bind to tissues of neuroectodermal origin.[18] The monoclonal antibody BA2, raised following immunization of mice with Nalm 6-M1-ALL cells, recognizes a cell surface glycoprotein of 24 kDa on both neuroblastoma and ALL cells.[19,20] As well as recognizing these malignant cells, BA2 binds to normal pre-B cells and normal fetal and adult brain.

Other examples of antibodies cross-reacting with hemopoietic cells and neural cells are Leu 7[21] and UCHT1.[22] Leu 7 binds to natural killer cells as well as neuroblasts and UCHT1 to a cell membrane glycoprotein on T lymphocytes and an intracellular protein present in Purkinje cells.[23]

Antibodies binding to neural cells that selectively cross-react with myeloid cells and platelets have also been described. The antibodies MIN1 and UJ308 raised against the human neuroblastoma cell line CHP 100 and human fetal brain repeatedly cross-react with promyelocytes and more mature cells of the granulocyte lineage.[24] Antibody M148 raised against human medulloblastoma tissue binds to the glycoprotein 11b/IIIa complex and also to neu-

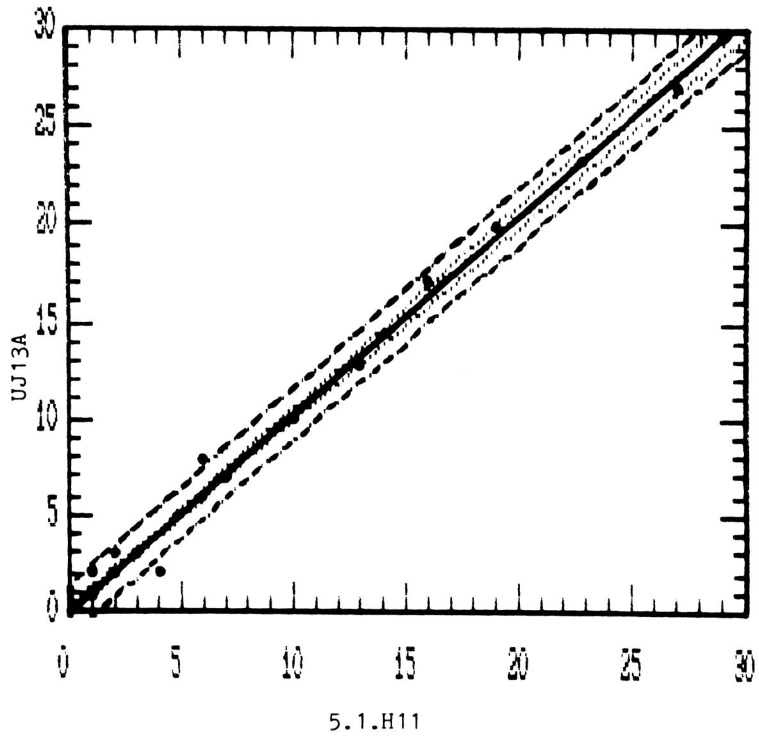

FIGURE 2. Scattergram plot of one antibody V per second. The reactivity of antibody one is plotted against antibody two. If the reagents recognize identical antigens, a line drawn between the points should lie at 45′ to the axis. This can be represented mathematically as the correlation coefficient. (···) 95% Confidence limit, (—) 95% prediction limit.

roblastoma cells.[25] Presumably, the latter illustrates an example of an antibody recognizing epitopes shared between two biochemically distinct antigens, as no reports of glycoprotein 11b/IIIa have been made on neural cells. However, for many of the antibodies described above, the biochemical characteristics of the antigen recognized by the reagent on either neural or hemopoietic cells remains unclear.

Antibodies with a more restricted specificity have been raised against human fetal brain as well as a variety of neuroectodermal tumors. UJ13A is one such antibody, of the IgG_{2a} isotype that binds to the majority of tissues/tumors derived from the neuroectoderm.[26] The exception to this reactivity is the antibody does not bind to melanoma. The reagent has proved extremely valuable in bone marrow purging studies, radioimmunolocalization, and targeted radiation therapy.[27] Looking more closely at the specificity of this antibody, it appears the reagent also binds to Wilms' tumors, hepatoblastoma, and embryonal rhabdomyosarcomas. This antigen is also expressed on the corresponding fetal tissues, although its neuroectodermal specificity is upheld in children and adults.[26]

The antigen that is recognized by antibody UJ13A is now thought to be a protein/glycoprotein, after preliminary investigations had indicated this to be a glycolipid. However, both cell surface labeling and immunoprecipitation as well as Western Blotting have failed to reveal the nature of the antigen. An antibody noted to have similar binding characteristics to UJ13A but raised against totally different immunogen is 5.1.H11.[28] This antibody of the IgG isotype was produced following immunization of mice with a primary culture of myoblasts. Comparison of the binding of these reagents on over 50 different tissues and several hundred samples suggests these may recognize the same antigenic structure. Statistical analysis of this binding data by scatter plot and regression analysis is a way of illustrating this similarity with a correlation coefficient of 0.994 being obtained (Figure 2).

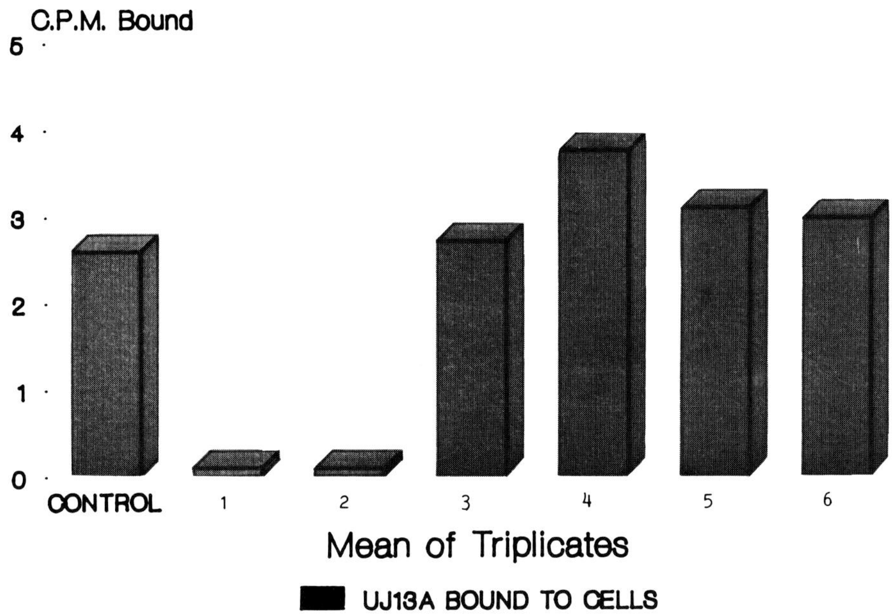

FIGURE 3. Blockade of radiolabeled UJ13A with an excess of nonradiolabeled antibody (UJ13A blocked with 5.1.H11; JR1. target cells 2.5 × 10E5). Radiolabeled and nonradiolabeled antibodies were mixed and then added to 2 × 10^5 target cells. After 30 min unbound isotope was washed from the cells and bound isotope counted. Control: No excess nonradiolabeled antibody. 1/2: Incubation with 125I UJ13A and 5μl and 50μl of unlabeled UJ13A ascites; blockade observed. 3/4: Incubation with 125I UJ13A and 5μl and 50μl of unlabeled 5.1.H11 ascites; no blockade observed. 5/6: Incubation with 125I UJ13A and 5μl and 50μl of unlabeled UJ127.11 ascites; not expected to block UJ13A.

Cross-blocking experiments to show that the two reagents bind to similar epitopes on the same antigen have not proved fruitful. While it is possible to block the binding of radiolabeled UJ13A to cells with a large excess of unlabeled antibody, this is not the case for an excess of antibody 5.1.H11 (Figure 3). This, however, does not mean the two reagents recognize different antigenic structures as one has to bear in mind the unique specificity of monoclonal antibodies. It is possible that the two antibodies may recognize different epitopes on the same antigen that are spatially separated so that cross-blocking does not occur.

While UJ13A has a broad spectrum of reactivity to neuroectodermally derived tumor tissues, other antibodies raised against human fetal brain have a much more restricted specificity. UJ181.4 binds to fetal brain, primitive neuroectodermal tumors such as medulloblastoma, neuroblastoma, and pineoblastoma, but not adult brain.[29] Again the antigen recognized by the monoclonal antibody is not known other than that it is a glycoprotein. Despite this, the antibody has been used for the intrathecal targeting of radiation to primitive neuroectodermal tumors.[30]

In addition to glycoproteins, glycolipids have also proved to be interesting antigenic determinants on neuroectodermally derived cells. The first monoclonal antibody described to a ganglioside expressed on neural cells was A2B5 raised following immunization of mice with chick retinal cells.[31] This antigen is highly conserved throughout the animal kingdom, being also expressed on human retinal cells as well as neuroblastoma.[32] While the antigen has a very restricted specificity, the antibody has been found to bind to epithelial cells in specific parts of the alimentary canal, and on occasion, to cells present in normal bone marrow. This latter reactivity may be due to Fc interaction with granulocytes, as the reagent can give ''high background staining'' on this particular cell type.

Several antibodies to the ganglioside GD_2 have been described.[33,34] This antigen is strongly expressed on neuroblastoma, melanoma, and small lung cell carcinomas. In addition, the antigen is present on brain and occasionally reported to be associated with Ewing's sarcoma. Whether this latter binding is due selectively to those Ewing's sarcomas that have other neuroectodermal characteristics remains to be evaluated. The number of GD_2 molecules per neuroblast has been calculated to be 110—270,000 depending on the cell line studied.[34] The high expression of this antigen on neuroblastic tissue makes this determinant useful for the diagnosis of tumor infiltration into bone marrow as well as targeted therapy. In addition to these roles, the antibody has been used to detect circulating GD_2 in the serum of children with metastatic disease.[35] Whether the shedding of antigen from the cell surface will interfere with targeted therapy still has to be ascertained, but this is obviously not an ideal situation.

2. *Cytoplasmic Antigens*

A comprehensive list of cytoplasmic markers is given in Tables 1 and 2 with selected illustrations discussed in more detail below.

a. Intermediate Filament Antigens

Intermediate filament proteins can be divided into five different groups, namely vimentin, desmin, cytokeratin, glial fibrillary acidic protein (GFAP) and neurofilaments. Within these groups subdivisions have been made. For example many different forms of cytokeratins have been identified. The precise function of intermediate filament proteins has to be elucidated, but it is thought that they play a structural role in the integrity of the cell. These proteins are composed of polymorphic subunits, and the expression of a particular intermediate filament type is restricted to a subset of tissues. In general the specific pattern of intermediate filament expression is maintained during transformation making the proteins useful as markers for malignant disease.

Within the small round cell tumors of childhood, desmin expression in rhabdomyosarcoma cells has proven to be the most reliable marker in our studies. This has been found to be present in all embryonal rhabdomyosarcoma (14/14) and 3/5 rhabdomyosarcoma cell lines examined.[36] No binding to neuroblastoma, Ewing's sarcoma, or lymphoblastic leukemia/lymphoma tissues of cell lines was identified. Coexpression of intermediate filament proteins can occur with vimentin also being identified in rhabdomyosarcoma (8/9). The specificity of vimentin expression in this group of tumors is weak as it has been identified in Ewing's sarcomas and leukemias/lymphomas (see Figure 5).

Neurofilament expression in tumors of neuroectodermal origin has also been used as a marker for neuroblastic malignancies. Approximately 50% of neuroblastomas bind a monoclonal antibody to neurofilament proteins in our experience. Neurofilament expression appears to be restricted to the mature cell phenotype indicating that immature anaplastic cells may not express this particular antigen. Most of the monoclonal antibodies to neurofilament proteins are directed against phosphorylated determinants on the molecules.[37] As phosphorylation may take place relatively late in the organization of subunits into neurofilament proteins, this may also explain why relatively immature cells do not bind antibodies to this structure.

GFAP and cytokeratins are expressed in groups of tumors other than the small round cell tumors of childhood (glial tumors and carcinomas, respectively). Studies on the expression of GFAP in the laboratory, however, illustrate two interesting points about intermediate filaments. While many glial tumors express GFAP when placed into primary culture, antigen expression is rapidly lost. This finding is obviously also true of glial cell lines that have been established, as the minority maintain GFAP expression. The other observation concerning GFAP and other intermediate filaments examined in the laboratory is that the molecules are subject to rapid proteolysis. This results in obtaining a "protein smear" on SDS polyacrylamide gel electrophoresis unless the most stringent purification procedures are applied. Limited proteolysis can make the biochemical characterization of intermediate filament proteins extremely difficult unless a technique such as Western Blotting is used. (See Table 2.)

b. Other Cytoplasmic Markers

Neuron specific enolase — This isoenzyme of enolase has been reported as being only expressed in cells of neuroectodermal origin. It is an acidic protein with a PI of 4.7 and a molecular weight of 78 kDa. The molecule consists of a dimer of 39 kDa subunits.[38] Antisera raised against neuron specific enolase do not cross-react with the other isoenzyme of enolase found in the brain NNE (non-neuronal enolase) which is also a dimeric protein consisting of 43.5 kDa subunits with a PI of 7.2. Hybrid molecules consisting of both subunits of NSE and NNE have also been found in the brain which may lead to confusion concerning the immunohistochemical characterization of cells expressing NSE. While neuron specific enolase has been described in neurons and neuroendocrine cells, non-neuronal enolase has been found in glia and non-neuronal cells.

NSE has also been identified in small lung cell carcinoma biopsies and neuroepitheliomas.[39] This finding along with other immunohistological studies has been used to differentiate neuroepitheliomas from Ewing's sarcomas and lymphomas. Whether or not NSE is expressed in Ewing's sarcomas remains a point of controversy. In addition, the specificity of NSE expression has been questioned, particularly as the antigen has been found in a small number of rhabdomyosarcomas (personal observation). Some doubt has been placed on these findings by some groups, particularly as immunohistological studies have had to rely on the use of heteroantisera to NSE. Monoclonal antibodies to the antigen have only just become available. However, biochemical analysis of rhabdomyosarcoma tissue has revealed a low expression of this isoenzyme of enolase.

Myosin and other "Muscle Associated Markers" — Myosin and myoglobin are generally accepted as cytoplasmic markers associated with skeletal muscle.[40,41] They have been used in attempts to characterize rhabdomyosarcoma cells, but in general are found to only be expressed in the more differentiated cell types. This somewhat avoids the diagnostic problem, as it is always the most anaplastic tumors that are the most difficult to classify. Titin and embryonic myosin heavy chain also fall into this category of markers, but do appear restricted in their specificity to rhabdoid tumors[42] (Table 1).

Terminal Deoxynucleotidyl Transferase (Tdt) — This enzyme is expressed in thymocytes, a small number of bone marrow cells, but not in mature lymphocytes. It is used as an early lymphoid marker, expressed in approximately 95% of acute lymphoblastic leukemias (ALL). Tdt has not been identified in neuroblastomas or rhabdomyosarcomas examined (unpublished observation) making the marker useful in the differential diagnosis of these diseases. Tdt is present in a larger number of ALLs than the CALLA cell membrane marker.[43] Analysis of Tdt is, therefore, a more reliable way of distinguishing ALL from acute myeloid leukemia which is mainly Tdt negative. As well as Tdt, cytoplasmic immunoglobulin has been used as a marker for distinguishing pre-B ALLs from common ALL, both of which are Tdt positive. New molecular techniques using B and T gene rearrangements as markers are making the classification of leukemias/lymphomas more precise — a topic discussed by W. Smith in Chapter 9.

3. Nuclear Antigens

A detailed discussion of the use of antisera and monoclonal antibodies to the N-myc oncogene product is presented by Garson in Chapter 10.

An antibody has been developed (KI 67) that binds to a nuclear antigen present in proliferating cells but absent in resting cells.[44] While all cell types have not been tested,

Table 1
CYTOPLASMIC MARKERS IDENTIFIED BY IMMUNOLOGICAL TECHNIQUES

Marker	Normal cell specificity	Tumor specificity	Ref.
Actin	Skeletal muscle	Rhabdomyosarcoma	48
Myosin	Skeletal muscle	Rhabdomyosarcoma	40
Embryonic myosin	Skeletal muscle	Rhabdomyosarcoma	49
Heavy chain myoglobin	Skeletal muscle	Rhabdomyosarcoma	50
Titin	Skeletal muscle	Rhabdomyosarcoma	42
B Enolase	Skeletal muscle	Rhabdomyosarcoma	51
NSE	Neurones Neuroendocrine cells	Neuroblastoma +	50
5A7 Antigen	Neurones	Neuroblastoma	52
S100 Protein	Schwann cells Glia	Neuroblastoma Ganglioneuroblastoma	53
Microtubule associated protein	Neurones	Neuroblastoma	54
Cytoplasmic Ig	Pre-B and B cells	Pre-B-ALL, ALL B cell lymphoma	6
Tdt	Pre-B and Pre-T lymphocytes	CALLA	43

Table 2
INTERMEDIATE FILAMENT PROTEINS

Protein	Molecular weight (kDa)	Ref.
Desmin	53	55
Vimentin	58	56
GFAP	55	57
Neurofilament	68 160 200	37
Cytokeratins	40—70	58

this specificity has been maintained for all cells examined to date. This reagent, while obviously not tumor specific, could be very useful in identifying the proliferation status of cells that have metastasized to bone marrow. This has implication for the use of clinical purging procedures in bone marrow harvested for autologous transplantation. To obtain efficient kill, cells need to be in cycle, particularly as many of the cyclophosphamide derivatives used for the chemical purging of bone marrow have a very short half-life in solution. Very preliminary data from our laboratory suggest that this may not be the case. The efficiency of purging techniques applied to marrow harvested for autologous transplantation is discussed by A. Gee, Chapter 7.

IV. PANELS OF ANTIBODIES FOR THE CHARACTERIZATION OF THE SMALL ROUND CELL TUMORS OF CHILDHOOD

Figure 4 illustrates that it is now easy to compile panels of antibodies that can be used for the differential diagnosis of neuroblastoma from acute lymphoblastic leukemia/lymphoma. Antibodies such as UJ13A, FMG25, UJ127.11, UJ181.4, A2B5, and 5.1.H11 bind

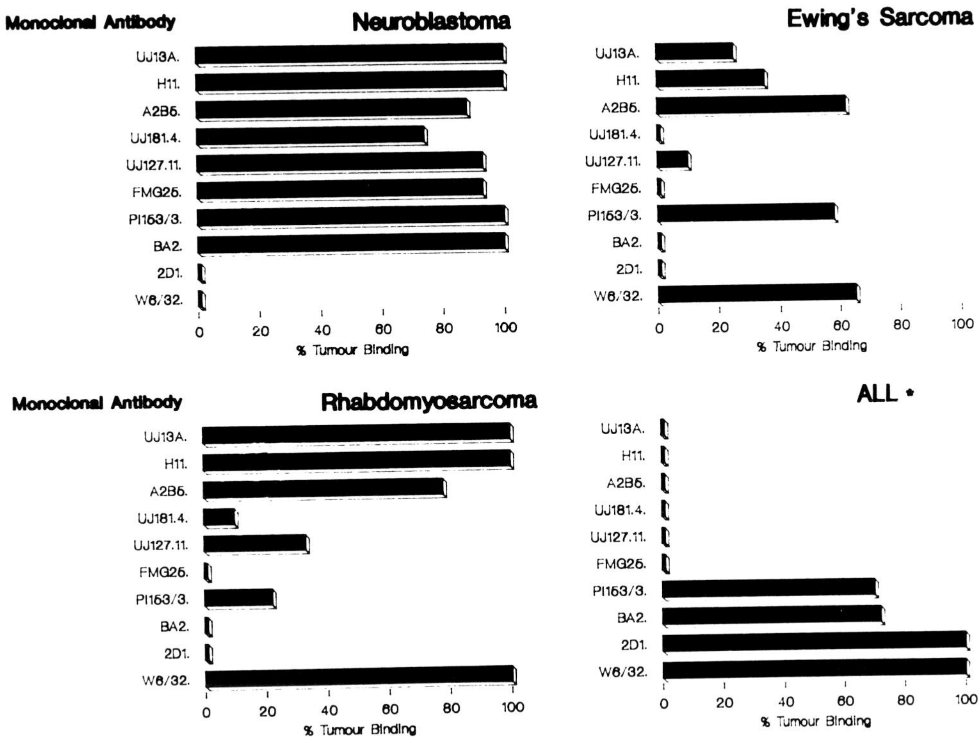

FIGURE 4. Monoclonal antibody profiles of the major small round cell tumors of childhood. Cell surface markers.

to a high proportion of neuroblasts but not to the majority of acute lymphoblastic leukemias examined. Although not illustrated, a variety of different markers can also be selected that bind to leukemias/lymphomas. These include antibodies to surface and cytoplasmic Ig, the C-ALLA antigen, and Tdt, all of which show no reactivity to neuroblastoma. It is beyond the scope of this review to extensively discuss the various different reagents used in the subtyping of leukemias/lymphomas, but it must be borne in mind that these malignancies can now be immunologically subgrouped.

In spite of the heterogeneity of antigen expression on tumor cells if samples are limited, antibodies UJ13A and 2D1 are capable in the vast majority of cases, of differentiating neuroblastoma and acute lymphoblastic leukemia. The 2D1 antigen has also not been found on rhabdomyosarcoma and Ewing's tumors although one has to exert care in the use of this reagent if tumors contain lymphoid infiltrates.

The differential diagnosis of neuroblastoma from rhabdomyosarcoma and Ewing's sarcoma is more problematical, as many of the reagents binding to neuroblastoma also recognize a population of rhabdomyosarcomas. The best reagents available in our studies for the differential diagnosis of neuroblastoma from rhabdomyosarcoma are FMG25, UJ181.4, and BA2. While the binding specificity of FMG25 and UJ181.4 has been confirmed in a recent workshop on the differential reactivity of antibodies to the small round cell tumors of childhood, that of BA2 has not.[59] This is possibly due to the confusion concerning BA2 binding to lymphocytes in tumor biopsies. If it were not for this problem, W6/32, an antibody recognizing a monomorphic determinant on HLA antigens, would also be useful in this differential diagnosis. HLA antigens appear weakly expressed on neuroblastoma tumors, but are detectable on both rhabdomyosarcomas and Ewing's sarcomas (see Figure 4).

The use of the above reagents, along with the selected expression of desmin in embryonal rhabdomyosarcomas, makes it possible to distinguish neuroblastoma from rhabdomyosar-

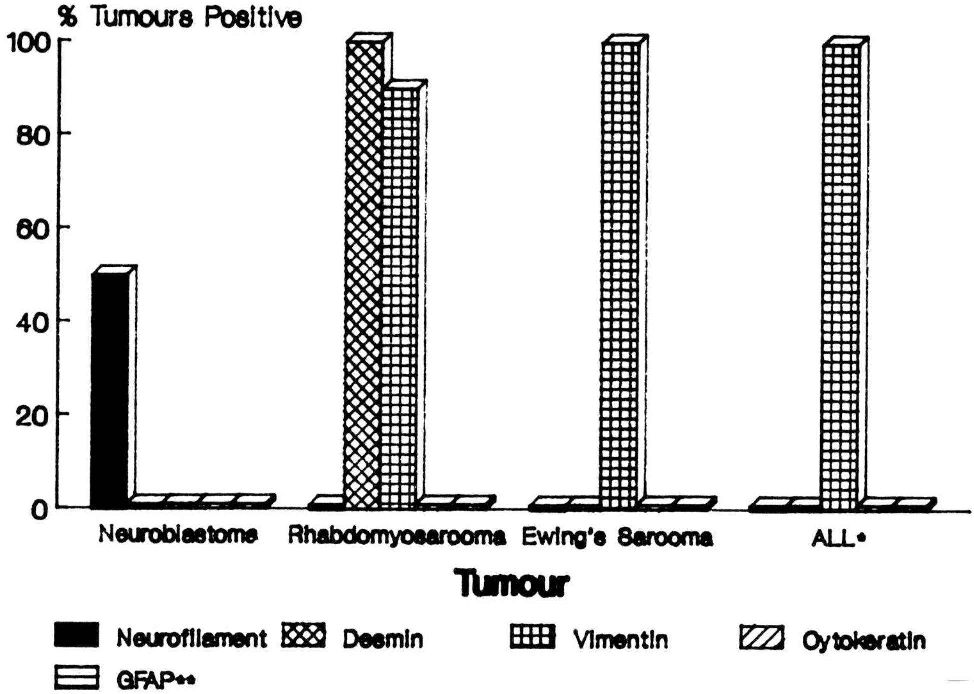

FIGURE 5. Monoclonal antibody profiles of the major small round cell tumors of childhood. Intermediate filament expression.

coma (Figure 5). It becomes more difficult to be sure of a differential diagnosis between neuroblastoma and Ewing's sarcoma because there is no antibody available that can positively and reproducibly recognize Ewing's sarcoma but not neuroblastoma. Obtaining a differential diagnosis on the basis of a one way selection of antibodies binding to neuroblastoma and not Ewing's sarcoma could be misleading. An additional problem here is the neuroepitheliomas which share many features in common with neuroblastoma. These tumors can be shown to contain neurosecretory granules and neurotubules, suggesting they are of neuroectodermal origin. In addition they express many cell membrane markers that are shared with neuroblastoma, e.g., UJ13A, 5.1.H11, UJ127.11, UJ181.4 (JTK, unpublished observation). The major differences between neuroblastoma and neuroepitheliomas are the expression of Class I HLA antigens and the synthesis of biogenic amines. HLA antigen has been reported as being more abundant on neuroepitheliomas as compared to neuroblastoma and the synthesis of biogenic amines in the two tumor types is different. In parallel with this latter observation, high levels of 3-4-dihydroxyphenylethylamine beta hydroxylase and tyrosine hydroxylase are found in neuroblastoma and not in neuroepitheliomas.[46] Neuroepitheliomas contain a chromosome translation (11:22) (q24:q12) that is indistinguishable from that found in some Ewing's sarcomas.[47] This has lead to the suggestion that at least a proportion of Ewing's sarcomas may be neuroectodermal in origin and may explain why in certain cases antibodies suggested as neuroectodermal markers react with the Ewing's sarcoma.

With the exception of desmin expression in rhabdomyosarcoma, no consistent marker has been identified that can differentiate between this tumor and Ewing's sarcoma. Multiple attempts in the laboratory to produce antibodies to Ewing's sarcoma have resulted in the generation of reagents binding extracellular matrix material associated with many different tumor types. More work is therefore necessary to resolve this diagnostic problem.

V. CONCLUSION

It has now been independently proven that monoclonal antibodies can play a role in the diagnosis of the small round cell tumors of childhood. In addition, they are useful in the identification of metastatic spread of tumor cells to bone marrow.

Antibodies form another approach to tumor diagnosis and must not be viewed in isolation. They rarely are the only approach to diagnosis. However, they offer cost and speed advantages over other more complex procedures that might be applied when a diagnosis is in doubt. Unfortunately, at the present time the use of monoclonal antibodies is limited by our need to have specially prepared tissues for examination. Frozen tissue is often not available, particularly when biopsy material is limited. Until recently, antibodies have been developed solely for their specificity. Such reagents have then found a wide use in both diagnostic and therapeutic procedures. However, it is apparent that reagents that are used for radioimmunolocalization studies may not be ideal for immunohistological procedures. The approach for the future will be to characterize antigens of interest and then develop monoclonals against the antigen that are selected for a particular purpose, e.g., recognizing the antigen in conventionally prepared pathological material. These reagents will form the next generation of monoclonal antibodies and will, hopefully, find a wider acceptance in the medical community.

REFERENCES

1. **Young, J. and Miller, R.,** Incidence of Malignant Tumours in US Children, *J. Paediatr.*, 86, 254, 1975.
2. **Erlandson, R.,** Diagnostic Immunochemistry of Human Tumours, *Am. J. Surg. Pathol.*, 8, 615, 1984.
3. **Malpas, J., Kemshead, J., Pritchard, J., and Greaves, M.,** Heterogeneity in Cell Surface Antigens on Neuroblastoma Cells, in *Proc. 13th Meet. Int. Soc. Paediatr. Oncol.*, Raybaud, C., Clement, R., and Lebreuil, G., Eds., Excerpta Medica, Amsterdam, 1983, 90.
4. **Ritz, J., Pesando, J., Notis-McConarty, J., Lazarus, H., and Schlossman, S.,** A Monoclonal Antibody to Human Lymphoblastic Leukaemia Antigen, *Nature*, 283, 583, 1980.
5. **Sugimoto, Y., Sawada, T., Negoro, S., Kidowaki, T., Morioka, H., Matsumura, T., Kemshead, J., and Seeger, R.,** Altered expression of cell surface membrane antigens in a common acute lymphoblastic leukaemia — associated antigen — expressing neuroblastoma cell line (SJ-N-CG) with morphological differentiation, *Cancer Res.*, 45, 358, 1985.
6. **Greaves, M., Janossy, G., Francis, G., and Minowada, J.,** Membrane phenotypes of human leukaemic cells and leukaemic cell lines. Clinical correlates and biological implications, in *Differentiation of Normal and Neoplastic Haemopoietic Cells*, Clarkson, B., Marks, P. A., Till, J., Eds., Cold Spring Harbor Laboratory, New York, 1978, 823.
7. **Sternberger, L.,** Tissue Preparation, in *Immunocytochemistry*, 3rd ed., J. Wiley & Sons, New York, 1986, chap. 4, 210.
8. **Casper, J., Borella, L., and Sen, L.,** Reactivity of human brain antiserum with neuroblastoma cells and non-reactivity with thymocytes and lymphocytes, *Cancer Res.*, 37, 1750, 1977.
9. **Seeger, R., Zeltzer, P., and Rayner, S.,** Onco-Neural Antigen: A New Neural Differentiation Antigen Expressed by Neuroblastoma, Oat Cell Carcinoma, Wilms Tumour and Sarcoma Cells, *J. Immunol.*, 122, 1548, 1979.
10. **Kemshead, J., Ritter, M., Cotmore, S., and Greaves, M.,** Thy-1 Expression on the Surface of Neuronal and Glial Cells, *Brain Res.*, 236, 451, 1982.
11. **Morris, R. and Williams, A.,** Antigens on Mouse and rat Lymphocytes Recognized by Rabbit Antiserum to Rat Brain; The Quantitative Analysis of a Xenogenic Serum, *Eur. J. Immunol.*, 5, 274, 1975.
12. **Hopp, T. and Wood, K.,** Production of Protein Antigenic Determinants from Amino Acid Sequences, *Proc. Natl. Acad. Sci.* U.S.A., 78, 3824, 1981.
13. **Evan, G., Lewis, G., Ramsey, G., and Bishop, J.,** Isolation of Monoclonal Antibodies Specific for Human C-Myc Proto-Oncogene Product, *Mol. Cell. Biol.*, 5, 3610, 1985.
14. **Hellstrom, K., Hellstrom, I., and Brown, J.,** Monoclonal Antibodies to Melanoma Associated Antigens, in *Monoclonal Antibodies and Cancer*, Ed. Wright, G. L., Ed. Marcel Dekker, New York, 1982, 31.

15. **Watanabe, J., Okabe, T., Fujisawa, M., Takaka, F., and Fukayama, M.,** Isolation of Small Lung Cell Cancer Associated Antigen from Human Brain, *Cancer Res.,* 47, 960, 1987.
16. **Kennett, R. and Gilbert, F.,** Hybrid Myelomas Producing Antibodies Against a Human Neuroblastoma Antigen Present in Foetal Brain, *Science,* 203, 1120, 1979.
17. **Momoi, M., Kennett, R., and Glick, M.,** A membrane glycoprotein from human neuroblastoma cells isolated with the use of a monoclonal antibody, *J. Biol. Chem.,* 225, 11914, 1980.
18. **Kemshead, J., Fritschy, J., Asser, U., Sutherland, R., and Greaves, M.,** Monoclonal antibodies defining markers with apparent selectivity for particular haemopoietic cell types may also detect antigens on cells of neural crest origin, *Hybridoma,* 1, 109, 1982.
19. **LeBien, T., Kersey, J., Nakazawa, S., Minato, K., and Minawada, J.,** Analysis of Human Leukaemia and Lymphoma Cells With Monoclonal Antibodies BA1, BA2 and BA3, *Leuk. Res.,* 6, 299, 1982.
20. **Kersey, J., Lebien, T., Abramson, C., Newman, R., Sutherland, R., and Greaves, M.,** P24: A human leukaemia associated and lympho-haemopoietic progenitor cell surface structure identified with monoclonal antibody, *J. Exp. Med.,* 153, 726, 1981.
21. **Abo, T. and Balch, C.,** A differentiation antigen of human NK and cells identified by a monoclonal antibody (HNK-1), *J. Immunol.,* 127, 1024, 1981.
22. **Beverley, P.,** Monoclonal Antibodies and Lymphoid Malignancies, *Haemat. Onc.,* 2, 139, 1984.
23. **Garson, J., Beverley, P., Coakham, H., and Harper, E.,** Monoclonal antibodies against human T cells stain Purkinje cells of many species, *Nature,* 298, 375, 1982.
24. **Kemshead, J., Bicknell, D., and Greaves, M.,** A Monoclonal Antibody Shared by Neural Cells and Granulocytic Cells, *Paediatr. Res.,* 15, 1282, 1981.
25. **Jones, D., Fritschy, J., Garson, J., Nokes, T., Kemshead, J., and Hardisty, R.,** A monoclonal antibody binding to human medulloblastoma cells and to the platelet glycoprotein IIb-IIIa complex, *Br. J. Haematol.,* 57, 621, 1984.
26. **Allan, P., Garson, J., Harper, E., Asser, U., Coakham, H., Brownell, B., and Kemshead, J.,** Biological characterization and clinical application of a monoclonal antibody recognizing an antigen restricted to neuroectodermal tissues, *Int. J. Cancer,* 31, 591, 1983.
27. **Kemshead, J.,** Monoclonal Antibodies: Their Use in the Diagnosis and Therapy of Paediatric and Adult Tumours Derived from the Neuroectoderm, in *Monoclonal Antibodies for Cancer Detection and Therapy,* Baldwin, R. W., Ed., Academic Press, London, 1985, 281.
28. **Hurko, O. and Walsh, F.,** Human Foetal Muscle Specific Antigen is Restricted to Regenerating Myofibres in Diseased Adult Muscle, *Neurology,* 33, 734, 1983.
29. **Bourne, S., Coakham, H. B., Kemshead, J., Brownell, B., Allan, P., and Davies, A.,** The role of monoclonal antibodies in the diagnosis and characterization of medulloblastoma, in *Medulloblastoma — Clinical and Biological Aspects,* Zeltzer, P. M., Ed., W. B. Saunders, Philadelphia, 1986, 87.
30. **Lashford, L., Davis, A., Richardson, R., Bullimore, J., Eckert, H., Coakham, H., and Kemshead, J.,** A Pilot Study of 131-I Monoclonal Antibodies in the Therapy of Leptomeningeal Tumour, submitted, 1987.
31. **LeBien, T., Kersey, J., Nakazawa, S., Minato, K., and Minawada, J.,** Analysis of Human Leukaemia and Lymphoma Cells With Monoclonal Antibodies BA1, BA2 and BA3, *Leuk. Res.,* 6, 299, 1982.
32. **Kemshead, J., Walsh, F., Pritchard, J., and Greaves, M.,** Monoclonal Antibody to Ganglioside Gq Discriminates Between Haemopoietic Cells and Infiltrating Cells in Bone Marrow, *Int. J. Cancer.,* 27, 441, 1981.
33. **Cheung, N., Saarinen, U., Neely, J., Landmeier, B., Donovan, D., and Coccia, P. F.,** Monoclonal antibodies to glycolipid antigen on human neuroblastoma cells, *Cancer Res.,* 45, 2642, 1986.
34. **Mujoo, K., Cheresh, D., Yang, H. M., and Reisfeld, R.,** Disialoganglioside GD2 on Human Neuroblastoma Cells: Target Antigen fort Monoclonal Antibody Mediated Cytolysis and Suppression of Tumour Growth, *Cancer Res.,* 47, 1098, 1987.
35. **Ladisch, S. and Wu, Z.,** Circulating gangliosides as tumour markers, in *Advances in Neuroblastoma Research,* Evans, A. E., D'Angio, G. J., and Seeger, R. C., Eds., Alan R. Liss, New York, 1985, 277.
36. **Clayton, J., Pincott, J., Van den Berghe, J., and Kemshead, J.,** Comparative studies between a new human rhabdomyosarcoma cell line, JR 1 and its tumour of origin, *Br. J. Cancer,* 54, 83, 1986.
37. **Wood, J. and Anderton, B.,** Monoclonal Antibodies to Mammalian Neurofilaments, *Biosci. Rep.,* 1, 263, 1981.
38. **Marangos, P.,** Clinical studies with neuron specific enolase, in *Advances in Neuroblastoma Research,* Evans, A. E., D'Angio, G. J., and Seeger, R. C., Eds., Alan R. Liss, New York, 1985, 285.
39. **Triche, T., Tsokos, M., Linnoila, R., Marangos, P., and Chaudrea, R.,** NSE in Neuroblastoma and Other Small Round Cell Tumours of Childhood, in *Advances in Neuroblastoma Research,* Evans, A. E., D'Angio, G. J., and Seeger, R. C., Eds., Alan R. Liss, New York, 1985, 295.
40. **Tsokos, M., Howard, R., and Costa, J.,** Immunohistochemical Study of Alveolar and Embryonal Rhabdomyosarcoma, *Lab. Invest.,* 48, 148, 1983.

41. **Brooks, J.**, Immunohistochemical Study of Soft Tissue Sarcomas: Myoglobin as a Marker for Rhabdomyosarcoma, *Cancer,* 50, 1757, 1982.
42. **Osborn, M., Hill, C., Altmannsberger, M., and Webb, K.**, Monoclonal Antibody to Titin in Conjunction with Antibodies to Desmin Separate Rhabdo from other Tumour Types, *Lab. Invest.*, 55, 101, 1986.
43. **Bollum, F.**, Terminal Deoxynucleotidyl Transferase as a Haemopoietic Marker, *Blood,* 54, 1203, 1979.
44. **Gerdes, J., Schwab, U., and Stein, H.**, Production of A Mouse Monoclonal Reactive With a Human Nuclear Antigen Associated with Cell Proliferation, *Int. J. Cancer,* 31, 13, 1983.
45. **Lampson, L., Whelan, J., and Fisher, C.**, HLA-A,B,C and B2-Microglobulin are expressed weakly by human cells of neuronal origin, but can be induced in neuroblastoma cell lines by interferon, in *Advances in Neuroblastoma Research,* Evans, A. E., D'Angio, G. J., and Seeger, R. C., Eds., Alan R. Liss, New York, 1985, 379.
46. **Israel, M.**, The Evolution of Clinical Molecular Genetics, *Am. J. Paediatr. Haematol. Oncol.*, 8, 163, 1986.
47. **Becroft, D., Pearson, A., Shaw, R., and Zwi, L.**, Chromosome Translocation in Extraskeletal Ewing's Tumour, *Lancet,* 2, 400, 1984.
48. **De-Yong, A., Van-Kessel, M., Albus-Lutter, C., Van-Raamsdonk, D., and Voure, P.**, Skeletal Muscle Actin as a Tumour Marker in the Diagnosis of Rhabdomyosarcoma in Childhood, *Am. J. Surg. Pathol.*, 9, 467, 1985.
49. **Schiaffino, S., Gorza, L., Sartore, S., Saggin, L., and Carli, M.**, Embryonic Myosin Heavy Chain as a Differentiation Marker of Developing Human Skeletal Muscle and Rhabdomyosarcoma, *Exp. Cell Res.*, 163, 211, 1986.
50. **Kodet, R., Kasthuri, N., Marsden, H., Coad, N., and Raafat, F.**, Gangliorhabdomyosarcoma: A Histological and Immunohistochemical Study of Three Cases, *Histopathology,* 10, 181, 1986.
51. **Royds, J., Varied, S., Timperley, W., and Taylor, C.**, Comparison of B Enolase and Myoglobin as Histological Markers of Rhabdomyosarcoma, *J. Clin. Pathol.*, 38, 1258, 1985.
52. **Gross, N., Beck, D., Carrel, S., and Munoz, M.**, Highly selective recognition of human neuroblastoma cells by mouse monoclonal antibody to a cytoplasmic antigen, *Cancer Res.*, 46, 2988, 1986.
53. **Shimada, H., Aoyama, C., Chiba, T., and Newton, W.**, Prognostic Subgroups for Undifferentiated Neuroblastoma: Immunohistochemical Studies With anti-S100 Protein Antibody, *Hum. Pathol.*, 16, 471, 1985.
54. **Artleib, U., Krepler, R., and Wiche, G.**, Expression of Microtubule Associated Proteins MAP-1 and MAP-2 in Human Neuroblastoma and Differential Diagnosis of Immature Neuroblasts, *Lab. Invest.*, 53, 684, 1985.
55. **Debus, E., Weber, K., and Osborn, M.**, Monoclonal Antibodies to Desmin The Muscle Specific Intermediate Filament, *EMBO J.*, 2, 2305, 1983.
56. **Lehtonen, E., Lehto, V., Paasivuo, R., and Virtanen, I.**, Parietal and Visceral Endoderm Differ in their Expression of Intermediate Filaments, *EMBO J.*, 2, 1023, 1983.
57. **Gown, A. and Vogel, A.**, Monoclonal Antibodies to Human Intermediate Filament Proteins. III. Analysis of Tumours, *Am. J. Clin. Pathol.*, 84, 413, 1985.
58. **Lane, E.**, Monoclonal Antibodies Provide Specific Intracellular Markers for the Study of Epithelial Tonofilament Organization, *J. Cell Biol.*, 92, 665, 1982.
59. **Kemshead, J. T.**, On behalf of the workshop; An International Study on Monoclonal Antibodies Binding to Pediatric Solid Tumours; A Forbeck Foundation Publication, 1987. (Details from J. T. K. or J. Forbeck, 17 Hilton Head Island, S. Carolina, 29928.)

Chapter 3

AN IMMUNOHISTOLOGICAL APPROACH TO THE DIFFERENTIAL DIAGNOSIS OF CHILDHOOD BRAIN TUMORS

Hugh B. Coakham and Stephen P. Bourne

TABLE OF CONTENTS

I. INTRODUCTION

Cerebral tumors are the commonest solid neoplasm affecting children, accounting for approximately 18% of childhood malignancy. The principal histological types of tumor are shown in Table 1; over 50% of these arise in the cerebellum or brain stem in contrast to adult brain tumors which largely occur in the cerebral hemispheres. A significant proportion of children's brain tumors are composed of small round cells and can, therefore, give rise to potential difficulties in pathological diagnosis. Brain tumors may be situated in deep and highly strategic brain areas which means that the surgeon may only be able to provide a small amount of biopsy material and this may be mechanically deformed by, for example, squeeze artifact by biopsy rongeurs. In the past, biopsies were not attempted for certain deep-seated tumors, but now the use of more refined and accurate techniques such as CT directed stereotactic biopsy[1] and endoscopic biopsy[2] means that small amounts of tissue will be more increasingly available for the diagnosis of such lesions. In addition, increased use of the newer techniques for tumor resection such as laser and ultrasonic aspirator[2] means that the pathologist might be denied adequate amounts of tissue in certain cases.

For the above reasons, the application of special techniques in tumor diagnosis is likely to become more widespread. These include the use of electronmicroscopy and immunocytochemical staining. This chapter will consider the use of monoclonal antibodies as diagnostic reagents for childhood brain tumors.

Immunohistological methods were introduced into neuropathology in the 1960s and involved the use of polyclonal antibodies against a small group of marker antigens. These included glial fibrillary acidic protein, (GFAP — an intermediate filament found in glial neoplasms), neuronspecific enolase (NSE), myelin basic protein, and S100 protein. The presence of these antigens was useful for answering basic diagnostic questions, although certain of them lacked specific tissue distribution. The most important and helpful were antisera against GFAP used in diagnosing tumors of the glioma group.[3-5]

In the past 5 years, the field of immunohistological diagnosis has significantly advanced with the development of monoclonal antibodies raised against neuroectodermal and other relevant antigens.[6,7] We describe here the use of such reagents in the diagnosis of pediatric solid tumor biopsies and also in the accurate characterization of malignant cells in the cerebrospinal fluid.

II. THE PRODUCTION AND CHARACTERIZATION OF MONOCLONAL ANTIBODIES FOR BRAIN TUMOR DIAGNOSIS

Many of the antibodies used in our immunohistological studies were raised following immunization with homogenates of fetal brain or cerebral tumors (medulloblastoma and astrocytoma). Screening the resulting clones of hybridoma cells for antibody production was carried out on frozen tissue sections since we were seeking useful immunohistological reagents. This was done by making compound frozen blocks of the immunizing tumor, normal adult brain, and fetal brain. Immunofluorescence was then used to detect monoclonal antibodies with potential tumor associated or oncofetal properties. These candidates were then reexamined by peroxidase to allow for greater interpretation of morphological detail. One great advantage of this approach is that unexpected reactivities were discovered which led to discovery of antibodies useful to investigators in other fields. For example, immunization with a medulloblastoma resulted in antibody M148 which reacted with the blood platelet glycoprotein IIB/IIIA, in addition to highly restricted activity against medulloblastoma and related tumors.[8] All the antibodies eventually used for prospective diagnosis were characterized by testing on a wide variety of normal tissues and tumors.

Table 1
INCIDENCE OF CHILDHOOD BRAIN TUMORS

	% of total
Astrocytomas (low grade)	36
Astrocytomas (high grade)	10
Medulloblastomas	21
Ependymomas	10
Craniopharyngiomas	6
Pineal region tumors	2.5
Choroid plexus tumors	1.5
Others	13

Note: In children under 16 years.

Table 2
COMPARISON OF PROPERTIES OF MONOCLONAL ANTIBODIES AND ANTISERA

Monoclonal antibody	Polyclonal antiserum
Total antigenic specificity	Requires absorption to achieve specificity
Unlimited supply	Supply limited
No variation between samples	Batch-to-batch variation
High titer	Titer variation
Tissue homogenates can be used routinely for immunization	Purification of antigen prior to immunization may be necessary
Novel antigens identified from complex antigenic mixtures	Good antisera against such antigens unlikely
Huge potential range of MCAs	Range of antisera more limited
Unexpected cross-reactivities can occur (due to duplicate epitopes on unrelated molecules)	No such problems

III. THE ADVANTAGES OF MONOCLONAL ANTIBODIES IN HISTOLOGY

As immunohistological reagents, monoclonal antibodies offer a number of considerable advantages over polyclonal heteroantisera (Table 2). Certain heteroantisera can be highly specific and are valuable in immunohistology but suffer from limitation of supply and batch-to-batch variation. However, a good MCA can be distributed in virtually unlimited quantities to laboratories throughout the world, thus permitting comparison of results. This might, hopefully, avoid discrepancies such as have arisen in the reporting of GFAP reactivity in certain types of tumors.

In addition, ''new'' antigens are continually being recognized by MCAs, as a result of being ''selected'' by the immune system of the immunized mouse. This avoids the biochemical purification of antigens necessary to produce a good antiserum. Indeed many of the new tumor-associated antigens defined by MCAs prove difficult to characterize biochemically.

This interesting phenomenon of duplicate antigenic sites (epitopes) recognized by MCAs can cause confusion. The single epitope to which a given MCA binds may be expressed on totally unrelated molecules and thus cause inappropriate staining patterns in tissues. For example, the antibodies UCHT1 and Leu-4 recognize an antigenic determinant which is present on the membrane of human T lymphocytes.[9] However, this determinant was also found in the cytoplasm of cerebellar Purkinje neurons of many species.[10] It is, therefore, important to remember that although each MCA is uniquely specific for its binding site, these reagents are not necessarily markers for molecular identity.[11] However, the diverse staining pattern displayed by some MCAs can be turned to advantage, provided the duplicate epitope phenomenon is recognized.

Human MCAs have been produced by harvesting human B lymphocytes from tumors and creating hybridomas by fusion with a human myeloma cell line.[12] While these reagents would be ideal for use *in vivo,* they may be limited in immunohistological use since the antihuman Ig second antibody will react with nonspecific tissue bound Ig thus creating a high background.

IV. BRAIN TUMOR ANTIGENS DEFINED BY MONOCLONAL ANTIBODIES

The ideal monoclonal antibody for diagnostic purposes is one that is tumor specific. Unfortunately, such reagents do not exist, and it is most unlikely that unique and restricted antigens are expressed by specific categories of tumor cells. However, there is a range of available monoclonal antibodies with sufficiently restricted reactivities to make them operationally specific. The most useful monoclonal antibodies are tissue specific, e.g., UJ13A[6] or preferentially react with tumors of a particular category, such as those showing neuronal differentiation (UJ181.4, M34O, M148).[13] The antibodies selected for diagnostic use react reasonably specifically with different categories of tumor; however, there are occasional instances when the target antigen is lacking or is ''inappropriately'' expressed on tumors of other types. It is, therefore, essential to use such antibodies as a panel rather than individually. This approach has already proved valuable in general histopathological practice,[14] and in general neuropathology.[15] The interpretation of immunostaining patterns produced by each antibody needs considerable experience, particularly when immunofluorescence is used, where familiarity with the staining intensity and background of each reagent is important. Obviously, as with all special pathological techniques, interpretations are more easily made with a knowledge of the routine histology and in the light of clinical information. The antigenic phenotype of major cerebral tumors defined by a panel of monoclonal antibodies is shown schematically in Figure 1.

Many of the antigens defined by diagnostically useful MCAs do not survive the process of routine fixation with formal-saline. It is, therefore, important to retain samples of fresh frozen tissue from each case, preferably snap-frozen in liquid nitrogen. However, strenuous attempts are being made to identify alternative methods of fixation and to produce new MCAs which react with fixed tissues.

The diagnostically important antigens expressed by brain tumors can be assigned to three broad categories — differentiation antigens, epithelial proliferation antigens, and oncofetal antigens.

A. Differentiation Antigens

These antigens are present on normal tissue and on neoplastic cells derived therefrom, and are extremely useful as markers for tissue-type or germ layer since they are consistently expressed even in highly anaplastic tumors. Differentiation antigens can be described in terms of their site, being either cytoplasmic or membrane-associated.

B. Cytoplasmic Differentiation Antigens

These include 7—11 nm intermediate-filament proteins which form part of the cytoskeleton. Five groups of these proteins have been described, four of which are reasonably tissue specific, and these have been comprehensively reviewed by Osborne and Weber.[16] These proteins were originally thought to be germ-layer specific and, therefore, would accurately reflect the origin of different tumor types. Inevitably, further research has revealed exceptions

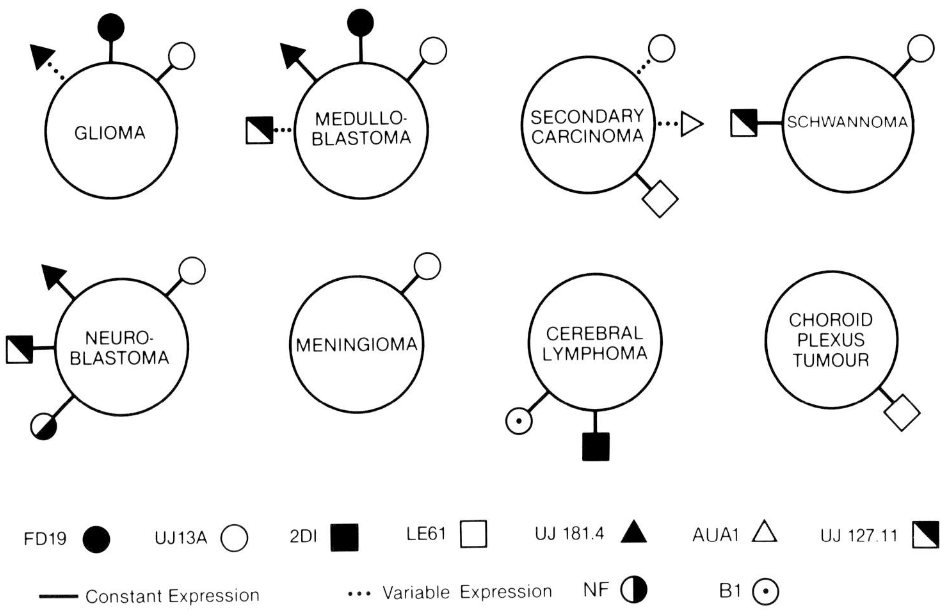

FIGURE 1. The antigenic phenotype of eight different cerebral tumors defined by the panel of MCAs. This summarizes the data obtained from testing 250 tumors. The majority of tumors had a distinctive phenotype and could be diagnosed by a small number of antibodies. Heterogeneity of antigen expression was not a major problem, but some variability was seen as shown here. The metastatic carcinomas expressing UJ13A antigen are brochogenic small-cell tumors.

to this rule and in addition examples of coexpression of two classes of intermediate-filament proteins within the same tissue have been discovered. Nevertheless, the basic pattern of tissue specificity holds well enough for these markers to play a useful diagnostic role. Table 3 shows the intermediate filament antigens together with examples of monoclonal antibodies used to identify them. In our experience, the antibodies which identify neurofilament protein and cytokeratin have been particularly useful. It will be seen that vimentin is a less specific marker, since, although it is constantly expressed by mesenchymal tumors, it is widely distributed among other cell types. Coexpression of vimentin and GFAP occurs in astrocytomas and medulloblastomas.

C. Cell Surface Differentiation Antigens

Cell surface differentiation antigens which are related to the cell surface and are relevant to brain tumor diagnosis are defined by antibodies UJ13A, UJ127.11, 2D1, B1, and UCHT1 (Table 4). Antibody UJ13A is a most useful reagent; immunohistologically, it will identify all tumors of neuroectodermal origin, both central and peripheral. The single exception is melanoma which does not express this antigen. Its principal role in our laboratories is in the diagnosis of anaplastic or small round cell tumors in which there is doubt as to the tissue of origin. This antibody has already been used clinically in the removal of neuroblastoma cells from bone marrow prior to autologous transplantation[24] and in radioimmunolocalization of neuroblastoma[25] and brain tumors.[26]

Antibody UJ127.11 recognizes an interesting antigen present on all normal neuroectodermal tissue but restricted to tumors of neuronal lineage and also Schwannomas. This curious reactivity pattern has yet to be fully explained.

The cell surface differentiation antigen of leukocytes recognized by antibody 2D1 provides a means of rapid identification of lymphoreticular CNS tumors which can be followed by more detailed typing of T and B cells by antibodies UCHT1 and B1. Finally, a detailed

Table 3
DIFFERENTIATION ANTIGENS USEFUL AS CNS TUMOR MARKERS — CYTOPLASMIC ANTIGENS[a]

Intermediate filament protein	Normal tissue	Neoplastic tissue	Monoclonal antibody	Ref.
Glial fibrillary	Astrocytes	Astrocytoma	FD19	17
Acid protein	Ependyma	Ependymoma		
		Medulloblastoma		
		Oligodendroglioma		
Neurofilament	Neurones	Neuroblastoma	BF10	18
		Medulloblastoma	RT97	
		Ganglioglioma		
Cytokeratin	Simple	Carcinoma	LE61	19
	epithelium		CAM5	20
Desmin	Muscle	Rhabdomyosarcoma	Anti-desmin	16
Vimentin	Mesenchyme	Sarcomas	Anti-vimentin[b]	21
	Astrocytes	Astrocytomas		
	Dura	Meningiomas		
	Melanocytes	Melanomas		
	Leukocytes	Lymphomas		

[a] Intermediate filament proteins.
[b] Polyclonal antiserum.

Table 4
DIFFERENTIATION ANTIGENS USEFUL AS CNS TUMOR MARKERS — CELL SURFACE ANTIGENS

Antigen	Normal tissue	Neoplastic tissue	Monoclonal antibody	Ref.
Pan-neuroectodermal antigen	Neuroectoderm	Neuroectodermal tumors[a]	UJ13A	6
Glycoprotein	Neuroectoderm	Neuroblastoma	UJ127.11	7
(220—240 kDa)		Medulloblastoma		
		Schwannoma		
HLe-11	Leukocytes	Lymphoma	2D1	22
(22 kDa)	T-lymphocytes	T-cell lymphoma	UCHT1	9
B1 antigen	B-lymphocytes	B-cell lymphoma	B1	23

[a] Except melanomas.

lymphocyte subset analysis can be carried out using appropriate markers for cytotoxic/suppressor cells, helper/inducer cells and natural killer cells. In addition to analyzing lymphoid tumors, this approach will also be valuable in studying tumor infiltrates.

D. Epithelial Proliferation Antigens

This term serves to describe a type of differentiation antigen which may be present in small amounts in normal epithelium, but is strongly expressed in proliferative states (Table 5). Antibodies which recognize antigens of this type, HMFG1 and AUA1[27] are, therefore, not specific for neoplasia, but are, nevertheless, of great practical use in identifying carcinoma cells, particularly when used in conjunction with antibodies for cytokeratin (unpublished observation).

Table 5
ANTIGENS EXPRESSED IN STATES OF DE-DIFFERENTIATION OR PROLIFERATION, USEFUL AS CNS TUMOR MARKERS

Antigen	Normal tissue	Neoplastic tissue	Monoclonal antibody	Ref.
Epithelial proliferation antigen	Proliferating epithelia	Carcinomas	AUA1	27
Human milk fat globule protein	Lactating breast	Carcinomas	HMFG1 HMFG2	27
Neuroblastic cell membrane antigen	Fetal brain	Neuroblastoma Medulloblastoma	UJ181.4	13
Carcinoembryonic antigen (CEA)	Fetal gut	Gastrointestinal and certain other tumors	MAB202	28

E. Oncofetal Antigens

Antigens of this type are restricted to fetal tissue but are reexpressed in adults by tissues that have undergone neoplastic transformation (see Table 5). While these antigens are closer to the ideal of "tumor-specific" marker, they appear to be expressed more heterogenously than do the other categories described here. Antibody UJ181.4 recognizes an oncofetal antigen expressed by fetal brain and by the neuroblastic tumors of all types. Carcinoembryonic antigen (CEA) is one of the earliest examples in this category, but very small amounts are present in normal tissues.

It is important to note that many antibodies now exist which recognize the categories of antigens described here, and that the examples given in their review are those with which we have personal experience.

V. IMMUNOHISTOLOGICAL DIAGNOSIS OF SOLID TUMOR BIOPSIES

The antigenic expression of each major tumor type will now be described. All pediatric tumors have been part of a prospective study of adult and childhood tumors examined by immunofluorescence and immunoperoxidase techniques for reactivity with a monoclonal antibody panel. The results of 252 cases are shown in Table 6.

A. Glioma

The commonest type of glial tumor in children is the well differentiated astrocytoma which occurs most commonly in the cerebellum but also in the cerebral hemispheres' diencephalon and optic chiasm. These tumors all express the pan-neuroectodermal UJ13A antigen (Figure 2) and contain large amounts of GFAP as detected by monoclonal antibody FD19 which was originally raised by immunizing with a cerebellar astrocytoma from a 6 year-old female. We have not yet found any reactivity in this group with the neuroblastoma cell markers UJ181.4, UJ127.11, M340, or M148. Neither is there expression of any other type of intermediate-filament protein such as neurofilament, cytokeratin, or vimentin. The tumor cells do not stain with the leukocyte marker 2D1 and 2D1 positive infiltrates are rare.

Less commonly, childhood gliomas are more malignant, and these usually occur in the cerebral hemispheres, thalamus, or brain stem. If deeply situated, they may be biopsied stereotactically, and the diagnosis of these tumors can then be difficult if only small amounts of tissue are available. Positivity with UJ13A shows them to be neuroectodermal, and they all contain small amounts of GFAP as shown by FD19 staining. Occasionally, the more malignant gliomas "inappropriately" express neuroblastic cell antigenic markers.

Table 6
REACTIVITY OF 252 CENTRAL NERVOUS SYSTEM TUMORS WITH A MONOCLONAL ANTIBODY PANEL

	No.	FD19	UJ13A	UJ127.11	UJ181.4	LE61	2D1	B1
Malignant glioma	55	+	+	2[a]	7	−	−	−
Astrocytoma	25	+	+	−	−	−	−	−
Oligodendro-glioma	16	+	+	−	3	−	−	−
Ependymoma	14	+	+	−	−	−	−	−
Schwannoma	10	−	+	−	−	−	−	−
Meningioma	25	−	22	−	−	−	−	−
Medulloblastoma	15	+	+	10	13	−	−	−
Cerebral neuroblastoma	2	−	+	+	+	−	−	−
Primitive neuroectodermal tumor	3	−	+	−	−	−	−	−
Choroid plexus tumor	4	−	−	−	−	+	−	−
Metastatic carcinoma	51	−	7	−	1	44	−	−
Primary brain lymphoma	22	−	−	−	−	−	+	+
Spinal extradural lymphoma	5	−	−	−	−	−	+	+
Metastatic melanoma	5	−	−	−	−	−	−	−

Note: +, All tumors positive; −, all tumors negative.

[a] The figure denotes the number of tumors positive out of the total of that tumor type.

B. Medulloblastoma

Medulloblastomas account for some 20% of pediatric brain tumors and constitute a group that is both biologically interesting and therapeutically challenging. The precise cell of origin remains to be determined and is at present the subject of controversy.[29,30] It is clear, however, that the primitive stem cell giving rise to the tumor retains its potential for differentiation, since these tumors are capable of showing both neuronal or glial phenotypes. Less frequently, evidence of more diverse differentiation into oligodendroglia, ependyma, and myoblasts is seen. However, a substantial proportion of medulloblastomas are of the undifferentiated hypercellular small round cell type, although careful examination of ultrastructure shows scattered areas of neuronal and glial differentiation. It is in these tumors that are undifferentiated at the light microscopic level that phenotyping with monoclonal antibodies is diagnostically useful and biologically interesting.

The results of testing 10 medulloblastoma biopsies with a panel of 12 MCAs are shown in Table 7.

All these tumors express the ubiquitous UJ13A antigen which signifies neuroectodermal origin. The antibodies recognizing neuroblast cell antigen stained the majority of tumors, with M148, M340, and UJ181.4 giving the most consistent results. Neuronal differentiation which included the production of neurofilament of intermediate molecular weight was seen in six of ten tumors and high molecular weight neurofilament in three of ten tumors (Figure 3). All tumors expressed glial fibrillary acidic protein in varying degrees. Therefore, in virtually all examples studied, these tumors showed simultaneous neuronal and glial differentiation by membrane antigen and intermediate filament expression. Although the numbers in this series are too small to permit conclusions regarding the relationship between the presence of cell membrane neuroblastic markers and the expression of cytoplasmic neurofilament, we found that the presence of neurofilament was usually associated with the expression of a complete set of neuroblastic surface antigens, indicating that full expression

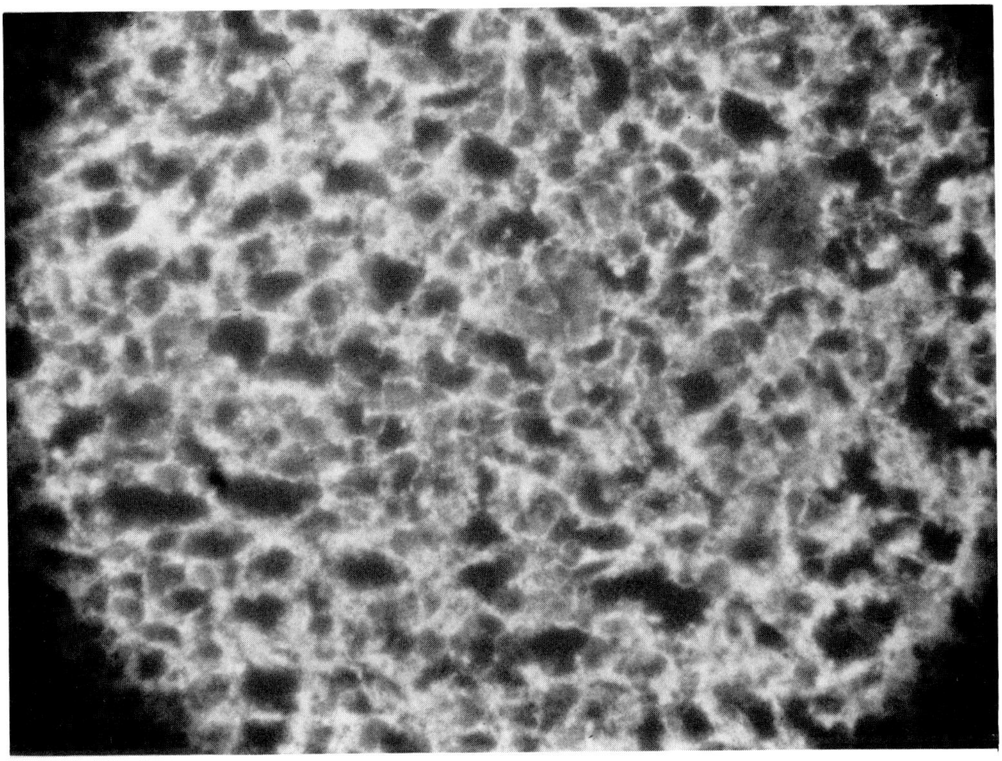

FIGURE 2. Frozen section of a high grade astrocytoma showing uniform membrane immunofluorescence with pan-neuroectodermal MCA UJ13A.

of these membrane determinants may be associated with a higher degree of neural differentiation.

It is still not clear whether the presence of differentiation at the light microscopic level is related to clinical prognosis; the literature on this point is itself divergent. Since it is now possible to demonstrate differentiation at a molecular level with monoclonal antibodies, it is hoped that future studies will reveal the biological significance of such a system of phenotyping.

C. Neuroblastoma

The monoclonal antibody profile of neuroblastomas have been previously described in this book. In the rare cases where this tumor involves the central nervous system, there are two principal sites (1) cerebral hemispheres, and (2) the anterior base of skull region, where the tumor takes origin from the olfactory bulb (esthesioneuroblastoma).

We have encountered one example of each and found the tumors to be antigenically similar to those occurring outside the CNS, i.e., lacking GFAP expression and reacting positively with UJ13A, UJ181.4, UJ127.11 and also expressing neurofilament antigens. In both cases the diagnosis was made by immunohistology, later confirmed by electron microscopy.

Case 1 — Previously reported by Kemshead and Coakham,[31] and Coakham and Brownell.[32] An 11-year-old girl presented with a large frontal tumor thought clinically to be an astrocytoma or ependymoma. Paraffin sections on this tumor stained routinely showed a monotonous small round cell tumor with no distinguishing features. However, positive staining by UJ13A and UJ181.4 showed this to be a primary neuroectodermal tumor with neuroblastic differentiation. Interestingly, no neurofilaments were detected in tumor sections (RT97 negative), however, the tissue culture was established which produced numerous

Table 7
ANTIGENIC PHENOTYPE OF MEDULLOBLASTOMA DEFINED BY A PANEL OF MONOCLONAL ANTIBODIES AND POLYCLONAL SERA

	Monoclonal antibodies											Serum	
Case	UJ13A	127.11	181.4	M148	M340	RT97	BF10	155	Vimentin	D19	LE61	GFAP	Histology
1	+	−	−	+	+	−	−	−	+	+	−	+	Rosettes, undifferentiated
2	+	−	+	+	+	−	−	−	−	+	−	+	Rosettes, undifferentiated
3	+	−	+	+	+	−	−	−	+	+	−	+	Rosettes, undifferentiated
4	+	+	+	+	+	−	−	−	+	+	−	+	Rosettes, undifferentiated
5	+	+	+	+	+	+	+	+	−	+	−	+	Rosettes, undifferentiated
6	+	+	+	+	+	−	+	+	+	+	−	+	Undifferentiated
7	+	+	+	+	+	+	+	+	−	+	−	+	Ologodendroglial diff. no.; neuronal diff.
8	+	+	+	+	−	−	+	+	+	+	−	+	Rosettes, undifferentiated
9	+	+	+	+	+	−	+	+	+	+	−	+	Rosettes, neuronal and glial diff.
10	+	+	+	+	+	+	+	+	+	+	−	+	Mature neurons, glial, and oligo diff.

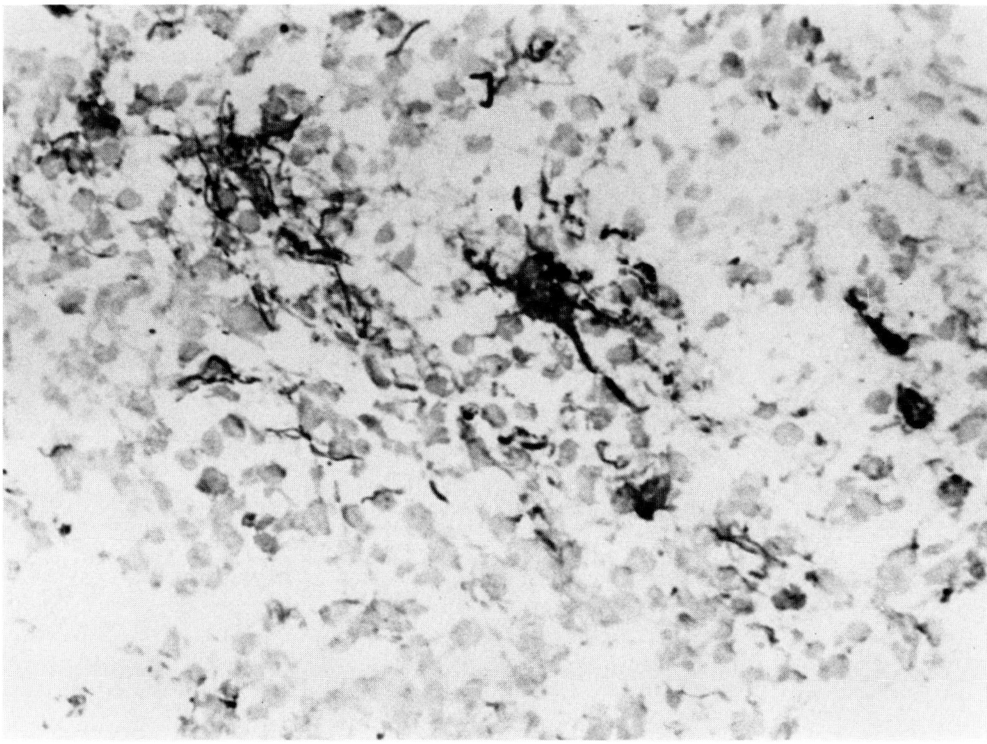

FIGURE 3. Frozen section of a medulloblastoma immunostained to show expression of 155 kDa neurofilament (immunoperoxidase).

cells of neuronal morphology, many of which expressed the 210,000 molecular weight neurofilament antigen and stained with RT97. In murine and human neuroblastomas morphological differentiation *in vitro* can be induced.[33] This appears to be the first demonstration of antigenic differentiation of a human neuroblastoma under routine tissue culture conditions. The patient received neuraxis irradiation and remains in remission at 6 years follow-up.

Case 2 — A 14-year-old boy presented with mass involving the nasal pharynx and sphenoid air sinus. When biopsied, this was reported as a possible lymphoma (Figure 4A), but immunohistologically the tissue had all the characteristics of a neuroblastoma: UJ13A+, UJ181.4+, BF10+, D19−, 2D1− (Figure 4B). The diagnosis of olfactory neuroblastoma was later confirmed by electron microscopy.

D. Schwannoma

Schwannomas growing from the 8th cranial nerve are uncommon in children, and when they occur in this group are a manifestation of neurofibromatosis (central type). The tumor does not generally cause difficulty in pathological diagnosis; however, it has been immunohistologically studied in the past. The polyclonal antibody has been previously used in anti-S100,[34-36] but this is not considered to be a reliable diagnostic indicator.[4] However, in our experience, Schwannoma may be characterized by a unique and consistent pattern of reactivity with UJ13A and UJ127.11. Monoclonal antibody UJ127.11 has previously been extensively used as a marker in neuroblastic tumor cells.[7] The postivity of this marker on Schwannoma is consistent with the neural crest origin of this tumor.

E. Choroid Plexus Tumor

Both benign and malignant forms of this tumor express low molecular weight keratin which is recognized by monoclonal antibody LE61 (Figure 5 A and B). This antigen is

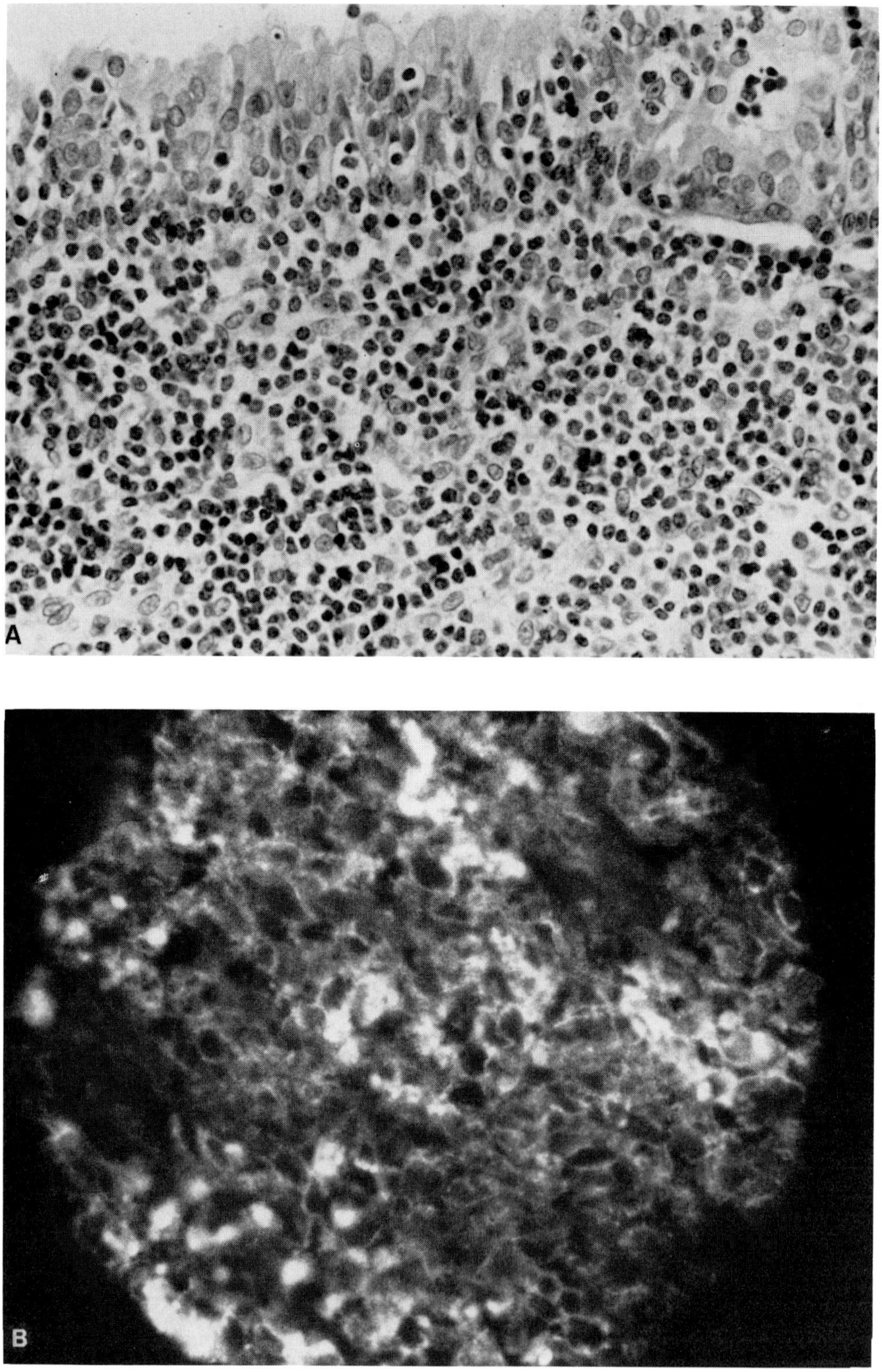

FIGURE 4. (A) A histological section of a tumor biopsied from the sphenoid sinus of a 14-year-old boy. A mass of undifferentiated small round cells is seen deep to the respiratory mucosa. Lymphoma was offered as the most likely diagnosis (H.E.). (B) Generalized membrane immunofluorescence is produced by UJ13A, indicating a neuroectodermal origin. Further immunophenotyping showed this to be a neuroblastoma.

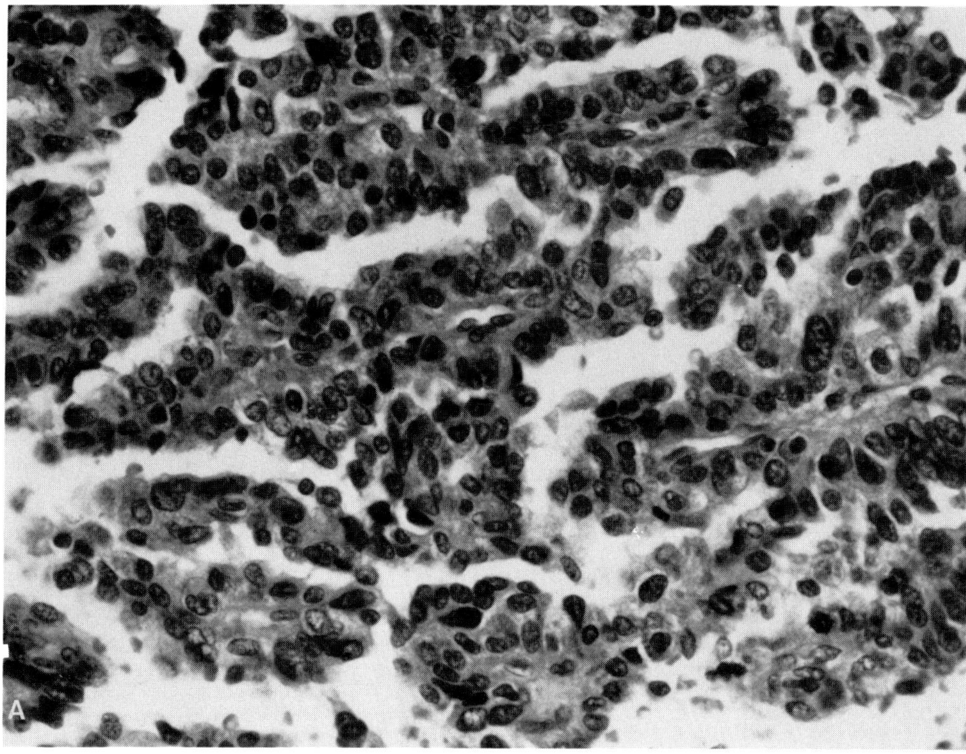

FIGURE 5. (A) Histological section of a poorly differentiated tumor with a papillary growth pattern and rosette formation. Biopsy from a large tumor of the lateral ventricle of a 10-month-old boy (H.E.). (B) A frozen section immunostained by LE61 to show cytokeratin expression, indicating a diagnosis of choroid plexus carcinoma (immunoperoxidase, no counterstain).

regularly expressed by carcinoma cells. However, choroid plexus tumors, unlike carcinomas, fail to express the milk fat globule and epithelial proliferation antigens recognized by HMFG1, HMFG2, and AUA1 antibodies. Choroid plexus tumors may occasionally be difficult to distinguish on purely histological grounds from ependymomas, especially papillary forms of the latter.[37] This diagnostic difficulty can easily be resolved, since ependymomas do not bind LE61. Interestingly, although choroid plexus develops from neuroectoderm, it fails to express the UJ13A antigen.

F. Teratoma

In common with teratomas from other sites, these tumors generally express antigens appropriate to the different germ layers represented histologically. Thus, differential tumors express cytokeratin in epithelial structures, vimentin in mesenchyme, and in neural areas, GFAP, neurofilament, UJ13A, and UJ181.4 expression is seen. The undifferentiated CNS teratomas also express some of these antigens but in a less organized manner (Figure 6A and B).

G. Pineal Tumors

Tumors of the pineal region in children are generally germ cell tumors which may be undifferentiated germinomas, yolk sac tumors, or various types of teratoma. Neoplasms arising from pineal cells are less common in this age group, but occasionally pineocytomas or pineoblastomas are seen. The germ cell tumors may stain with antibodies against human chorionic gonadatrophin, carcinoembryonic antigen, or alpha-fetoprotein. Pineocytoma and

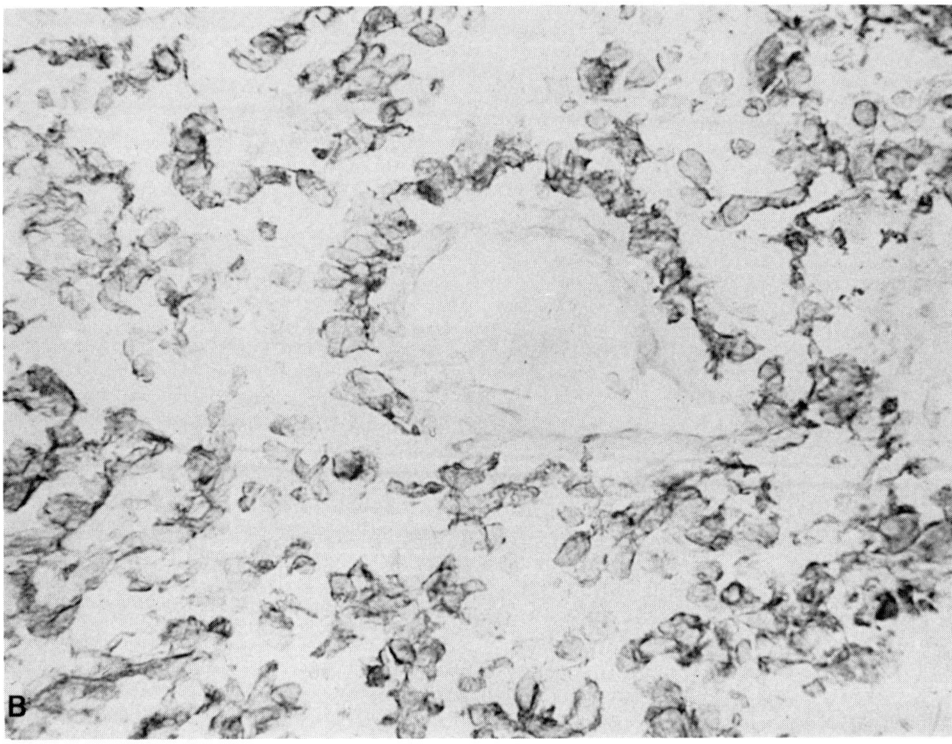

FIGURE 5B.

pineoblastoma express UJ13A antigen and can also demonstrate neuronal and glial differentiation in the same manner as medulloblastomas. In a rare case of pineoblastoma metastatic to the bone marrow, we were able to demonstrate cells expressing UJ13A and GFAP antigens.

H. Primitive Neuroectodermal Tumors (PNETs)

These tumors are uncommon and generally occur in the cerebral hemispheres. They are composed of undifferentiated small round cells, and in our experience they stain with only UJ13A but fail to express GFAP or the neuronal differentiation antigens. This phenotype supports the view that these tumors arise from primitive, uncommitted neuroectodermal stem cells.[38]

I. Cerebral Lymphoma and Leukemia

These uncommon lesions can be readily characterized by antibodies against a pan-leukocyte antigen (2D1 and Dako LC) which will stain them uniformly. Further phenotyping is carried out using antibodies directed against surface antigens of B cells, T cells or CALLA.

J. Metastatic Carcinoma

It is extremely uncommon to find children presenting with metastatic carcinoma lesions in the brain, in contrast to adults where such lesions are at least as common as primary brain tumors. We have shown that the use of antibodies LE61 and AUA1 in combination will accurately detect 98% of cerebral metastatic carcinomas in adults. Adult small cell bronchogenic carcinomas also express UJ13A, signifying a neuroectodermal phenotype. This antigen has also been detected on pediatric Wilms' tumors (Dr. J. Berry, personal communication).

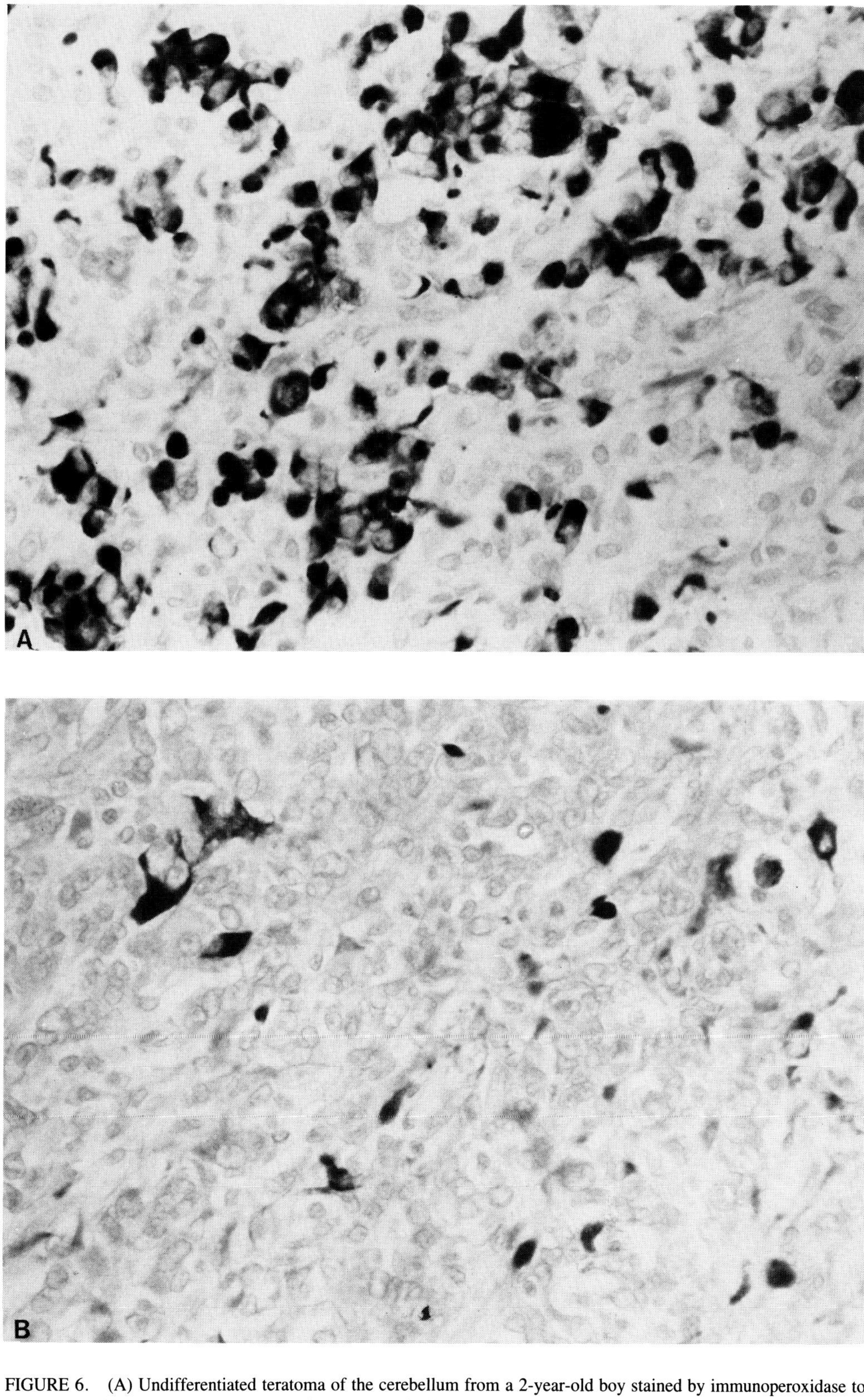

FIGURE 6. (A) Undifferentiated teratoma of the cerebellum from a 2-year-old boy stained by immunoperoxidase to show glial differentiation (GFAP expression). (B) A similar section showing neuronal differentiation (155 kDa neurofilament expression).

VI. CEREBROSPINAL FLUID IMMUNOCYTOLOGY

Problems encountered in the histological diagnosis of undifferentiated cerebral tumors are amplified in the examination of CSF from malignant cells. Here the principal difficulties consist of:

1. Distinguishing neoplastic cells from the reactive lymphoreticular cells
2. Paucity of neoplastic cells in the sample
3. Deterioration of morphological appearance with time
4. Precise diagnosis of the malignant condition when neoplastic cells are seen in the absence of any known primary tumor

We have developed methods of immunostaining CSF cytological preparations and applied panels of MCAs in order to characterize the cells.

A. Immunocytological Method

Cytological preparations were made from fresh CSF samples with a Shandon Elliott Cytospin. The cells were centrifuged at 1150 revolutions per min for 10 min on the gelatin-coated slides, a separate slide being used for test with each antibody. Slides for positive and negative control MCAs were also prepared. Immunological testing with the screening panel could be accomplished with a minimum of six slides, and small volumes of CSF. If cell counts were low, larger volumes were preconcentrated by low-speed centrifugation for 5 min. After being washed in phosphate buffered saline (PBS) a monoclonal antibody, at the appropriate dilution, was added to each slide and incubated for 30 min at room temperature in a humid chamber. After further washing in PBS and incubation with affinity purified fluorescein conjugated goat anti-mouse Ig for 30 min, slides were mounted in 90% glycerol and were examined with a Zeiss standard microscope fitted with epifluorescence using a "Planapochromat" 40 × oil immersion objective. Immunoperoxidase or alkaline phosphate methods can also be used.

We have recently been using an improved technique, having shown that rapid air drying and acetone fixation enables virtually all important marker antigens to be preserved (Bourne, unpublished observation). This allows for testing at leisure and transportation of acetone fixed slides to special centers for antibody analysis. If smears are first prepared from CSF that has been preconcentrated by centrifugation, the yield of cells is greater than that obtained by cytocentrifugation.

Immunocytology with a panel of monoclonal antibodies provides a powerful means of accurately characterizing tumor cells in CSF samples. A suitable panel of antibodies is shown in Table 8, where it will be seen that in 28 cases of all ages an accurate diagnosis has been made in 96% of cases. In pediatric practice the commonest problem is to distinguish between the small round neoplastic cell of neuroblastoma and those of leukemia or lymphoma. This may be easily accomplished by testing with UJ13A and antibodies against common leukocyte antigen (Figure 7). The results of testing CSF from nine cases of neuroectodermal tumors are shown in Table 9. In four of nine cases, immunocytology with the MCA panel was responsible for the correct diagnosis, later confirmed histologically from biopsy or autopsy material.

The technique is particularly valuable in accurately characterizing cells that have malignant features on routine cytological staining, but reveal no clue as to their origin. An example is seen in Figure 8A and B, where the neoplastic cells were shown to contain GFAP and thus be of glial origin.

Table 8
CSF IMMUNOCYTOLOGY USING A MONOCLONAL ANTIBODY PANEL (28 CASES)

Monoclonal antibody	Carcinoma	Neuroectodermal tumor	Lymphoma	Melanoma
LE61	+	−	−	−
AUA1[a]	+	−	−	−
UJ13A	−	+	−	−
UJ181.4	−	+	−	−
2D1	−	−	+	−
B1	−	−	+	−
UCHT1	−	−	+	−
9.2.27	−	−	−	+
Positive immunodiagnosis	8/9	9/9	5/5[b]	5/5

Note: I-reactive leukocytes which stain positively with 2D1 are not scored.

[a] AUA1 not used in all cases.
[b] 3 cases of B-cell lymphoma diagnosed by B1; 1 case of T-cell lymphoma diagnosed by UCHT1.

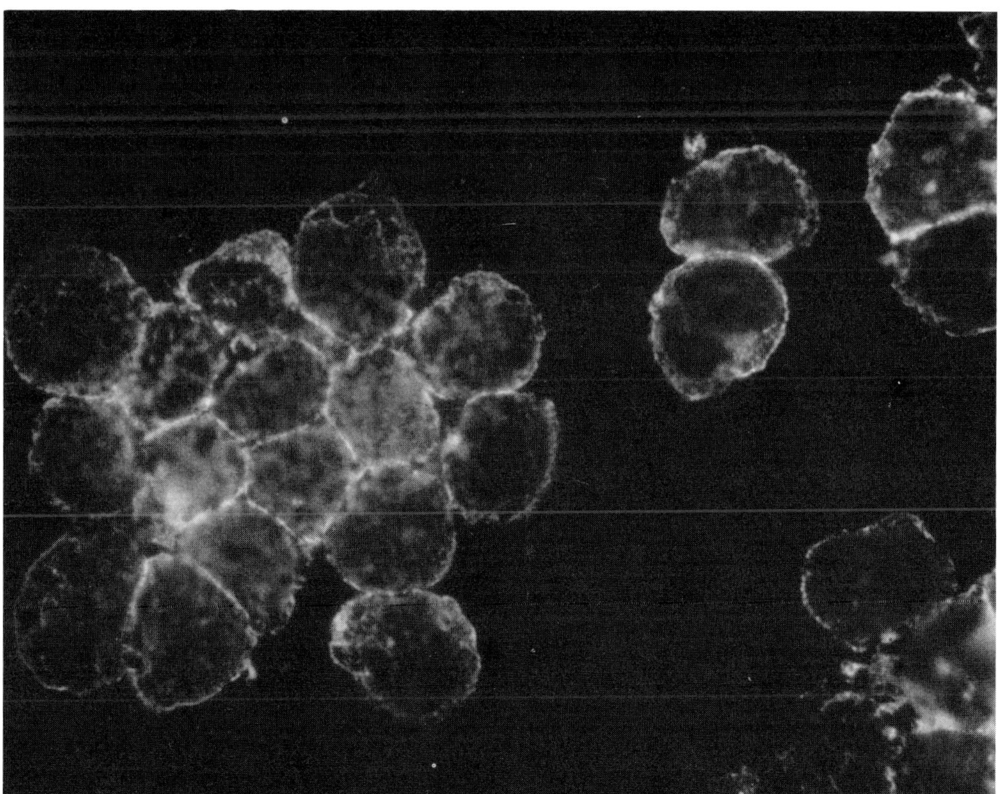

FIGURE 7. Neuroblastoma cells from CSF showing bright membrane fluorescence with antibody UJ13A. This finding excluded the alternative diagnosis of lymphoma suggested in this case.

Table 9
RESULTS OF CSF IMMUNOCYTOLOGICAL TESTING IN CASES OF NEUROECTODERMAL TUMOR

Case	Clinical diagnosis prior to CSF examination	CSF diagnosis		Screening panel				Additional antibodies
		Cytology	Immunocytology	LE61	UJ13A	UJ181.4	2D1*	
1	Medulloblastoma	N.D.	Medulloblastoma	–	+	+	+	
2	Medulloblastoma	N.D.	Medulloblastoma	–	+	+	+	
3	Medulloblastoma	Malignant cells	Medulloblastoma	–	+	+	+	
4	Neuroblastoma	Malignant cells	Neuroblastoma	–	+	+	+	M340+, UJ127.11+
5	Pineoblastoma	N.D.	Pineoblastoma	–	+	+	+	F7(A)+ UJ127.11+
6	? Neuroblastoma ? Lymphoma	Malignant cells	Neuroblastoma	N.D.	+	–	+	
7	Malignant intrinsic tumor	Malignant cells	PNET	–	+	–	+	FD19–
8	Carcinomatous meningitis	Carcinoma	Neuroectodermal tumor	–	+	–	+	FD19+
9	Pineal germinoma	Malignant cells	Pineocytoma	–	+	+	–	M340+

Note: N.D., not determined.

* Antibody 2D1 stains all white cells that form the accompanying leukocytes.

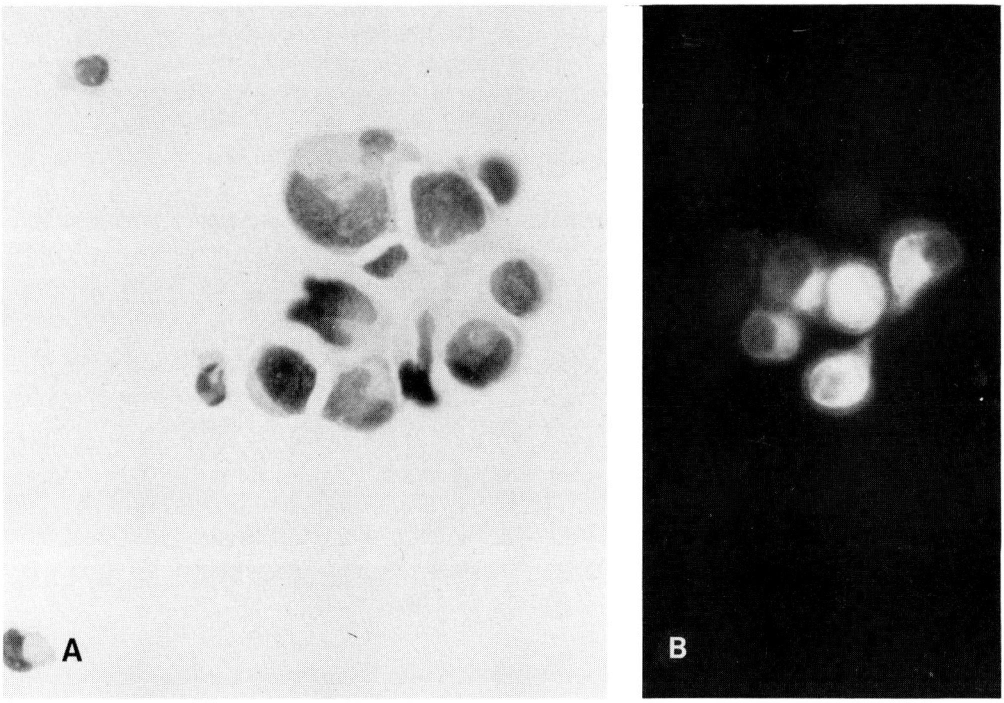

FIGURE 8. (A) A group of obviously malignant cells from CSF in a case with no known primary tumor. (B) Positive immunofluorescence shows the cells to be GFAP positive, thus indicating a primary glial neoplasm. Subsequent investigation revealed an ependymoma of the cervical cord which was surgically removed.

VII. CONCLUSION

The application of monoclonal antibody techniques to solid tumor and cytological diagnosis is already becoming established in both general pathology[39,40] and in neuropathology.[41] The techniques are straightforward and suitable antibodies are becoming increasingly available, many on a commercial basis. The costs per case are not high. The majority of useful antibodies do not react with fixed tissues, but the use of immunological markers is considered so important that refrigeration facilities are being made available in many centers. This also results in a valuable tissue bank for research. We hope that the panel of antibodies described here will eventually be replaced by similar reagents which react with fixed tissues. This will have the obvious advantage of more widespread clinical application and the ability to examine embedded material retrospectively. At least two such reagents have been produced which can be substituted for the members of our current panel. These are CAM-5 which recognizes an antigen of epithellial cytokeratin and Dako LC, a cocktail of two monoclonal antibodies, which recognizes a common leukocyte antigen.[20,42]

From the time of Bailey and Cushing's monograph of 1926[43] there has been interest in the concept that many cerebral tumors originate from neuroectodermal stem cells. Immunophenotyping of cerebral tumors with monoclonal antibodies has only just begun. However, just as lymphoreticular malignancies can be classified according to their lineage from stem cells, it may soon be possible to achieve a biological classification of primary cerebral tumors by identifying antigenic phenotypes which relate to differentiation from the neuroectodermal stem cell.

Currently available monoclonal antibodies are valuable probes for examining the nature of the neoplastic process. However, a new generation of monoclonals will soon be produced which have even more exciting implications. These are antibodies which will recognize the presence of growth factor receptors and oncogene products in tissue sections.[44] Not only might such markers come closer to the ideal of tumor specific antibodies, but it might be possible to define regions of abnormal oncogene expression prior to an obvious malignant change within the tissues.

The studies of antibody *in vitro* described above have led to attempts at *in vivo* targeting of radiolabeled monoclonal antibodies in patients with neoplasms of the CNS.[26,45] The use of antibody guided irradiation in therapeutic amounts seems a promising technique for cleaning the CSF of malignant cells in childhood tumors which are predisposed to CSF seeding, such as medulloblastoma and leukemia. This will be further described in Chapter 6.

ACKNOWLEDGMENTS

We are grateful to Drs. D. B. Brownell, T. Moss, and J. Berry for collaboration and for referring material. Antibodies were generously donated by P. C. L. Beverley, B. Anderton, E. B. Lane, J. Taylor-Papadimitriou, C. Makin, C. Woodhouse, S. Carrel, and J. P. Mach. Mrs. G. Wenczek expertly prepared the manuscript. Funding is acknowledged from the Bristol Brain Cancer Research Fund, The Imperial Cancer Research Fund, the Newman Foundation, and the Cancer and Leukaemia in Children Trust.

REFERENCES

1. **Thomas, D. G. T., Anderson, R. E., and DeBoulay, G. H.,** CT guided stereotactic neurosurgery, *J. Neurol. Neurosurg. Psychiatry,* 47, 9, 1984.
2. **Coakham, H. B.,** Brain Tumours — recent advances in diagnosis and treatment, in *Progress in Surgery,* Vol. 2., Taylor, I., Ed., Churchill Livingstone, Edinburgh, 1986, 223.
3. **Bignami, A., Eng, L. F., Dahl, D., and Uyeda, C. T.,** Localisation of the glial fibrillary acidic protein in astrocytes by immunofluorescence, *Brain Res.,* 43, 429, 1972.
4. **Bonnin, J. M. and Rubinstein, L. J.,** Immunochemistry of central nervous system tumours, *J. Neurosurg.,* 60, 1121, 1984.
5. **Esiri, M.,** Immunohistological techniques in neuropathology, in *Recent Advances in Neuropathology,* Vol. 2, Smith, W. T. and Cavanagh, J. B., Eds., Churchill Livingstone, Edinburgh, 1982, 1.
6. **Allan, P. M., Garson, J. A., Harper, E. I., Asser, U., Coakham, H. B., Brownell, D. B., and Kemshead, J. T.,** Biological characterisation and clinical applications of a monoclonal antibody recognising and antigen restricted to neuroectodermal tissues, *Int. J. Cancer,* 31, 591, 1983.
7. **Kemshead, J. T., Fritschy, J., Garson, J. A., Allan, P. M., Coakham, H. B., Brown, S., and Asser, U.,** Monoclonal antibody UJ127.11 detects a 220,000—240,000 M. W. glycoprotein present on a subset of neuroectodermally derived cells, *Int. J. Cancer,* 31, 187, 1983.
8. **Jones, D., Fritschy, J., Garson, J. A., Nokes, T. J. C., Kemshead, J. T., and Hardisty, R. M.,** A monoclonal antibody binding to human medulloblastoma cells and to the platelet glycoprotein IIb-IIIa complex, *Br. J. Haematol.,* 57, 621, 1984.
9. **Beverley, P. C. L. and Callard, R. E.,** Distinctive functional characteristics of human T-lymphocytes defined by E-rosetting or a monoclonal anti-T-cell antibody, *Eur. J. of Immunol.,* 11, 329, 1981.
10. **Garson, J. A., Beverley, P. C. L., Coakham, H. B., and Harper, E. I.,** Monoclonal antibodies against human T lymphocytes label Purkinje neurons of many species, *Nature,* 298, 375, 1982.
11. **Lane, E. B. and Koprowski, H.,** Molecular recognition and the future of monoclonal antibodies, *Nature,* 296, 200, 1982.
12. **Sikora, K., Alderson, T., and Ellis, J.,** Human hybridomas from patients with malignant disease, *Br. J. Cancer,* 47, 135, 1983.
13. **Bourne, S. P., Coakham, H. B., Kemshead, J. T., Brownell, D. B., Allan, P. M., and Davies, A. G.,** The role of monoclonal antibodies in the diagnosis and characterization of medulloblastoma, in *Medulloblastomas in Children,* Zeltzer, P. M., and Pochedl, C., Eds., Praeger, New York, 1986, 87.
14. **Gatter, K. C., Abdulaziz, Z., Beverley, P., Corvalan, J. R. F., Ford, C., Lane, E. B., Mota, M., Nash, J. R. G., Pulford, K., Stein, H., Taylor-Papadimitriou, J., Woodhouse, C., and Mason, D. Y.,** Use of monoclonal antibodies for the histopathological diagnosis of human malignancy, *J. Clin. Pathol.,* 35, 1253, 1982.

Table 1
SEROLOGIC-DEFINED MARKERS FOR NEUROBLASTOMA

Marker	Tissue	Serum	Ref.
NSE	+	+	10—12
Ferritin	+	+	13
CK-BB	+	+	14,21
LDH	+	+	15—17
CEA	+	+	18—21
S-100	+	−	
Neurofilament	+	nt	23
Thy-1	+	nt	24,25
INMA	+	nt	27
MBA-2	+	nt	29
HB	+	nt	28
FONA-1	+	nt	36
FONA-2	+	nt	36
ONA	+	nt	37
OFA-1	+	nt	38
GFAP	−	nt	22,23
Fibronectin	−	nt	51

Note: See also Table 4. nt, Not tested.

Table 2
SERUM NSE VALUES AT DIAGNOSIS BY SEX AND AGE RANGE IN PATIENTS WITH STAGE IV NEUROBLASTOMA

Serum NSE	Number		Number aged			
(ng/ml)	Male	Female	<1 yr[a]	1—5 yr[b]	>5 yr	Total %
<15	4	1	0	3	2	4
15—50	14	15	3	22	4	24
51—100	21	10	4	21	6	25
101—500	22	23	6	35	4	37
>500	8	4	2	9	1	10
Total	69	53	15	90	17	—

[a] Normal means serum NSE: 8·0 ± 2·8 ng/ml (n = 15).
[b] Normal means serum NSE: 7·0 ± 1 ng/m. (n = 15)

From Zeltzer, P. M., Marangos, P. J., Parmma, A. M., Sather, H., Dalton, A., Hammond, D., Siegel, S. E., and Seeger, R. C., *Lancet*, 2, 361, 1983. With permission.

at diagnosis could be prognostic for survival, and they were ($p = 0.009$). The strongest correlation was for infants less than 1 year of age ($p = 0.0003$) when a serum level of greater than and less than 100 ng/ml was used: 7/7 infants having serum NSE less than 100 ng/ml survived while 7/8 infants with levels greater than 100 ng/ml died within 12 months of diagnosis. (Figure 1.)[11]

When we analyzed the survival of all patients diagnosed before 1 year of age in CCSG studies over the past 10 years, there was a precipitous decline in the first year with a plateau at 2 years with a 50% long-term survival.[10,11] These data independently suggested that there were two subsets of infants with stage IV disease whose survival may be predicated by initial serum NSE level.

In collaboration with Drs. Audrey Evans and Paul Marangos, we studied additional stage

Table 3
SERUM NEURON SPECIFIC ENOLASE IN DIFFERENT STAGES OF NEUROBLASTOMA

Stage of disease	N	NSE in Serum (Mean ± SD[a])	Range	% (with >100ng/ml)	% Survivors
I	6	20 ± 4	14—23	0	100
II	19	34 ± 33	5—114	5	90
III	36	195 ± 514	8—3012	34	37[b]
IV	168	245 ± 353	6—7500	54	10[b]
IV-s	10	50 ± 14	4—114	10	90

[a] ng of NSE per ml of serum.
[b] Estimated survival.

From Zeltzer, P. M., Marangos, P. J., Sather, H., Evans, A. E., et al., *Prog. Clin. Biol. Res.*, 175, 319, 1985. With permission.

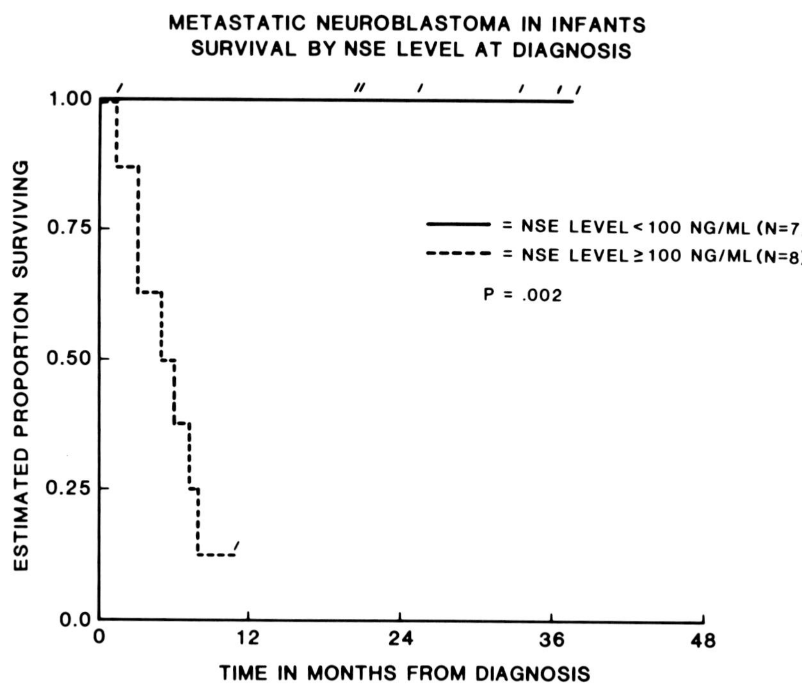

FIGURE 1. Serum NSE in infants with stage IV neuroblastoma. Survival in infants less than 1 year of age at diagnosis with stage IV disease by serum NSE values > and < than 100 ng/ml. (p, 0.002). (From Zeltzer, P. M., Marangos, P. J., Parmma, A. M., Sather, H., Dalton, A., Hammond, D., Siegel, S. E., and Seeger, R. C., *Lancet*, 2, 361, 1983. With permission.)

IV-s infants to determine if their serum levels mimicked the older patients with metastatic disease or lower stage patients.[12] To our surprise, 9/10 patients with metastatic stage IV-s had serum NSE less than 100 ng/ml, i.e., in the range seen with lower stage disease. However, one patient with a 270 ng/ml level with stage II continues disease free and all four stage II patients who progressed had initial serum levels less than 100 ng/ml. Thus, factors other than NSE level alone contribute to tumor progression in lower stage disease. (See Table 3.)

We quantitated serial serum specimens at diagnosis, in remission, and at relapse in 17

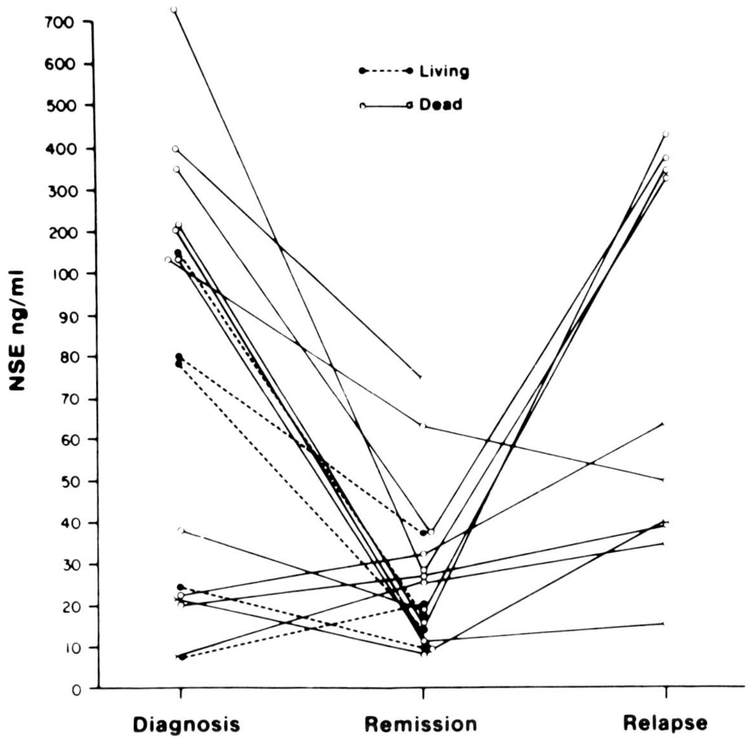

FIGURE 2. Serum NSE levels in remission and relapse. Survival and changes in serum NSE levels in 17 patients with stages II, III, IV neuroblastoma at diagnosis, in remission, and at relapse. (From Zeltzer, P. M., Marangos, P. J., Evans, A. E., and Schneider, S. L., *Cancer,* 57, 1230, 1986. With permission.)

patients. Four of nine patients with initial levels less than 100 ng/ml are disease free. Of five who relapsed, one had a raised level and four were slightly higher but less than 100 ng/ml at the time of relapse. Of eight patients with initial levels greater than 100 ng/ml, all had near-normal levels during remission. Of seven who relapsed, three had levels greater than 100 ng/ml, two were low, and two were not measured. Thus only 4/12 had serum levels greater than 100 ng/ml at relapse (Figure 2).

In summary, serum NSE levels at diagnosis are prognostic for survival in infants with Stage III and IV disease, and NSE is a sensitive marker to detect neuroblastoma in all stage III and IV patients (> 85% have raised levels). However, it is not recommended as a sole screening test to detect relapse.

3. *Ferritin*

Serum ferritin levels have been conclusively demonstrated to be prognostic for survival in children with neuroblastoma.[13] Ferritin is not a tumor specific marker, since immunoreactive ferritin is also found in hematologic conditions with iron overload. Hann and coworkers found that 50% and 65% of stage III and IV patients had abnormally raised serum levels.[13] A low serum ferritin was prognostic for good survival (75% vs 15%) in all ages of stage III patients. For stage IV, patients had a survival advantage if low serum levels were present at diagnosis. However, the survival effect was greatest in the infant group less than 1 year of age (55% vs 25%). Multivariate analysis using both NSE and ferritin will no doubt yield a more rational approach for allocating patients into more appropriate treatment programs (P. Zeltzer and R. Seeger, personal communication, 1988).

4. CK-BB

This isoenzyme is found in normal brain and other tissues, in brain tumors,[14] in neuroblastoma cell lines,[10,14] and in sera of neuroblastoma patients. Its usefulness for diagnosis and prognosis has not been studied.

5. Lactate Dehyrogenase (LDH)

LDH is a glycolytic enzyme widely distributed in normal and neoplastic tissues and is released into the blood from injured or dying cells. At least five isoenzymes exist. Prognosis for neuroblastoma has been associated with both elevated total LDH[15] and raised isoenzymes LDH-2 and -3.[16] Raised levels also have been found in yolk sac tumors, lymphomas, and Wilms' tumors.[17]

6. Carcinoembryonic Antigen (CEA)

CEA is a cell surface protein found predominantly on fetal endodermal tissues in the second trimester. Seventy-five percent of gastrointestinal neoplasms are associated with serum levels greater than 2.5 ng/ml. Patients with head and neck tumors and 20% of smokers may also have raised levels (reviewed in Reference 18). Raised serum levels have been reported with neuroblastoma.[19,20] Most workers do not feel that its sensitivity is sufficient for screening, although its originally elevated serum levels may reflect disease response. The CEA from neuroblastoma has been characterized as the nonspecific cross-reacting antigen (NCA).[21] No data exist for its use in monitoring for relapse.

7. Other markers

Additional markers of neuroblastoma cells have been defined using heterologous antisera or by biochemical techniques (see Table 1). Some were detected only on cultured cell lines. Though none of these other markers has been adapted for monitoring antigen levels in serum or urine, they hold promise for future application. A brief description of each follows. The intermediate filaments (IF) like neurofilament (NF), desmin, vimentin, and GFAP are normal cytoskeletal proteins. Cell type expression of IF may be useful for diagnosis of human tumors.[22]

Monoclonal antibodies to NF were raised against bovine spinal cord and tested on CNS and peripheral nervous system (PNS) tumors.[23] NF was found only in tumors of putative neuronal origin: neuroblastoma and pheochromocytomss have been identified on the basis of NF content.[23] Thus, histogenesis of neural tumors might be inferred with the use of these proteins.

The Thy-1 antigen originally described on human T lymphocytes, has been detected on neural tissue of all mammalian species, but its functional significance remains unknown. Thy-1 was detected on human neuroblastoma, astrocytoma, and medulloblastoma cell lines and fresh tumors of neural origin using F(ab)2 antiserum.[24,25] Thy-1 is not detected on normal bone marrow cells and has been used to detect and remove tumor cells from marrow prior to autologous marrow transplantation.[26]

Nervous system specific membrane antigens on cultured murine neuroblastoma cells have been shown to be "interspecies" antigens also found on human neuronal cells.[27,28] An interspecies neural membrane antigen (INMA) was produced by sequential immunization with rabbits using IMR-32 (human) and NK-119 and N18 (murine) neuroblastoma cell lines. INMA was found on some cultured human and murine neuroblastoma cells and on normal brain of both species.[27]

The mouse brain antigen-2 (MBA-2) was defined by a naturally occurring antibody in normal mouse sera,[29] and it has been detected on normal brain and kidney of both human and murine tissue. This interspecies antigen was detected on neuroblastoma cell lines, but not glioma or retinoblastoma lines. INMA and MBA-2 are not identical, since their distribution is different on human and murine neuroblastoma cell lines.[27,29]

Antifetal brain (HB) serum reacted with a neuroblastoma cell line, tumor, and 5—10% of lymphocytes.[28] This antigen was lacking on thymocytes, human, murine, and guinea pig brain, liver, or kidney.[30-34] HB differs from mouse brain markers NS-4 and Thy-1.[35]

First trimester human fetal brain was the immunogen for the rabbit antiserum which identified fetal onconeural antigens, FONA-1 and FONA-2.[36] The former is expressed on normal human fetal brain, neuroblastoma, and other tumor cells. FONA-2 is expressed by fetal brain and neuroblastoma cells only. These antigens differ from HB which reacts with adult brain.[36]

Human neuroblastoma cell line, LAN-1, was the immunogen used to generate the rabbit antiserum which defined the onconeural antigen (ONA). It is common to adult human brain, neuroblastoma, oat cell carcinoma, Wilms' tumor, and sarcomas. This differentiation antigen is expressed by neuroectodermal and mesodermal tumors and some leukemias.[37]

Oncofetal antigen (OFA) is a human tumor associated antigen which shares determinants with fetal brain tissue.[38] OFA-1 is not detected on adult brain or fetal liver, spleen, thymus, or small intestine. Melanoma cell line M14 expresses OFA-1, and sera from melanoma patients reactive with M14 was used to characterize the distribution of OFA-1 in human tumors: melanomas (87%), lung carcinomas (71%), sarcomas (61%), brain tumors (58%), breast carcinomas (53%). OFA-1 recognizes an antigen of ectodermal and mesodermal origin, and unlike CEA, is not present on fetal digestive organs.

8. Monoclonal Antibodies to Neuroblastoma

The approach to prepare neuroectodermal specific monoclonal antibodies (MAb) has been to use fetal or adult neural tissue as immunogens. Tumor cell extracts and cell lines also have been used to prepare mouse/human and human/human hybridomas with neuroectodermal specificity.[39-40] The majority of MAb to neuroectodermal tumors share antigens with normal fetal and adult brain tissue. MAb raised against normal[40-41] and transformed hematopoietic cells[42-46] share reactivity with neuroectodermal tumors as well. Over 25 MAb with these characteristics have been described and were recently reviewed.[47]

B. Brain Tumors

1. Introduction

At least 22 markers for brain tumors have been described. Tables 1 and 4 contain a summary of the markers and their expression within tumor groups. As yet no marker is unique for neural neoplastic cells and most are expressed by normal cells. All except two have been defined strictly by immunohistologic or biochemical methods. Only NSE and the BB isoenzyme of creatine kinase (CK-BB), have been assayed and found in sera and cerebrospinal fluid (CSF)[14] (Table 5). Wasserstrom et al. have reviewed additional biochemical markers for brain tumors which are not included in this review.[48]

2. Medulloblastomas

a. Neuron Specific Enolase (NSE)

Tumor tissue levels of NSE ranged from 600 to 7400 ng/mg protein (normal brain = 13,500 ng/mg protein and were six-fold higher than that found in other brain tumors[14] (Table 6). Raised serum levels were found in 7/11 patients tested. CSF levels also were raised in 7/11 patients, though these were not all the same patients with raised serum levels (see Table 5).

The CK-BB tissue levels were 700 to 7900 ng/mg protein with normal being 14,700 ng/mg protein and no differences were noted between medulloblastomas and other brain tumors (see Table 6). Five of eight cases had raised serum levels, but 0/7 had raised CSF levels (see Table 5). Too few cases were studied to know if serum or CSF levels are prognostic for treatment response or reflect response to therapy.

Table 4
MARKERS FOR BRAIN TUMORS

Markers[b,c]	Neural Tumor Type[a] Medulloblastoma	Astrocytoma	Schwannoma	Oligo	Ependy	Other[d]	Ref.
NSE (C)	+(*) (**)	+	+	+	+	M,CP	14
CK-BB	+(*)	+	+	N.D.	N.D.	M	14
Polyamines	+	N.D.	N.D.	N.D.	N.D.	N.D.	49,50
α-2 glycoprotein	−	+/−	N.D.	+	−	N.D.	
S-100 (C)	+	+	+	+(−*)	+	CP,AN	
CNPase (S)	N.D.	+	+	+	+	M,CP,AN	
GFAP (C)	+	+	+	+	+	GG,T	52-57
Fibronectin (S)	N.D.	−	N.D.	N.D.	N.D.	N.D.	51
Neurofilament (C)	+	−	N.D.	N.D.	−	GG,GN,T,P	23
Desmin (C)	N.D.	N.D.	−	N.D.	N.D.	R	22
Vimentin (C)	N.D.	N.D.	+	N.D.	N.D.	R,L	22
Thy-1 (S)	(*)	+*	+*	N.D.	N.D.	(T,R,W,L)*	24,25
HB (S)	N.D.	N.D.	N.D.	N.D.	N.D.	R	28
FONA-1 (S)	N.D.	N.D.	N.D.	N.D.	N.D.	T,R,W,O,C,E,Ly,H	36
ONA (S)	+*	N.D.	N.D.	(R,W,O)*	N.D.		37
OFA-1	+	N.D.	N.D.	N.D.	N.D.	(T,W,M)[e],B,S	38

Note: N.D., not done

[a] Neural tumor cell types — medulloblastoma; astrocytoma; glioblastoma multiform; schwannoma; oligodendroglioma; ependymoma, melanoma. Studies using: + or - = histology cell lines of human neuroectodermal tumors (*); sera (**).

[b] Neural tumor markers — CK-BB: BB enzyme of creatine kinase; CNPase: 2′,3′-cyclic nucleotide 3′-phosphohydrolase; FONA: fetal onconeural antigen: GFAP: glial fibrillary acidic protein; GSMA: glioma specific membrane antigen; HAAA: human astrocytoma associated antigen; HB: human fetal brain antigen; IMMA: intraspecies neural membrane antigen; MBA-2: mouse brain antigen; NSE: neuron specific enoclase; OFA: oncofetal antigen or M14 melanoma-associated antigen; ONA: onconeural antigen; S-100: nervous system specific protein.

[c] Location — cytoplasmic (c); surface (s).

[d] Tumor types — AN: acoustic neuroma; B: breast; C: colon carcinoma; CP: choroid plexus papilloma; E: Ewing's sarcoma; GG: ganglioglioma; GN: ganglioneuroma (blastoma); H: Hodgkin's lymphoma; L: leiomyosarcoma; Ly: lymphoma; M: meningioma; O: oat cell carcinoma; P: pheochromocytoma; R: rhabdomyosarcoma; S: sarcoma; T: teratoma; W: Wilms'.

[e] Positive in one case.

Derived from data in Schneider, S. L., Sasaki, F., and Zeltzer, P. M., *CRC Crit. Rev. Oncol./Hematol.*, 5, 199, 1987.

Table 5
NEURON SPECIFIC ENOLASE AND CREATINE KINASE ISOENZYME LEVELS IN SERUM AND SPINAL FLUID (CSF) FROM PATIENTS AT TIME OF DIAGNOSIS

	NSE				CK-BB			
	N	Mean	(range)	No. abnormal	N	Mean	(range)	No. abnormal
Serum								
Medulloblastoma	11	21 ± 6	(10—78)	7/11	8	12 ± 2	(4—26)	5/8
Astrocytoma (III-IV) (glioma)	9	10 ± 1	(8—11)	0/9	2	109 ± 102	(8—210)	1/2
Astrocytoma (I-II)	9	13 ± 13	(8—18)	3/9	8	10 ± 1	(6—15)	3/8
Other	6	29 ± 8	(13—52)	4/6	5	13 ± 6	(6—35)	1/5
Control	52	12 ± 1	(2—16)		44	3 ± 3	(1—12)	
Acute stroke/ trauma	9	13 ± 13	(3—64)		15	24 ± 6	(14—39)	
CSF								
Medulloblastoma	7	28 ± 16	(4—123)	4/7	7	2 ± 1	(0—5)	0/7
Astrocytoma (III-IV) (glioma)	1	118		1/1	1	16		1/1
Astrocytoma (I-II)	2	21 ± 19	(2—40)	1/2	2	142 ± 137	(6—278)	1/2
Other	1	11		1/1	1	2		0/1
Adult control	5	2 ± 0			11	7 ± 2	(0—12)	
Acute stroke	10	10 ± 6	(3—25)		15	34 ± 9	(6—140)	

Note: Mann-Whitney U (Two-Tailed) contrasts of serum and cerebrospinal fluid NSE and CK-BB. Serum NSE contrast are as follows: medullo vs. control $p < .01$; medullo vs. glioma not significant (N.S.); medullo vs. astro $p < .1$; medullo vs. other $p < .02$; glioma vs. control N.S.; glioma vs. astro N.S.; glioma vs. other $p < .05$; astro vs. control N.S.; astro vs. other $p < .05$. Serum CK-BB contrast are as follows: medullo vs. glioma N.S.; medullo vs. astro N.S.; medullo vs. other N.S.; glioma vs. astro N.S.; glioma vs. other N.S.; astro vs. other N.S. CSF NSE contrast is as follows: medullo vs. astro N.S. CSF CK-BB contrast is as follows: medullo vs. astro $p < .10$.
ng/ml Expressed as mean ± standard error of the mean. Normal serum and CSF NSE values are < 16 and < 2 ng/ml, respectively. Normal Serum and CSF CK-BB values are < 10 and < 12 ng/ml, respectively.

Derived from Zeltzer, P. M., Schneider, S. L., Marangos, P. J., and Zweig, M. H., *J. Natl. Cancer Inst.*, 77, 625, 1986.

b. Polyamines

The polyamines, putrescine and spermidine, were evaluated as tumor markers for diagnosis and monitoring of medulloblastomas. Strictly speaking they are not tumor markers, but are metabolic products of nucleic acids reflecting cellular growth and proliferation. The assay technique uses chromatography and amino acid analysis. Approximately 30-40% of tumors have raised levels (> 184 and 150 pmol/ml for putrescine and spermidine, respectively, at diagnosis). Marton et al. found that 15/16 patients had a raised level correlating with response to therapy.[49]

Recurrent tumors were also associated with raised levels. In a follow-up study, 15/15 cases associated with raised levels all had recurrent disease and three false negative results were noted.[50] Thus, polyamines are a helpful adjunct to monitor for relapse.

3. Astrocytomas/Gliomas

a. NSE and CK-BB

Malignant astrocytomas were found to express low levels of NSE (89-386 ng/mg protein) while a larger range was found for CK-BB (74 to 26,000 ng/mg protein; N = 4)[14] (see Table 6).

Table 6
QUANTITATION OF NEURON SPECIFIC ENOLASE AND CREATINE KINASE CONTENT IN BRAIN TUMORS AT DIAGNOSIS

	NSE[a]			CK-BB[a]		
Tumor	N	Mean ± S.E.M.	Range	N	Mean ± S.E.M.	Range
Medulloblastoma	11	3137 ± 572	(604—7356)	10	3155 ± 772	(723—7913)
Glioma (III-IV)[b]	4	219 ± 63	(89—386)	3	6757 ± 5050	(74—26,320)
Astrocytoma (I-II)	9	514 ± 167	(94—1488)	9	1434 ± 346	(352—9347)
Other	3	933 ± 542	(414—2056)	3	12,626 ± 6557	(4842—25,396)

Note: The % cell viability for medulloblastoma (tumors) was 20 to 40% (2), 50 to 80% (2), and >90% (7). For all other tumors it was 0 to 10% (2), 20 to 40% (3), 50 to 80% (3), and >90% (8). Mann-Whitney U (two-tailed) contrasts for tumor NSE and CK-BB. Tumor NSE contrasts are as follows: medullo vs. glioma p <0.01; medullo vs. astro p <0.01; medullo vs. other, not significant (N.S.); glioma vs. astro, N.S.; glioma vs. other p <0.02; astro vs. other, N.S. Tumor CK-BB contrasts are as follows: medullo vs. glioma, N.S.; medullo vs. astro N.S.; medullo vs. other p <0.10; glioma vs. other N.S.; astro vs. other p < 10.

[a] As ng/mg protein. Normal brain NSE is 13,500 and for CK-BB is 14,700 ng/mg protein.
[b] Kernohan classification.

Derived from Zeltzer, P. M., Schneider, S. L., Marangos, P. J., and Zweig, M. H., *J. Natl. Cancer Inst.*, 77, 625, 1986.

b. Fibronectin

Fibronectin (FN) is an extracellular matrix glycoprotein found in normal fetal and adult brain but restricted to the vascular endothelium.[51] It is rarely detected in gliomas, although GFAP positive glioma cell lines express FN, and these tumors grown in athymic mice shed human FN into the serum.[51]

c. Glial Fibrillary Acidic Protein (GFAP)

GFAP is expressed by neoplastic, reactive, and normal astrocytes.[52] Well-differentiated astrocytomas stain intensely, while glioblastoma and astrocytoma of higher grade malignancy stain poorly or only in focal areas.[53]

GFAP also has been identified in medulloblastoma and embryonic CNS tumors.[54] Cerebellar astrocytomas and malignant glioma have been differentiated from other tumors by their GFAP content.[55] Prognostically, astrocytic differentiation in medulloblastoma was associated with extended survival in one study,[56] although another report suggests any differentiation is associated with a poorer prognosis.[57] Thus the predictive value of GFAP is unknown.

d. CEA

Raised levels of CEA were reported with neuroblastoma[21] and with brain tumors.[58] Most of the raised levels were found in adults with metastases. None of the patients with primary brain tumors had significantly raised levels.

All of the other markers (except CNPase) were immunohistologically defined and none have been prospectively studied for their diagnostic or prognostic features. A review of their tumor distribution is found under neuroblastomas.

4. Markers Defined by Monoclonal Antibodies

With the exception of the intermediate filament proteins, no single MAb-defined marker has been accepted as useful for diagnosis or monitoring. The MAb, their immunogens, and tissue distribution have been extensively reviewed.[47]

Table 7
AFP IN MALIGNANT AND NONMALIGNANT CONDITIONS

Type of cancer	Range[a]	Percentage of patients >20 ng/ml
Endodermal sinus	390—210,000	100
Teratocarcinoma	20—130,000	75
Seminoma	20	0
Hepatocellular carcinoma	20—5,000,000	70
Pancreatic, gastric carcinoma with liver metastases	20—500	15
Noncancerous conditions		
Hepatitis		
Neonatal (0—3 months)	40,000—290,000	100
Viral	21—4400	31
Chronic active	23—4210	33
Persistent	21—267	10
Chronic hepatitis B antigenemia	33—36	18
Primary biliary cirrhosis	20	0
Ataxia telangiectasia	44—2800	95
Cystic fibrosis	56—8800	?
Tyrosinemia	20,000—300,000	100

[a] Range of serum alpha-fetoprotein values in cancer and noncancerous conditions.

Derived from Zeltzer, P. M., *Manual of Allergy and Immunology, Diagnosis, and Therapy,* Lawler, G., and Fischer, T., Eds., Little, Brown, Boston, 1987, 336.

III. MARKERS ON OTHER PEDIATRIC TUMORS

A. Germ Cell/Endodermal Sinus Tumors

1. Noncentral Nervous System

Tumors of germ cell origin can be found anywhere in the body from the cranium to the coccyx or testicle. They may contain either germ cell (endodermal sinus or yolk sac) or extra embryonic (dysgerminoma) elements, or both (malignant teratocarcinoma). Regardless of site, 85% of these tumors secrete either one or both of the markers alpha fetoprotein (AFP) and human chorionic gonadotrophin (hCG).

AFP is a normal product of the yolk sac during fetal development. Peak serum levels are reached during the second trimester (1000 μg/ml) of fetal life[59] and gradually fall to 100 μg/ml at birth and then fall to less than 20 ng/ml by four months of postnatal life.[60] It is reexpressed by hepatomas, endodermal sinus tumors, a minority of gastrointestinal tumors, and in other nonmalignant hepatic conditions[61] (Table 7).

Human chorionic gonadothrophin (hCG) is another marker useful for diagnosis and monitoring these tumors. It is secreted by those tumors which have histologic evidence of trophoblastic tissue, such as choriocarcinomas and malignant teratocarcinomas. The cells secreting AFP and hCG are different. Normal levels of hCG are <1 IU by radioimmunoassay. It is important to specify the beta unit assay of hCG because the alpha chain may cross-react with lutinizing hormone. The presence of both hCG and AFP is strong evidence of a mixed tumor even if the biopsy only demonstrates endodermal sinus tumor.

In adults, 75% of these tumors are associated with raised serum AFP levels greater that 40 ng/ml.[62] In 55 benign testicular lesions, no raised levels were found. For clinical staging, raised levels were found in those patients with nodal and distant metastases.[63]

In a series of 101 men with malignant nonseminomatous tumors, serum levels of both AFP and hCG were raised in 58%, 17% had raised AFP alone, 14% had raised hCG alone, and neither marker was raised in 11%. Thus, the true positive rate was 89% and true negative rate equalled only 11%. Therefore, assay of both markers will accurately assess 89% of the patients. Occasionally, both markers can be raised at the beginning of therapy, but, only one may be raised at relapse. This implies that the recurrence is taking place in a limited number of tumor cell clones.[63]

Serial serum levels are of value in monitoring response to therapy. In a review of the literature, Waldmann notes that no false positives occurred and the false negative rate was only 10%. For patients in whom the tumor persisted but the markers remained low, maturation to a benign teratoma was noted.[63]

2. Central Nervous System

Both AFP and hCG have been raised in the CSF when the tumor is primary or metastatic to the CNS.[64,65] The exact incidence of positive markers for CNS disease is unknown, though it appears to approximate the systemic malignancy. CSF levels up to 1000 ng/ml of AFP and up to 400,000 IU/ml for hCG have been reported.[65] Importantly, the CSF to serum ratio is raised with primary CNS disease. Normal serum levels were found in 2/2 patients in the face of raised CSF levels. Also, marker levels from lumbar fluid were five- to thirteen-fold higher than ventricular levels.[65] Thus, to accurately evaluate tumor status with germ cell tumors, both CSF from a spinal tap and serum levels are mandatory.

In summary, AFP and hCG are useful for both diagnosis and monitoring of these neoplasms within the CNS. Some investigators have advocated that the presence of one or both of these markers may even obviate the need for biopsy of the lesion.[48]

B. Hepatoblastoma

1. Incidence of Markers

The incidence of raised serum AFP in children with malignant hepatic tumors is 97% using a radioimmunoassay.[66] This differs from the data in adults where 72% were positive.[62] In the former study, there were no differences among individual histologic types. Recently, higher levels were found among embryonic hepatoblastomas compared with hepatocarcinomas (P. Rogers, personal communication, 1987).

There is a differential avidity of AFP for the lectin concanavalin between hepatic and yolk sac tumor derived AFP. About 5% of normal hepatic AFP binds to the lectin, while 50% of tumor AFP binds. This is due to the carbohydrate portion of the yolk sac AFP having an additional N-acetylglucosamine residue. This test is not yet available commercially.

Other tumors of the liver such as hamartomas or metastatic lesions, may be associated with slightly raised serum AFP levels. No data is available on the prognostic value of serum levels of AFP at diagnosis.

2. Usefulness of Monitoring

Serum levels (using a less sensitive gel diffusion technique) paralleled the clinical response to therapy in adults.[67] The incidence of false positive and false negative serum levels have not been studied but is probably low. Confusion in interpreting raised serum levels may exist in the clinical situation where a chemical or infectious hepatitis coexist with recurrent tumor. Serial sampling would be helpful in elucidating this problem.

C. Wilms' Tumor

There are no commercially available tests for antigens or tumor products specific for Wilms' tumor. Fetuin is an antigen found on tumor extracts, but, there have been no additional clinical reports on its use.[68] Serum LDH may be raised from either tumor breakdown or hemorrhage.[16,17] Serum NSE was raised in one patient.[12] Several of the antigens found on neuroblastoma (see Table 1) also were reactive with Wilms' tumor specimens: FONA-1, ONA, HB, OFA.[36-38] Their cross-reactivity raises the question of neuroectodermal derivation for Wilms' tumor cells. But sarcomas also reacted with these antibodies. This suggests that these antigens reflect either a more primitive cell of origin or aberrant expression by the malignant cells.

D. Rhabdomyosarcoma

Rhabdomyosarcomas contain desmin and vimentin, while vimentin alone is found in schwannomas and lymphomas.[22,23] Thus, the IF type can be useful in differentiating among small cell tumor types. No serum tests using desmin have been described.

Antibodies reactive with Wilms' tumor also react with many sarcomas.[36,37] Human sera from adult patients with sarcomas react with their own tumor cells (autologous reactivity/ private antigen), with other sarcomas (allogeneic reactivity/public antigen), or with other tumor types. At least 14 antigens have been so defined. Only two have restricted reactivity, and none have been tested prospectively as to their diagnostic, prognostic, or monitoring capabilities. Questions as to the specificity and prevalence in the normal population of these antibodies has been raised.[69]

E. Conclusion

Over the past 25 years, serologic techniques have been helping clinicians confirm diagnoses and monitor only a minority of childhood neoplasms. The next 5 to 10 years will not see only development of additional markers, but clinical studies testing the sensitivity and specificity of these markers. This will follow similar studies of leukemia markers performed by the large European (SIOP) and North American cooperative clinical groups (CCSG and POG).

ACKNOWLEDGMENTS

Dr. Zeltzer acknowledges support from the Robert J. and Helen C. Kleberg Foundation, the Concern II Foundation, and Dr. Bela Bodey for review of the manuscript.

REFERENCES

1. **Silverberg, E. and Lubera, J.,** Cancer Statistics, 1986, *CA — A Cancer J. Clin.*, 36, 9, 1986.
2. **Seeger, R. C., Brodeur, G. M., Sather, H., Dalton, A., Siegel, S. E., Wong, K. Y., and Hammond, D.,** Association of multiple copies of the n-myc oncogene with rapid progression of neuroblastomas, *N.Engl. J. Med.*, 313, 1111, 1985.
3. **Belasco, J. and D'Angio, G.,** Wilms Tumor, *CA — A Cancer J. Clin.*, 31, 258, 1981.
4. **Hellstrom, I. E., Hellstrom, K. E., Pierce, G. E., et al.,** Demonstration of cell bound and humoral immunity against neuroblastoma cells, *Proc. Natl. Acad. Sci. U.S.A.*, 60, 1231, 1968.
5. **Coakham, H. B., Garson, J. A., Brownell, B., and Kemshead, J. T.,** Monoclonal antibodies as reagents for brain tumor diagnosis, a review, *J. R. Soc., Med.*, 77, 780, 1984.
6. **Siegel, S. E., Laug, W., et al.,** Patterns of urinary catecholamine metabolite excretion in neuroblastoma, in *Advances in Neuroblastoma Research,* Evans, A., Ed., Raven Press, New York, 1980, 22.
7. **Marangos, P. J. and Zomzeley-Neurath, C.,** Immunological studies of a nerve specific protein (NSP), *Arch. Biochem. Biophys.*, 190, 289, 1975.
8. **Bock, E. and Dissing, J.,** Demonstration of enolase activity connected to the brain specific protein, 14-3-2, *Scand. J. Immunol.*, 4(Suppl. 2), 31, 1975.
9. **Marangos, P. J. and Schmechel, D.,** The neurobiology of the brain enolases, *Essays Neurochem. Neuropharmacol.*, 4, 211, 1980.

10. **Zeltzer, P. M., Marangos, P. J., Sather, H., Evans, A. E., et al.,** Prognostic importance of serum neuron specific enolase in local and widespread neuroblastoma, *Prog. Clin. Biol. Res.*, 175, 319, 1985.
11. **Zeltzer, P. M., Marangos, P. J., Parmma, A. M., Sather, H., Dalton, A., Hammond, D., Siegel, S. E., and Seeger, R. C.,** Raised neuron specific enolase in serum of children with metastatic neuroblastoma, *Lancet,* 2, 361, 1983.
12. **Zeltzer, P. M., Marangos, P. J., Evans, A. E., and Schneider, S. L.,** Serum neuron specific enolase in children with neuroblastoma: relationship to stage and disease course, *Cancer,* 57, 1230, 1986.
13. **Hann, H.-W., Evans, A. E., Siegel, S. E., Wong, K. Y., Sather, H., Dalton, A., Hammond, D., and Seeger, R. E.,** Prognostic importance of serum ferritin in patients with stages III and IV neuroblastoma: the childrens cancer study group experience, *Cancer Res.*, 45, 2843, 1985.
14. **Zeltzer, P. M., Schneider, S. L., Marangos, P. J., and Zweig, M. H.,** Differential expression of neural isoenzymes by human medulloblastomas and gliomas and neuroextodermal cell lines, *J. Natl. Cancer Inst.*, 77, 625, 1986.
15. **Quinn, J. J., Altman, A. J., and Frantz, C. N.,** Serum lactic dehydrogenase: an indicator of tumor activity in neuroblastoma, *J. Pediatr.*, 97, 89, 1980.
16. **Kinumaki, K., Takeuchi, H., and Ohmi, K.,** Serum lactate dehydrogenase isoenzyme pattern in neuroblastoma, *Eur. J. Pediatr.*, 123, 83, 1976.
17. **Tsuchida, Y.,** Markers in childhood solid tumors, in *Pediatric Surgical Oncology,* Hays, D., Ed., Grune & Stratton, New York, 1985.
18. **Zeltzer, P. M.,** The immune system and neoplasia, in *Manual of Allergy and Immunology,* Lawlor, G. and Fischer, T., Eds., Little, Brown, Boston, 1987.
19. **Frens, D. B., Bray, P. F., Wu, J. T., et al.,** The carcinoembryonic antigen assay: prognostic value in neural crest tumors, *J. Pediatr.*, 88, 591, 1976.
20. **Helson, L., Ghavimi, F., Wu, C. J., Fleisher, M., and Schwartz, M. K.,** Carcinoembryonic antigen in children with neuroblastoma, *J. Nat. Cancer Inst.*, 57, 725, 1976.
21. **Helson, L., Nisselbaum, J., Helson, C., Majeranowsk, A., and Johnson, G. A.,** Biological markers in neuroblastoma and other pediatric neoplasms, in *Human Cancer: Its Characterizations and Treatment,* Proc. 8th Int. Symp. Biological Characterization of Human Tumors, Vol. 5, Davis, W., Harrap, K. R., and Stathopoulos, G., Eds., Excerpta Medica, Princeton, 1980, 85.
22. **Osborn, M. and Weber, K.,** Tumor diagnosis by intermediate filament typing: a novel tool for surgical pathology, *Lab. Invest.*, 48, 372, 1983.
23. **Trojanowski, J. Q., Lee, V. M-Y., and Schlaepfer, W. W.,** An immunohistochemical study of human central and peripheral nervous system tumors, using monoclonal antibodies against neurofilaments and glial filaments, *Hum. Pathol.*, 15, 248, 1984.
24. **Seeger, R. C., Danon, Y. I., Rayner, S. A., and Hoover, F.,** Definition of a Thy-1 determinant on human neuroblastoma, glioma, sarcoma and teratoma cells with a monoclonal antibody, *J. Immunol.*, 128, 983, 1982.
25. **Kemshead, J. T., Ritter, M. A., Cotmore, S. F., and Greaves, M. F.,** Human Thy-1: expression on the cell surfaces of neuronal and glial cells, *Brain Res.*, 236, 451, 1982.
26. **Seeger, R. C., Reynolds, C. P., Vo, D. D., Ugeistad, J., and Wells, J.,** Depletion of neuroblastoma cells from bone marrow with monoclonal antibodies and magnetic immunobeads, *Prog. Clin. Biol. Res.*, 175, 443, 1985.
27. **Akeson, R. and Seeger, R. C.,** Interspecies neural membrane antigens on cultured human and murine neuroblastoma cells, *J. Immunol.*, 118, 1995, 1977.
28. **Casper, J. T., Borella, L., and Sen, L.,** Reactivity of human brain antiserum with neuroblastoma cells and non-reactivity with thymocytes and lymphoblasts, *Cancer Res.*, 37, 1750, 1977.
29. **Martin, S. E. and Martin, W. J.,** Expression by human neuroblastoma cells of an antigen recognized by naturally occurring mouse anti-brain autoantibody, *Cancer Res.*, 35, 2609, 1975.
30. **Brown, G. and Greaves, M. F.,** Expression of human T and B lymphocytic cell-surface markers on leukaemic cells, *Lancet,* 2, 753, 1974.
31. **Brown, G. and Greaves, M. F.,** Cell surface markers for human T and B lymphocytes, *Eur. J. Immunol.*, 4, 303, 1974.
32. **Greaves, M. F. and Brown, G.,** Letter: antigenic correlation between brain and thymus, *Lancet,* 1, 455, 1974.
33. **Takada, A., Takada, Y., Ito, U., and Minowada, J.,** Shared antigenic determinants between human brain and human T-cell line, *Clin. Exp. Immunol.*, 18, 491, 1974.
34. **Whiteside, T. L. and Rabin, B. S.,** Surface immunoglobulin on activated human peripheral blood thymus-derived cells, *J. Clin. Invest.*, 57, 762, 1976.
35. **Schachner, M., Wortham, K. A., Carter, L. D., and Chaffee, J. K.,** NS-4 (Nervous System antigen-4), a cell surface antigen of developing and adult mouse brain and sperm, *Dev. Biol.*, 44, 313, 1975.
36. **Danon, Y. L., Seeger, R. C., and Maidman, J. E.,** Fetal neural antigens on human neuroblastoma cells, *J. Immunol.*, 124, 2925, 1980.

37. **Seeger, R. C., Zeltzer, P. M., and Rayner, S. A.,** Onconeural antigen: a new neural differentiation antigen expressed by neuroblastoma, oat cell carcinoma, Wilms tumor, and sarcoma cells, *J. Immunol.*, 122, 1548, 1979.
38. **Irie, R. F., Irie, K., and Morton, D. L.,** A membrane antigen common to human cancer and fetal brain tissues, *Cancer Res.*, 36, 3510, 1976.
39. **Boss, B. D.,** An improved *in vitro* immunization procedure for the production of monoclonal antibodies against neural and other antigens, *Brain Res.*, 291, 193, 1984.
40. **Kung, P. C., Talle, M. A., DeMaria, M. E., Butler, M. S., Lifter, J., and Goldstein, G.,** Strategies for generating monoclonal antibodies defining human T-lymphocyte differentiation antigens, *Transplant Proc.*, 12(Suppl 1), 141, 1980.
41. **Reinherz, E. L., Kung, P. C., Goldstein, G., and Schlossman, S. F.,** A monoclonal antibody with selective reactivity with functionally mature human thymocytes and all peripheral human T cells, *J. Immunol.*, 123, 1312, 1979.
42. **Abramson, C. S., Kersey, J. H., and LeBien, T. W.,** A monoclonal antibody (BA-1) reactive with cells of human B lymphocyte lineage, *J. Immunol.*, 126, 83, 1981.
43. **Kersey, J. A., Lebien, T. W., Abramson, C. S., Newman, R., Sutherland, R., and Greaves, M.,** A human leukemia-associated and lymphohemopoietic progenitor cell surface structure identified with monoclonal antibody, *J. Exp. Med.*, 153, 726, 1981.
44. **LeBien, T. W., Boue, D. R., Bradley, J. G., and Kersey, J. H.,** Antibody affinity may influence antigenic modulation of the common acute lymphoblastic leukemia antigen *in vitro*, *J. Immunol.*, 129, 2287, 1982.
45. **Trowbridge, I. S. and Omary, M. B.,** Human cell surface glycoprotein related to cell proliferation is the receptor for transferring, *Proc. Natl. Acad. Sci. U.S.A.*, 78, 3039, 1981.
46. **Abo, T., Cooper, M. D., and Balch, C. M.,** Characterization of HNK-1 + (Leu-7) human lymphocytes, *J. Immunol.*, 129, 1752, 1982.
47. **Schneider, S. L., Sasaki, F., and Zeltzer, P. M.,** Normal and malignant neural cells: a comprehensive survey of human and murine system markers, *Crit. Rev. in Oncol. Hematol.*, 5, 199, 1986.
48. **Wasserstrom, W. R., Scheartz, M. K., Fleisher, M., and Posner, J. B.,** Cerebrospinal fluid biochemical markers in the central nervous system: a review. *Ann. Clin. Lab. Sci.*, 11, 239, 1981.
49. **Marton, L. J., Edwards, M. S., Levin, V. A., Lubich, W. P., and Wilson, C. B.,** Predictive value of cerebrospinal fluid polyamines in medeloblastomas, *Cancer Res.*, 39, 993, 1979.
50. **Marton, L. J., Edwards, M. S., Levin, V. A., Lubich, W. P., and Wilson, C. B.,** CSF Polyamines: a new and important means of monitoring patients with medulloblastoma, *Cancer*, 47, 757, 1981.
51. **Jones, T. R., Ruoslahti, E., Schold, S. C., and Bigner, D. D.,** Fibronectin and glial fibrillary acidic protein expression in normal human brain and anaplastic human gliomas, *Cancer Res.*, 42, 168, 1982.
52. **Eng, L. F. and Rubinstein, L. J.,** Contribution of immunohistochemistry to diagnostic problems of human cerebral tumors, *J. Histochem. Cytochem.*, 26, 513, 1978.
53. **Tascos, N. A., Parr, J., and Gonatas, N. K.,** Immunocytochemical study of the glial fibrillary acidic protein in human neoplasms of the central nervous system, *Hum. Pathol.*, 13, 454, 1982.
54. **Palmer, J. O., Kasselberg, A. G., and Netsky, M. G.,** Differentiation of medulloblastoma: studies including immunohistochemical localization of glial fibrillary acidic protein, *J. Neurosurg.*, 55, 161, 1981.
55. **DeArmond, S. J., Eng, L. F., and Rubinstein, L. J.,** The application of glial fibrillary acidic protein (GFA) immunohistochemistry in neurooncology, *Pathol. Res. Pract.*, 168, 374, 1980.
56. **Camins, M. B., Cravioto, H. M., Epstein, F., and Ransohoff, J.,** Medulloblastoma: an ultrastructural study — evidence for astrocytic and neuronal differentiation, *J. Neurosurg.*, 6, 374, 1980.
57. **Packer, R. J., Sulton, L. N., Rorke, L. B., Littman, P. A., Sposto, R., Rosenstock, J. G., Bruce, D. A., and Schut, L.,** Prognostic importance of cellular differentiation in medulloblastoma of childhood, *J. Neurosurg.*, 61, 296, 1984.
58. **Schold, C., Wasserstrom, W. R., Fleisher, M., Schwartz, M. K., and Posner, J. P.,** Cerebrospinal fluid biochemical markers of central nervous system disease, *Ann. Neurol.*, 8, 597, 1980.
59. **Hyvarinen, M., Zeltzer, P. M., Oh, W., and Stiehmm, E. R.,** Influence of gestational age on serum levels of alpha-1 fetoprotein, 1gG globulin, and albumen in newborn infants, *J. Pediatr.*, 82, 430, 1973.
60. **Tsuchida, T., Endo, Y., and Sato, S.,** Evaluation of alpha fetoprotein in early infancy, *J. Pediatr. Surg.*, 13, 155, 1978.
61. **Zeltzer, P. M.,** The immune system and neoplasia, in *Manual of Allergy and Immunology, Diagnosis, and Therapy*, Lawler, G. and Fischer, T., Eds., Little, Brown, Boston, 1987, 336.
62. **Waldmann, T. A. and McIntire, R. K.,** The use of radioimmunoassay for alphafetoprotein in the diagnosis of malignancy, *Cancer*, 34, 1510, 1974.
63. **Waldmann, T. A. and McIntire, R. K.,** The use of sensitive assays for alpha fetoprotein in monitoring the treatment of malignancy, in *Immunodiagnosis of Cancer, Part I*, Herberman, R. B. and McIntire, R. M., Eds., Immunology Series, N. Rose, Ed., Marcel Dekker, New York, 1979.

64. **Sundaresan, N., Vugrin, D., Nisselbaum, J., Galicich, J. H., Cvitkovic, E., and Schwartz, M. K.,** Cerebrospinal fluid markers in central nervous system metastases from testicular carcinoma, *J. Neurosurg.*, 4, 292, 1979.
65. **Allen, J. C., Nisselbaum, J., Epstein, F., Rosen, G., and Schwartz, M. K.,** Alpha fetoprotein and human chorionic gonagotrophin determination in cerebrospinal fluid, *J. Neurosurg.*, 51, 368, 1979.
66. **Tsuchida, T. and Saito, S.,** Pediatric malignant tumors, in *Tumor Markers,* Urushizaki, I. and Hattori, N., Eds., Igaku-shoin, Ltd., Tokyo, 1984, 242.
67. **Matsumoto, Y., Suzuki, T., Ono, H., Nakase, A., and Honso, I.,** Response of alpha-fetoprotein to chemotherapy in patients with hepatomas, *Cancer,* 34, 1602, 1974.
68. **Wise, K. S., Allerton, S. E., Trump, G., et al.,** A fetuin-like antigen from human nephroblastoma, *Int. J. Cancer,* 16, 199, 1975.
69. **Hirshaut, Y.,** Immunodiagnosis of human sarcomas, in *Immunodiagnosis of Cancer, Part II,* Herberman, R. B. and McIntire, K. R., Eds., Marcel Dekker, New York, 1979.

Chapter 5

GANGLIOSIDE G_{D2} SPECIFIC ANTIBODIES IN THE DIAGNOSIS AND THERAPY OF HUMAN NEUROBLASTOMA

Nai-Kong V. Cheung and Floro D. Miraldi

TABLE OF CONTENTS

I. INTRODUCTION

Neuroblastoma (NB), one of the more common solid tumors in the pediatric age group, accounts for 7—14% of all childhood malignancies.[1] It is a malignant neoplasm originating in the paraspinal sympathetic ganglia or adrenal medulla that metastasizes to lymph nodes, bone marrow, liver, and bones. Two thirds of children with neuroblastoma present with metastatic disease at the time of diagnosis. Although metastatic neuroblastoma is often responsive to chemotherapy initially, drug resistance usually develops within 12 months, and long-term survival in older children is rare.[2] Aggressive chemotherapy using high-dose cis-platinum, VM26 or VP16,[3,4] melphalan,[5] cyclophosphamide, or their combinations has added to the overall response rate of these patients. Ablative doses using these drug combinations in patients who achieved complete remissions, followed by autologous or allogeneic bone marrow transplantation have been encouraging.[6] Although many patients achieved complete remissions after aggressive chemotherapy, less than 40% of this favorable group are long-term survivors.[6]

II. DIAGNOSIS OF NEUROBLASTOMA *IN VITRO* USING G_{D2}-SPECIFIC ANTIBODIES

A. Detection of Microscopic Disease in Bone Marrow

Ganglioside G_{D2} is a glycolipid antigen present on most neuroblastomas tested.[7,8] It is a surface antigen estimated at 10 million molecules per cell. Except for the brain, this antigen is present only at low levels in restricted tissues of the normal body. We have described murine monoclonal antibodies (MAb) specific for this ganglioside,G_{D2}, that bind strongly to human NB irrespective of whether they are from established cell lines, fresh patient tumors, or tumors xenografted and passaged in athymic nude mice.[9] None of the non-NB bone marrow samples we tested reacted with these antibodies.[10] Using conventional fluorescent microscopy, as few as 0.01% tumor cells can be detected. The detection of metastatic NB by these MAb correlates with the results of *in vitro* clonogenic assays.[10] Histochemical staining using Wright-Giemsa and Hematoxylin-Eosin have thus far been unable to monitor microscopic disease quantitatively so as to be able to measure the impact of intensive chemotherapy. The detection of micrometastasis in the bone marrow will be a convenient method to evaluate the overall metastatic disease in the patient. Our antibodies to G_{D2} seem useful in detecting extremely low levels of metastatic disease in the bone marrow of patients with NB. They may allow a quantitative measure of the extent and the chemoresponse of microscopic disease. They may also be useful in identifying the time of minimal disease for optimal bone marrow transplantation as well as for adjuvant monoclonal antibody immunotherapy.

B. Use of Serum G_{D2} as a Tumor Marker

The ganglioside G_{D2} is present in the blood of patients with neuroblastoma.[11,12] Since this antigen is present only at low levels in normal people, it is a useful tumor marker for diagnosis and may be for prognosis of NB. Two tenths to 0.4 ml serum is used for extracting G_{D2} which is then assayed by an *ELISA* inhibition assay.[9,11] Normal volunteers have less than 13 ng/ml of serum G_{D2} while patients with stage IV neuroblastoma have elevated levels at the time of active disease (Figure 1). When these patients achieve remission, their serum G_{D2} becomes normal. Patients with ganglioneuroma and other malignancies usually have G_{D2} levels in the normal range. When the serum G_{D2} of individual patients was followed, the level correlated with the extent of the disease (Figure 2). An example is a 12-year-old patient diagnosed with Stage IV neuroblastoma involving bone and bone marrow. She was treated with combination chemotherapy (melphalan, cyclophosphamide, DTIC, and vin-

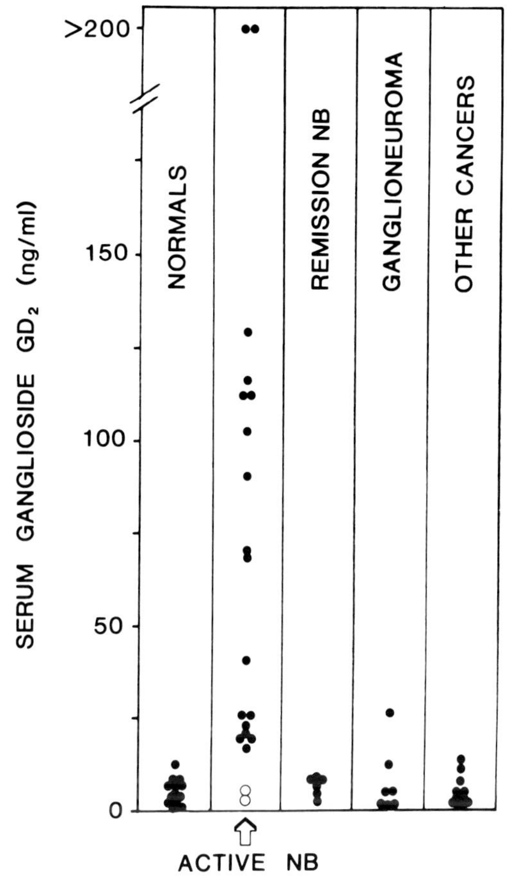

FIGURE 1. Serum ganglioside G_{D2} in normals and in patients with neuroblastoma with active disease and in remission, ganglioneuroma, and other malignancies. G_{D2} was extracted, assayed with an *ELISA* inhibition method, and expressed as ng/ml concentrations. NB, neuroblastoma.

cristine). Her clinical tumor response correlated with the decreasing levels of serum G_{D2} marker. She was restaged at 115 days after the beginning of therapy and showed small residual disease in bone, bone marrow, left adrenal, and neighboring lymph nodes. However, her serum G_{D2} and urine catecholamines were in the normal range. She received high dose melphalan and total body irradiation followed by allogeneic bone marrow transplantation from her matched brother. She continued to have residual bone and bone marrow disease post transplantation and was treated with the MAb 3F8 specific for the ganglioside G_{D2}. Her bone marrow and bone disease completely cleared posttreatment, and her serum G_{D2} remained normal. She is an example of a patient demonstrating the usefulness as well as the limitation of serum G_{D2} as a tumor marker for patients with neuroblastoma.

C. Differentiation of Neuroblastoma from other Small Round Cell Tumors of Childhood

The ganglioside G_{D2} is present on neuroblastoma but absent from lymphoblastic leukemias, myelogenous leukemias, and lymphomas.[9] By immunofluorescence as well as by immunoperoxidase staining of fresh tumor samples, it is found on the cell surface as well as the cytoplasm. Normal peripheral blood lymphocytes have no detectable G_{D2} by immunofluorescence. When activated with phytohemagglutinin *in vitro,* a small percent (<5%) of the lymphocytes becomes faintly surface positive. Among solid tumors, osteogenic sarcomas react strongly with these MAb while Wilms' tumor and Ewing's sarcomas do not.[9] Since

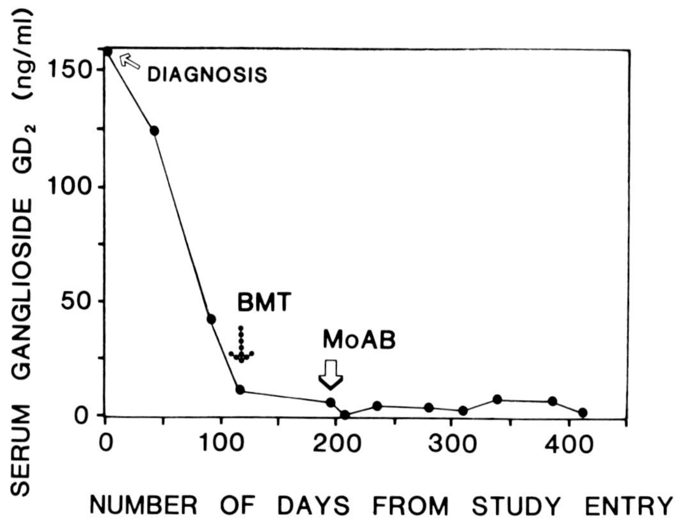

FIGURE 2. Serum ganglioside G_{D2} levels in a patient with stage IV neuroblastoma from the time of diagnosis. BMT indicates the time when this patient underwent supralethal therapy with allogeneic bone marrow transplantation. MAb indicates the time when she received the monoclonal antibody 3F8.

some rhabdomyosarcomas are also strongly positive, the utility of these MAb in differentiating NB from certain sarcomas may be limited.

III. DIAGNOSIS OF NEUROBLASTOMA *IN VIVO*

A. Nuclear Imaging with ^{131}I Labeled Antibody

The IgG_3 MAb 3F8 can be radiolabeled with ^{131}I using the chloramine T method with retention of immunoreactivity.[13] When injected into patients, this antibody localizes to human neuroblastoma with optimal tumor to nontumor ratios of 20:1.[14] It has advantages over other MAb because of absence of nonspecific uptake in the liver, spleen, or lymph nodes, and the high percentage injected dose per gram uptake into tumors.[13,14] It is able to detect NB in the primary sites (abdomen), as well as when metastatic to lymph node, bone marrow, bone (axial as well as appendicular), and liver. Figure 3 shows the antibody scans of a patient with active stage IV neuroblastoma 1 day after antibody injection. While patients with no metastatic disease showed only homogeneous organ distribution, this patient demonstrated focal uptakes at various sites in her skull, spine, pelvis, and extremities. Her left proximal femur was irradiated because of bone pain one week prior to the antibody study. This may explain the lack of metastatic disease at this site in the antibody scans (Figures 3D and 3F).

B. Dosimetry Calculations

Using known dosimetry standards, the tumor radiation dose can be estimated from serial imaging studies of patients with metastatic NB[13] and compared to doses delivered to normal organs. As shown in Table 1, an ablative tumor dose of 4000 rad can be delivered with less than 500 rad to normal tissues if 110 mCi of ^{131}I labeled antibody is infused. Even higher tissue doses may be possible if *in vivo* de-iodination can be decreased. Preliminary results with nude mice NB xenografts show that tumors can be ablated completely with ^{131}I labeled MAb 3F8.[15]

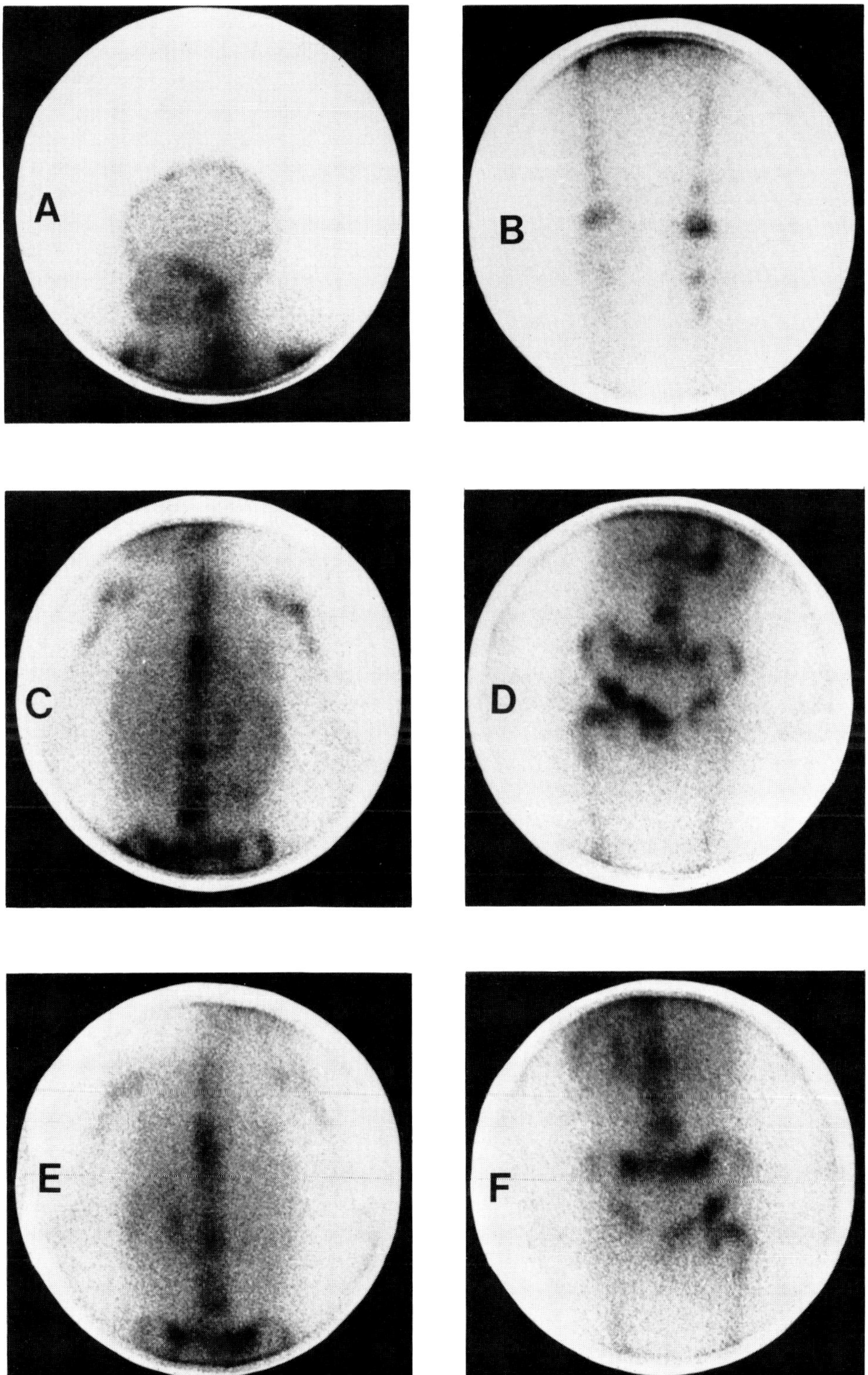

FIGURE 3. Multiple gamma images of a patient with state IV neuroblastoma 24 h after injection with 3 mCi of ^{131}I labeled monoclonal antibody 3F8. (A) Lateral skull; (B) femurs, knees, and tibias; (C) anterior chest; (D) anterior pelvis; (E) posterior chest (F) posterior pelvis. Focal uptakes of radioactivity identify sites of metastatic neuroblastoma in the cranium, humeri, scapula, spine, pelvis, femurs, and tibia.

Table 1
APPROXIMATE ^{131}I-3F8 CONCENTRATIONS AND RADIATION DOSE

Tissue	24 h after MAb injection percent administered ^{131}I-3F8 dose/g	Average ^{131}I radiation	
		Dose (rad/mCi)	Gy/MBq × 10^{-4}
Tumor	80×10^{-3}	36.6	100
Blood	21×10^{-3}	3.4—5.2	9.2—14.1
Brain	2.2×10^{-3}	0.6	1.6
Liver	7.5×10^{-3}	2.1	5.7
Lung	5.7×10^{-3}	1.5	4.1
Kidney	10.0×10^{-3}	3.3	8.9
Muscle	7.7×10^{-3}	2.0	5.4

Modified from Miraldi, F. D., Nelson, A. D., Kraly, C., et al., *Radiology,* 161, 413, 1986. With permission.

IV. ANTITUMOR EFFECTS MEDIATED BY MAb TO G_{D2} *IN VITRO*

A. Complement Mediated Cytotoxicity

Both the IgM and the IgG_3 MAb to G_{D2} activate human complement efficiently in tumor cytotoxicity.[20,25] Using the Hoechst stain method[20] to monitor the rare tumor cells, as many 10% tumor cells in the bone marrow can be eliminated without damaging normal marrow stem cells. Normal human cells are resistant to complement lysis because of the presence of decay-accelerating factor (DAF) on their cell surface.[16] However, neuroblastomas and many melanomas have low to absent expression of this protein and, therefore, are very sensitive to human complement. This sensitivity of human neuroblastoma cells to complement has important therapeutic implications. With the activation of human complement, anaphylatoxic and chemotactic properties of activated complement fragments can play an important role in the formation of local inflammatory response as well as the influx of important effector cells to tumor sites. Complement receptors for C3b and C3bi are present on granulocytes and natural killer cells. Since C3b and C3bi are deposited on tumor cells after MAb activation of human complement, they may enhance such cell mediated tumor cytotoxicity.

B. Antibody-Dependent Cell-Mediated Tumor Cytotoxicity (ADCC)

Human peripheral blood contains at least two effector cell populations that can mediate ADCC with the MAb 3F8, namely the granulocytes and the NK cells. They both possess the IgG FcRIII receptor recognized by the Leu 11 MAb[17]. Human NB is sensitive to ADCC, as well as NK and LAK cells (lymphokine activated killer cells). Interleukin-2 (IL-2) is a potent stimulator of ADCC/NK[18,19] as well as lymphokine activated killer (LAK). However, more lytic units of ADCC/NK than LAK can be generated with lower doses of IL-2. In addition, activated ADCC/NK can be maintained for at least 4 days with low doses of IL-2. Preclinical studies using nude mice xenografts suggest that G_{D2} bearing tumors can be effectively eradicated using such approaches.[19]

C. Purging of Autologous Marrow with MAb

The IgM antibodies to G_{D2} have been used in the purging of autologous marrows before cryopreservation.[20,26] Since the antigen G_{D2} is present in most of the NB cells, a single antibody 3G6 has been used. After one cycle of MAb and human complement, no detectable tumor cells are seen by immunofluorescence using antibodies of both G_{D2} and other NB

Table 2
CLINICAL FEATURES AND TUMOR RESPONSES IN NB PATIENTS TREATED WITH ^{131}I-3F8

Patient	Age (years)	Sex	Primary site	Prior therapy	Sites of disease	Response
1	3.5	M	Right adrenal	ADRIA/CPPD VCR/CPM XRT	BM, bone	Decreased NB in BM
2	9.5	M	Adrenal	DTIC/CPM/VCR XRT	BM, bone mediastinal mass	Decreased NB in BM, Decreased tumor mass with calcifications
3	3.5	M	Right Adrenal	L-PAM/VCR/CPM DTIC/CPPD ADRIA/NM/VR16	BM, bone, right Adrenal	Decreased NB in BM, normalized bone scan

Note: VCR, vincristine; CPM, cyclophosphamide; L-PAM, melphalan; CPPD, cis-platinum; ADRIA, adriamycin; NM, nitrogen mustard; BM, bone marrow.

specificities. The estimated $\log_{10}$ kill is at least three.[20] Preliminary results suggested that there was no significant difference between the number of days required for bone marrow engraftment for patients receiving purged vs. unpurged marrows after high dose ablative therapy.

V. ANTITUMOR EFFECTS *IN VIVO*

A. Immunotherapy with Unmodified MAb 3F8

In a phase I study, MAb 3F8 was given intravenously to 17 patients with metastatic, G_{D2} positive NB, or malignant melanoma.[21] Among the eight patients with metastatic stage IV neuroblastoma, two patients (5 years and 12 years old) achieved complete bone marrow and bone remission after antibody 3F8 treatment. They both received one single dose of 3F8 and did not receive further chemotherapy or other systemic treatments. Their duration of remission were 28 weeks and 63 weeks, respectively. Although the acute side effects were significant (pain, hypertension, and urticaria), none of the patients had long-term neurological side effects or noticeable pigmentary changes. Most MAb reported to date have been primarily useful for *in vitro* diagnosis. When given as the native antibody to patients, the majority did not demonstrate antitumor effects.[22] The ability to effect major tumor responses with a small dose of MAb is uncommon.[23-24] Some have suggested that the usefulness of MAb may be best realized in patients with minimal disease. All the patients in the phase I study had gross metastatic disease, many with disease in bone and bone marrow. Nevertheless, more than one-third of them experienced tumor regression. Given the reversibility of all the side effects during treatment, the antibody 3F8 is potentially useful in the selective eradication of microscopic metastatic disease in the hope of achieving longer survival.

B. Therapy with ^{131}I labeled MAb 3F8

Based on preclinical studies using NB xenografted nude mice and the dosimetry studies from NB tumor imaging in patients, a pilot study was carried out using ^{131}I labeled 3F8 in three patients with refractory stage IV NB and metastatic disease to the bone marrow. Their clinical features and tumor responses are summarized in Table 2. All three patients had failed prior combination chemotherapy with rapidly progressive disease in bone marrow, bone, and soft tissue sites (mediastinal nodes and adrenals). All three patients showed selective uptake of the ^{131}I-3F8 in areas of metastatic disease. Their heavy bone marrow involvement was evident on their antibody scans. Before treatment, their thyroids were protected with oral SSKI. Iodination was performed using chloramine T and the radiolabeled antibody purified through sephadex G-25 and Ag-1-X8 resin. Each patient received a single dose of 100 mCi ^{131}I-3F8 infused intravenously over 1 h. In contrast to the native MAb 3F8, none of the three patients experienced severe pain, hypertension, or urticaria, even though they all received more than 10 mg of ^{131}I-3F8 protein. All three patients tolerated the infusions without any other acute side effects. They were followed without further systemic therapy until they developed progressive disease.

The major toxicity was marrow hypoplasia. All three patients developed thrombocytopenia nadiring around 25 days after ^{131}I-3F8. All three required frequent platelet transfusions for about 3 to 4 weeks before recovery of platelet counts to above 50,000. Neutropenia (ANC or absolute neutrophil count $<1000/mm^3$) was also evident during the same period. The degree of neutropenia varied among the three patients (ANC nadirs of <100, 300, and 900/mm^3, respectively). All three required 55 to 70 days to recover their pretreatment ANC level. Absolute lymphocyte counts decreased rapidly within the first 6 days and then quickly recovered. None of the three patients had bleeding or infectious complications that required hospitalization.

All three patients had a subjective response with resolution of bone pain and achieving a general feeling of well being for at least 1 month after the antibody treatment. Patient #1 had initial bone marrow with 65% cellularity and 40% tumor involvement. Six days post treatment, the tumor count by immunofluorescence using MAb decreased by 40-fold. Both the aspirates and biopsies on day 6 and day 14 revealed only scant tumors. However, bone marrow was hypoplastic with fibrosis noted. One month after treatment, progression of NB was observed in the bone marrow. Two months after treatment, a new pelvic mass was discovered. In patient #2, bone marrow involvement by tumor decreased from 65% replacement to scattered foci 1 week and 5 weeks after treatment. At 1 week, these tumor foci showed necrosis with infiltration by neutrophils. At Week 5, 10% of marrow was noted to be fibrotic on biopsy. Small foci of ganglion-like cells and schwanoma tissues were found. Again, marrow hypoplasia was seen. His anterior mediastinal mass showed calcifications on follow up CT scans. Although the follow-up CT study at Week 1 showed tumor shrinkage, by Week 5 the tumor had regrown. The abnormal uptakes in his bone scan did not show any significant change. For Patient #3, 1 month after treatment, the bone marrow showed clearing with scattered tumor clumps and some ganglion-like cells suggestive of maturation. The previous abnormal uptakes in the ribs and spines on bone scan showed complete clearing, but the adrenal mass showed slight increase in size with two new nodes noted. In general, tumor responses in all three patients were observed after the ^{131}I-3F8 treatment. However, these responses tended to be short-lived.

VI. CONCLUSIONS

The ganglioside G_{D2} appears to be a useful target antigen for human NB. It may be a useful serum tumor marker and bone marrow tumor marker for metastatic disease. The *in vitro* immunological functions mediated by murine antibodies specific for G_{D2} may have many therapeutic applications. The preliminary Phase I study using the native MAb 3F8 has clearly demonstrated its antitumor effects. Further research into the use of these antibodies as an adjuvant for patients with early relapse or minimal disease is underway. The combined use of these antibodies and lymphokine activated effector cells will shed further light on the host mechanisms of tumor surveillance. Although preliminary, both the Phase I, as well as the *in vitro* bone marrow purging studies, demonstrate that antibodies to G_{D2} do not damage stem cells in bone marrow. The utility of these antibodies in an antibody cocktail for NB tumor removal from autologous marrow is obvious. Our *in vivo* imaging studies have clearly demonstrated the targeting potentials of the antibody 3F8 both in nude mice xenografts as well as in patients. The therapeutic studies using ^{131}I-3F8 are encouraging in nude mice xenograft experiments. However, in patients with widespread bone marrow disease, the toxicity to the bone marrow is severe. In addition, the tumor response has been of short duration. Further optimization in the use of ^{131}I-3F8 is needed before their general clinical application can be realized. Although most of our experience has been gathered in neuroblastomas, the reactivity of these G_{D2} specific MAb with other solid tumors, like osteogenic sarcoma,[27] brain tumors,[28,29] other sarcomas,[29] melanoma,[29,30] and small-cell carcinoma of the lung,[29,30] suggests their potential broader applications in the diagnosis and therapy of human malignancies.

ACKNOWLEDGMENTS

This work was supported in part by grants from the American Cancer Society (CDA85-7, RD-226), National Institutes of Health (CA-39320), and the Ireland Cancer Cener, Cleveland, Ohio. We want to thank Dr. P. F. Coccia, Dr. S. Strandjord, Dr. P. Warkentin, Dr. S. Susan, Dr. M. Gordon, Dr. B. Gordon, Dr. J. Stein, Ms. N. Albanese and nurses, and residents of Rainbow Babies and Childrens Hospital, Cleveland, Ohio for their excellent care of patients in these studies. We are grateful for the technical assistance of Ms. B. Landmeier, Mr. D. Donovan, Mr. W. Smith-Mensah, Ms. S. Ellery, Ms. C. Kraley, and Mr. B. Adams; dosimetry calculations by Dr. Dennis Nelson; the expert advice and collaborations with Dr. E. Medof in complement cytotoxicity studies.

REFERENCES

1. **Evans, A. E.,** Natural history of neuroblastoma, in *Advances in Neuroblastoma Research,* Raven, New York, 1980, 3.
2. **Rosen, E. M., Cassady, J. R., Frantz, C. N., Kretschmar, C., Levey, R., and Sallen, S. E.,** Neuroblastoma: the joint center for radiation therapy/Dana Farber Cancer Institute/Children's Hospital experience, *J. Clin. Oncol.,* 2, 719, 1984.
3. **Hayes, F. A., Green, A. A., Casper, J., Cornet, J., and Evans, W. E.,** Clinical evaluation of sequentially scheduled cisplatin and VM26 in neuroblastoma, *Cancer,* 48, 1715, 1981.
4. **Philip, T., Ghalie, R., Pinkerton, R., Zucker, J. M., Bernard, J. L., Leverger, G., and Hartmann, O.,** A phase II study of high dose cis-platinum and VP-16 in neuroblastoma, *J. Clin. Oncol.,* in press, 1986.
5. **Pritchard, J., McElwain, T. J., and Graham-Pole, J.,** High dose melphalan with autologous marrow for treatment of advanced neuroblastoma, *Br. J. Cancer,* 45, 86, 1982.
6. **Seeger, R. C., Lenarsky, C., Moss, T., Feig, S., Selch, M., Ramsey, N., Harris, R., Reynolds, P., Siegel, S., Sather, H., Hammond, D., and Wells, J.,** Bone marrow transplantation for poor prognosis neuroblastoma, Proc. American Society of Clinical Oncology, (abstr.), 1987.
7. **Wu, Z-L., Schwartz, E., Seeger, R., and Ladisch, S.,** Expression of G_{D2} ganglioside by untreated primary human neuroblastomas, *Cancer Res.,* 46, 440, 1986.
8. **Schengrund, C.-L., Repman, M. A., and Shochat, S.,** Ganglioside composition of human neuroblastomas: correlation with prognosis, a pediatric oncology group study, *Cancer,* 56, 2640, 1985.
9. **Cheung, NK. V., Saarinen, U. M., Neely, J. E., Landmeier, B., Donovan, D., and Coccia, P. F.,** Monoclonal antibodies to a glycolipid antigen on human neuroblastoma cells, *Cancer Res.,* 45, 2642, 1985.
10. **Cheung, NK. V., Von Hoff, D. D., Strandjord, S. E., and Coccia, P. F.,** Detection of neuroblastoma cells in bone marrow using G_{D2} specific monoclonal antibodies, *J. Clin. Oncol.,* 4, 363, 1986.
11. **Schultz, G., Cheresh, D. A., Varki, N. M., Yu, A., Staffileno, L. K., and Reisfeld, R. A.,** Detection of ganglioside G_{D2} in tumor tissues and sera of neuroblastoma patients, *Cancer Res.,* 44, 5914, 1984.
12. **Ladisch, S. and Wu, Z-L.,** Detection of a tumor-associated ganglioside in plasma of patients with neuroblastoma, *Lancet,* 1, 136, 1985.
13. **Miraldi, F. D., Nelson, A. D., Kraly, C., Ellery, S., Landmeier, B., Coccia, P. F., Strandjord, S. E., and Cheung, NK. V.,** Diagnostic imaging of human neuroblastoma with radiolabeled antibody, *Radiology,* 161, 413, 1986.

14. **Miraldi, F. D., Nelson, A. D., Ellery, S., Adams, R., Landmeier, B., Kallick, S., Kraly, C., Berger, N., and Cheung, NK. V.,** Imaging of malanoma, osteogenic sarcoma, and neuroblastoma using G_{D2} specific I-131 labeled monoclonal antibody, *J. Nucl., Med.*, 27, 881, 1986.
15. **Cheung, NK. V., Landmeier, B., Neely, J., Nelson, D., Abramowsky, C., Ellery, S., Adams, R. B., and Miraldi, F. D.,** Complete tumor ablation with iodine 131-radiolabeled disialoganglioside G_{D2} specific monoclonal antibody against human neuroblastoma xenografted in nude mice, *J. Natl. Cancer Inst.*, 77, 739, 1986.
16. **Cheung, NK. V., Walter, E., Smith-Mensah, H., Ratnoff, W., Tykocinski, M., and Medof, M. E.,** Decay accelerating factor (DAF) protects tumor cells from complement mediated cytotoxicity, *J. Clin. Invest.*, 81, 1122, 1988.
17. **Trinchieri, G. and Perussia, B.,** Biology of disease: human natural cells: biologic and pathologic aspects, *Lab. Invest.*, 50, 489, 1984.
18. **Munn, D. H. and Cheung, NK. V.,** Interleukin-2 (IL-2) enhances monoclonal antibody-mediated cellular cytotoxicity (ADCC) against human melanoma, *Cancer Res.*, 47, 6600, 1987.
19. **Honsik, C. J., Jung, G., and Reisfeld, R. A.,** Lymphokine-activated killer cells targeted by monoclonal antibodies to the disialogangliosides G_{D2} and G_{D3} specifically lyse human tumor cells of neuroectodermal origin, *Proc. Natl. Acad. Sci. U.S.A.*, 83, 7893, 1986.
20. **Saarinen, U. M., Coccia, P. F., Gerson, S. L., Pelley, R., and Cheung, NK. V.,** Eradication of neuroblastoma cells *in vitro* by monoclonal antibody and human complement: method for purging autologous bone marrow, *Cancer Res.*, 45, 5969, 1985.
21. **Cheung, NK. V., Lazarus, H., Miraldi, F., Abramowsky, C., Kallick, S., Saarinen, S., Spitzer, T., Strandjord, S., Coccia, P., and Berger, N.,** Ganglioside G_{D2} specific monoclonal antibody 3F8: a phase I study in patients with neuroblastoma and malignant melanoma, *J. Clin. Oncol.*, 5, 1430, 1987.
22. **Oldham, R. K., Foon, A., Morgan, C., Woodhouse, C. S., Schroff, R. W., Abrams, P. G., Fer, M., Schoenberger, C. S., Farrell, M., Kimball, E., and Sherwin, S. A.,** Monoclonal antibody therapy of malignant melanoma: *in vivo* localization in cutaneous metastasis after intravenous administration, *J. Clin. Oncol.*, 2, 1235, 1984.
23. **Houghton, A. N., Mintzer, D., Cordon-Cardo, C., Welt, S., Fliegel, B., Vadhan, S., Carswell, E., Melamed, M. R., Oettgen, H. F., and Old, L. J.,** Mouse monoclonal IgG_3 antibody detecting G_{D3} ganglioside: a phase I trial in patients with malignant melanoma, *Proc. Natl. Acad. Sci. U.S.A.*, 82, 1242, 1985.
24. **Meeker, T. C., Lowder, J., Maloney, D. G., Miller, R. A., Thielemans, K., Warnke, R., and Levy, R.,** A clinical trial of anti-idiotype therapy for B cell malignancy, *Blood,* 65, 1349, 1985.
25. **Mujoo, K., Cheresh, D., Yang, H. M., and Reisfeld, R.,** Disialoganglioside G_{D2} on human neuroblastoma cells: target antigen for monoclonal antibody-mediated cytolysis and suppression of tumor growth, *Cancer Res.*, 47, 1098, 1987.
26. **Stein, J., Strandjord, S., Saarinen, U., Warkentin, P., Gerson, S., Lazarus, H., Van Hoff, D., Coccia, P., and Cheung, NK. V.,** *In vitro* treatment of autologous bone marrow (BM) from neuroblastoma (NB) patients with anti-G_{D2} monoclonal antibody (MoAb) and human complement: a pilot study, in *Advances in Neuroblastoma Research,* Evans, A., D'Angio, G., and Seeger, R. C., Eds., Alan R. Liss, New York, 1987.
27. **Kallick, S., Miraldi, F., Neely, J., Makley, J., and Cheung, NK. V.,** Successful radiolocalization of human osteogenic sarcoma using iodine 131 labeled monoclonal antibody specific for the ganglioside G_{D2}, *Proc. Am. Assoc. Cancer Res.*, 27, 334, 1986.
28. **Zeltzer, P.,** personal communications.
29. **Cordon-Cardo, C.,** personal communications.
30. **Cheresh, D., Rosenberg, J., Mujoo, K., Hirschowitz, L., and Reisfeld, R.,** Disalogangliosiode G_{D2} on human melanoma serves as a relevant target antigen on small cell lung carcinoma for monoclonal antibody-mediated cytolysis, *Cancer Res.*, 46, 5112, 1986.

Chapter 6

THE DEVELOPMENT OF TARGETED RADIOTHERAPY FOR THE TREATMENT OF THE SMALL ROUND CELL TUMORS OF CHILDHOOD

L. S. Lashford

TABLE OF CONTENTS

I. INTRODUCTION

The concept of "targeting" radiotherapy extends a principle of chemotherapeutic practice to radiation oncology. By coupling a radionuclide to a carrier, the investigator attempts to exploit a physiological difference between tumor and normal tissue. Through a property of the vector, the aim is to selectively accumulate the radionuclide at a tumor site. Systemic administration of the conjugate offers potential for treatment of disseminated disease.

Two types of conjugates have excited interest in the small round cell tumors of childhood: the low molecular weight radiopharmaceutical meta-iodobenzylguanidine (mIBG), and radiolabeled monoclonal antibodies.

mIBG is a radioiodinated aralkylguanidine, which bears a structural relationship to the sympathetic ganglion blocker guanethidine. Like guanethidine, the compound actively accumulates in sympathetic nervous tissue.[1] The striking affinity of the compound for chromaffin storage granules has led to its use as a radiotracer for normal and abnormal sympathetic nervous tissue.[2,3] A number of neural crest tumors also accumulate mIBG and include pheochromocytoma, neuroblastoma, and carcinoid.

Monoclonal antibodies (MAb) are potentially useful in a wider setting. The relative ease of hybridoma technology has led to a plethora of antibodies being raised against a large number of tumors. Consequently, a variety of agents are available for investigation. The antibody 3F8,[4] an IgG_3 murine monoclonal raised against the disialoganglioside G_{D2}, and UJ13A, an IgG_{2a} murine monoclonal raised against 16-week human fetal brain, have both been investigated in neuroblastoma. The antibody UJ13A has been chosen to represent the problems of radiation targeting with MAb and reflects the experience of the author.

II. THE MONOCLONAL ANTIBODY UJ13A — RATIONALE FOR USE

A. The Conjugate

As with all biologically active proteins, care is required in the storage and handling of UJ13A. Purified antibody is kept at a constant temperature of −20°C in phosphate buffered saline. Loss of immunoreactivity may occur as a result of temperature fluctuation and prolonged storage.

Radiolabeling with ^{131}I by a modified chloramine T method produces a conjugate that is stable *in vitro* for several days. A high specific activity of radiolabeling diminishes the biological activity of the compound, but satisfactory levels of immunoreactivity may be achieved at a specific activity of 5 μCi/μg of protein.

B. Antigen Expression

The antigen recognized by UJ13A is widely expressed on neuroblastoma tissue, both at primary and metastatic sites. Greater than 90% of tumors express the antigen at diagnosis, and there is little evidence to support a changing antigenic profile at relapse (J. T. Kemshead, personal communication).

Examination of multiple sections of human tissues by indirect immunofluorescence has demonstrated that the UJ13A antigen expression is confined to tissues of neuroectodermal origin.[5] The major site of expression is the central nervous system. Fortunately, the antibody is excluded from this site following intravenous injection, by an intact blood brain barrier.[6]

C. Uptake of UJ13A into Tumor Xenografts

The uptake of ^{131}I/UJ13A has been investigated in the nude mouse model.[7] Mice bearing xenografts of the human neuroblastoma cell line TR14 have received approximately 1 μg of radiolabeled UJ13A. Tumors have been resected, and antibody uptake into the xenograft calculated. It has been possible to demonstrate that a mean of 6% of the injected dose per gram of tumor is present in the xenografts at 24 h. The half life of the conjugate in the tumor lies between 2 and 4 days.

Using the dual label technique is Pressman and Day, it has been possible to show that the uptake of UJ13A is specific. Nude mice bearing tumor xenografts were simultaneously injected with equal amounts of ^{131}I radiolabeled UJ13A and ^{125}I radiolabeled FD_{44}. FD_{44} is a murine monoclonal of the same isotype as UJ13A, but does not bind to any antigen expressed in mice or human neuroblastoma. The concentration of radiolabeled UJ13A in the xenograft reached a median of seven times that of FD_{44}.

These experiments have been extended to show that tumor ablation may be achieved by increasing the amount of ^{131}I/UJ13A. Intravenous administration of 150μCi of conjugate (specific activity 15 μCi/μg protein) produced regression of neuroblastoma xenografts in the nude mice. Over a period of 21 days, tumors of approximately 1 cm^3 regressed to 10% of their original volume. Repeated injection caused tumors to apparently disappear, but regrowth at the original site always occurred. At relapse, xenografts continued to express the UJ13A antigen.

The experimental system was controlled and developed to demonstrate that tumor ablation had been produced by a specific targeting effect of the antibody. First, neither a ten-fold excess of unlabeled antibody or isotope alone could induce tumor regression. Second, the therapeutic effect of ^{131}I/UJ13A was blocked by administering a 50-fold excess of unlabeled UJ13A 24 h before. Third, only ^{131}I labeled antibody produced tumor regression. Neither ^{125}I or ^{123}I labeled conjugate produced the same effect. This suggests that it is the B emissions of the isotope that produces the therapeutic effect.

These studies in the nude mouse model provide encouraging data for the continuing investigation of the ^{131}I/UJ13A as a therapeutic conjugate. However, the model system is limited in several areas.[8] First, the antibody is itself murine derived, and as such does not induce the same immunological response it would in a second species. Second, no murine tissues, including those neuroectodermally derived, express the UJ13A antigen. Third, the artificially produced xenograft growing on the flank of mouse may have very special characteristics facilitating access of antibody into tumor. In particular, the blood supply to the tumor is murine derived.

To understand whether there is a clinical potential for the conjugate, it is necessary to examine the behavior of the monoclonal antibody in patients.

III. PATIENT STUDIES

A. Biodistribution of UJ13A in Children with Neuroblastoma

In a study established at the Hospital for Sick Children, London, a total of 14 children with neuroblastoma received tracer amounts of ^{131}I/UJ13A (Dose 10 μg/kg s.a. 15 μCi/μg protein). The detailed biodistribution of the compound was studied, using a combination of the gamma camera and venepunture. In seven patients it was possible to study the early biodistribution of the conjugate by imaging the thorax and abdomen in 30 × 1 min sequential scans. In all patients a minimum of three further sequential static scans were performed over a period of 6 days from injection. These data gave information on both organ uptake of isotope and organ half-life, from which radiation dose estimates could be obtained. Blood sampling was undertaken sequentially from 30 min to 48 h.

All children were imaged in the context of other staging procedures for their disease, and as such received a combination of Tc^{99} MDP bone scans, TC^{99} "Nanocoll" colloidal bone marrow scans, abdominal ultrasound, CXR, skeletal survey, and CAT scan. Interpretation of true positive sites took place against this background.

Following intravenous injection of antibody, the conjugate clears relatively slowly from the vascular compartment. The decline in blood activity follows typical biexponential clearance kinetics. The major influence on the first clearance component are factors influencing distribution of the antibody. The rate of fall of activity during this phase is principally influenced by factors which increase reticuloendothelial uptake. These include the degree of protein aggregation of the injected product, the level of circulating antimouse immunoglobulin, and the presence of circulating tumor shed antigen. In this series, the quality of the injected product was rigidly controlled (less than 3% aggregated protein on all occasions) and this was the first exposure of the children to murine protein. The mean biological half life of the conjugate during this first phase was estimated at 1.2 h.

The second clearance phase is largely influenced by metabolism of the conjugate, and appears to be significantly faster in children than in adults. In nine adults with brain tumors, the second phase had a mean half-life of 53 h compared with 29 h in children with neuroblastoma. It is not known whether this reflects an intrinsic difference in metabolic rate between adults and children, or reflects the different tumor system. However, age specific differences in rates of immunoglobulin clearance have been previously documented.[9]

The rate of clearance of the conjugate from blood has two important aspects. The radiation dose delivery to bone marrow is dependent on the vascular clearance of antibody. In this series, dose delivery from blood to marrow was estimated at 0.6 rad/mCi of infused conjugate. This figure assumes no specific uptake of ^{131}I/UJ13A by the marrow, and will clearly depend upon the degree of marrow infiltration by tumor. Consequently, in relapsed metastatic neuroblastoma, it may be assumed that marrow dosage will be in excess of this figure.

The major organs involved in vascular clearance and metabolism of the antibody are liver and spleen. In the scintigraphic studies, isotope was demonstrated to accumulate in these tissues. As neither organ expresses the UJ13A antigen, this represents the nonspecific mechanisms for protein clearance. The magnitude of the uptake influences bioavailability of antibody for radiation targeting, and radiation dose to the organ.

For a first exposure to a tracer amount of ^{131}I/UJ13A, the estimated liver and splenic uptake varies between 2 to 20% for liver and 0.2 to 7.7% for spleen. Using the mIRD formalism, radiation dosage to these organs was estimated as between 0.8 to 6.8 rad/mCi for liver, and 1.2 to 17.9 rad/mCi for spleen.

In a small number of children undergoing multiple scanning studies, it has been apparent that a change in biodistribution occurs on second exposure to antibody. This phenomenon has been studied in detail in a study of the biodistribution of ^{123}I/UJ13A in nonhuman primates.

B. Repeat Administration of UJ13A; Immunoglobulin and Fragments

A colony of 12 marmosets was established to systematically investigate the effect of repeated administration of UJ13A immunoglobulin (Ig) on the biodistribution of antibody. Several workers in the field have established that changing kinetics may be attributable to the development of anti-mouse immunoglobulin in the host.[10,11] Whether the anti-mouse Ig response is directed against the Fc component or idiotype of the antibody may be a characteristic of the individual antibody. To investigate this aspect of the relationship between immunogenicity and biodistribution, Fab_2 and Fab fragments of UJ13A were prepared.

Administration of whole antibody into marmosets on four separate occasions 4 to 6 weeks apart, produced a progressive increase in the rate of clearance of isotope from blood. This was true for both aspects of the biexponential clearance curve. However, the most profound change occurred in the first clearance component. A dynamic acquisition series taken over the first 15 min from injection demonstrated that liver was a major site of isotope uptake. A sequential rise in hepatic uptake occurred at each administration. The change in pharmacokinetics correlated with a rise in circulating anti-mouse Ig.

The biodistribution of fragments vary from that observed for whole Ig. In particular, renal mechanisms play an additional part in their clearance and metabolism. Repeat administration of fragments did not induce any change in pharmacokinetics, despite a small but variable rise in anti-mouse immunoglobulin. Consequently, it does seem possible to maintain a stable biodistribution of UJ13A on repeat exposure by the use of fragments, and suggests that the anti-mouse activity generated is not anti-idiotype.

C. Toxicity of High Dose ^{131}I/UJ13A *in Vivo*

To date, the administration of potentially therapeutic doses of UJ13A has been undertaken in six children with chemoresistant neuroblastoma.[12] In an attempt to establish toxicity, doses of between 35 to 55 mCi of ^{131}I radiolabeled conjugate have been administered over a period of 45 min. The administration of the conjugate has been well tolerated. Acute toxicity has been restricted to relatively minor symptoms of nausea and pyrexia. However, in one patient, an acute anaphylactic reaction occurred. This patient had an atopic history and had had a previous allergic response to VM26. The anticipated change in pharmacokinetics occurred, with a rapid elimination of conjugate and rise in anti-mouse Ig titer.

Major toxicity was confined to bone marrow aplasia. In two patients receiving 50 mCi of ^{131}I/UJ13A, a transient depression in lymphocytes or platelets was observed. Neither cytopenia was sufficient to require supportive therapy. Both patients receiving 55 mCi developed a profound marrow aplasia. In the first patient, this was irreversible and persisted until the patient died with progressive disease at 6 weeks. The second patient to receive 55 mCi also developed a pancytopenia which spontaneously reversed. No further escalation in dosage has been undertaken beyond this level. However, the availability of purged autologous marrow for transplantation renders continued dose escalation a possibility.

D. Tumor Uptake in Patients

Initial observations on the scintigraphy of neuroblastoma using ^{131}I/UJ13A suggested that greater than 70% of primary and metastatic sites accumulate UJ13A. In a larger series conducted over a 3-year period, this result has not been maintained, with only 45% of tumor sites taking up conjugate.[13]

Estimates of radiation dose delivery to tumor using scintigraphic techniques are notoriously inaccurate. The calculation suffers from errors caused in assessment of the volume of viable tumor, the choice of region interest and background subtraction, variations in the geometry and homogeneity of tracer uptake, and assumptions concerning decay kinetics. For a small series of tumors, it has been possible to make some estimate of radiation dose delivery. In a series of tumor sites, radiation dose delivery was assessed with a mean value of 37 rad/mCi within a range of 21 to 88. Even allowing for the uncertainty of the accuracy of these measurements, it seems likely that sufficient isotope may be delivered to some tumors to effect therapy. This has been observed in one out of the six patients entering the Phase I toxicity study.

The patient remained with two active bony deposits of neuroblastoma, and a bone marrow infiltrate despite intensive chemotherapy. 55 mCi of ^{131}I/UJ13A was administered with clear scintigraphic evidence of tumor localization. Radiological and biopsy evidence of bony healing was obtained in addition to clearance of marrow disease. This response was maintained for a period of 8 months.

This encouraging result makes it important to understand why 55% of tumors fail to accumulate isotope. All patients failing to image active disease expressed the UJ13A antigen either in tumor metastatic to bone marrow, or at the primary site. Although this does not exclude the possibility that antigenic heterogeneity explains the result, it strongly suggests that additional factors are important. These are yet to be defined, but will probably reflect a combination of factors influencing bioavailability of antibody at tumor sites and the preservation of immunoreactivity of the conjugate. To date, the best figures from tissue resection studies, in a variety of antibody tumor systems, suggests that only 10^{-3}% of

Table 1
PATIENTS STUDIED

No.	Age	Tumor	Antibody used in diagnostic study		Antibody used in therapy
1	62	Pineoblastoma	UJ181.4	(ICRF)	UJ181.4
			HMFG2	(ICRF)	
2	54	Cerebral lymphoma	F8.111	(J. Faber)	F8.111
			HMFG2		
3	3	Spinal teratoma	—		UJ181.4
4	30	ICL neuroblastoma	UJ181.4		UJ181.4
			HMFG2		
5	32	Melanoma	Mel 14	(J. P. Mach)	Mel 14
			4C6	(D. Bigner)	
6	16	Ependymoma	FD32	(ICRF)	No
			UJ181.4		

injected dose per gram of tissue is retained in tumor.[14] This is insufficient conjugate to deliver effective radiotherapy from ^{131}-I at a bulky tumor deposit. Consequently, at the current level of technological development of MAb/isotope conjugates, the best chance for effective radiation delivery is in the treatment of small volume or minimal residual disease, or in the special situation where tumor is confined to an accessible body cavity. This latter approach is illustrated by the application of ^{131}I MAb to the treatment of leptomeningeal tumor.

E. Experience with Intrathecally Administered Antibody

Direct instillation of the radiolabeled antibody into a tumor lined cavity maximizes the opportunity for tumor targeting. The volume of distribution of the conjugate is reduced, as is the effect of reticuloendothelial uptake. Moreover, the influence of vascular barriers in tumors are minimized.

A study has been established to study the biodistribution and toxicity of this approach to therapy using ^{131}I MAb.[15] As a variety of tumors are amenable to this mode of therapy, a heterogenous group of neoplasms have been included in the study. Consequently, the choice of MAb reflects the antigenic expression of the tumor type (Table 1). Patients eligible for the study demonstrate persistent or relapsed tumor despite maximal conventional therapy. A suitable MAb for radiation targeting is chosen and has been defined as one which is immunoreactive with the patients tumor, but not with normal CNS constituents. In addition, the isotype should be such that it is not capable of complement mediated cytolysis.

To date, seven patients have been enrolled in the study. Information on the biodistribution of intrathecally administered antibody and the specificity of the approach has been sought in a dual label study. Each patient has received tracer amounts of ^{131}I radiolabeled tumor specific antibody and ^{125}I radiolabeled nonspecific antibody. The kinetics of both have been followed by direct CSF, blood, and urine sampling. Although the rate of clearance of radiolabled conjugate is variable from patient to patient, there has been good evidence of the selective retention of the ^{131}I tumor specific antibody. The retained ^{131}I "relevant antibody" is not accounted for by preferential liver or splenic uptake and appears to have delayed excretion into the vascular compartment. Examination of CSF indicates that the antibody is not free within the CSF and so implies that it is bound. Scintigraphy has shown accumulation of ^{131}I MAb at known tumor sites (Figure 1). Supportive evidence that this approach represents specific targeting was provided in one patient with free-floating malignant cells (pineoblastoma) within the CSF. Examination of cell pellets following injection of tracer amounts of relevant and irrelevant antibody showed a progressive rise in the ration of relevant:irrelevant antibody associated with tumor. This reached a maximum of 10:1 at 3 days.

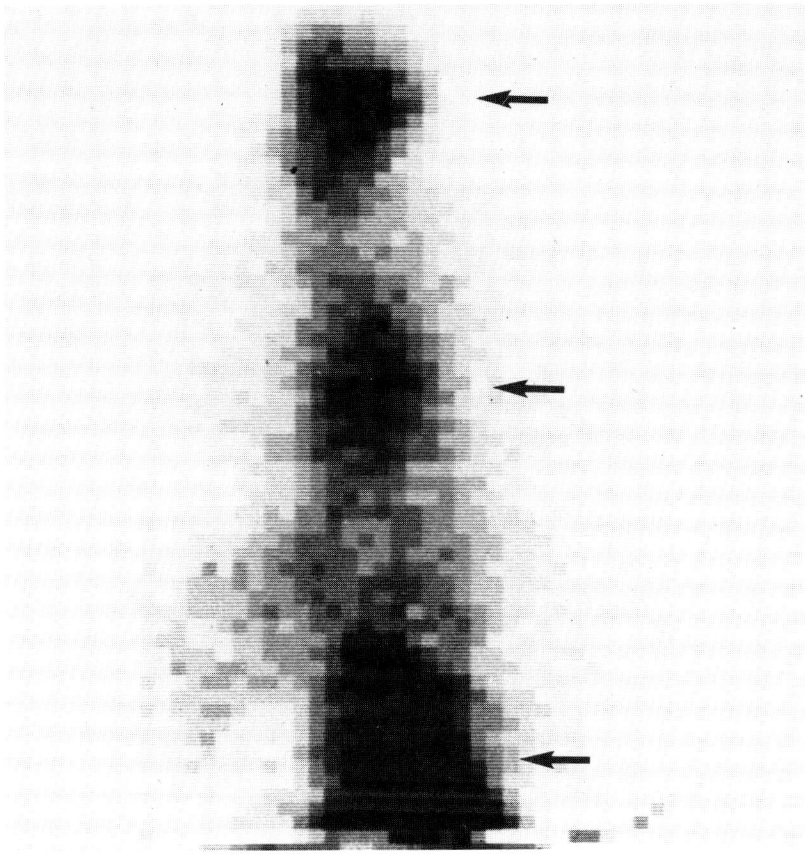

FIGURE 1. Scintigram of thoraco-lumbar spine 7 days after injection of ^{131}I/UJ181.4. This patient had active medulloblastoma disseminated throughout the spinal column. Arrows indicate known areas of tumor.

Six of seven patients who have been enrolled within the study were considered suitable for high-dose ^{131}I MAb. The administered dose has steadily increased from 12.5 mCi in a child aged 3 years to 45 mCi in an adult patient. Evidence of tumor localization has been demonstrated by scintigraphy in four of the patients following intrathecal therapy, and tumor half lives of between 79 to 310 h observed. In three of these four patients, a complete response has been documented (defined as clearance of all measurable disease) and in the fourth, a partial response (defined as greater than 50% disease clearance). In the remaining two patients in whom tumor localization was not observed, no therapeutic effect has been gained (Table 2).

This study is important because it gives the clearest evidence yet that effective targeted radiotherapy can be achieved when conditions are optimal.

IV. mIBG — AN ALTERNATIVE AGENT FOR DELIVERING RADIOTHERAPY IN NEUROBLASTOMA

A. Tumor Uptake of mIBG

The systematic study of mIBG as a targeting agent has been hampered by a lack of suitable models. Only one human neuroblastoma cell line, SK-N-SH, has demonstrated the ability to accumulate mIBG *in vitro*. To date it has been possible to demonstrate that mIBG uptake in SK-N-SH occurs by an energy-dependent mechanism that is inhibited by cocaine and the tricyclic antidepressants. Animal data looking at the distribution of mIBG within the adrenals

Table 2
ANTIBODY-GUIDED IRRADIATION: RADIATION DOSES AND RESULTS

Case	Diagnosis	Antibody	Radio nuclide	Dose mCi	Site effects[a]	Results
1	Pineoblastoma	UJ181.4	^{131}I	24	Minimal[a]	Complete remission for 22 months; died at 24 months
2	Lymphoma	F8-11-13	^{131}I	43	Minimal	Complete remission with neurological improvement; died at 12 months of systemic disease
3	Teratoma	UJ181.4	^{131}I	11	Minimal	Died at 6 weeks
4	ICL Neuroblastoma	UJ181.4	^{131}I	45	Minimal	Complete remission with clinical improvement, sustained for 9 months
5	Melanoma	Mel-14	^{131}I	38	Minimal	Partial remission with clinical improvement; followed to 6 months

[a] mild meningism or perineal paresthesia.

have shown that mIBG is associated with the chromaffin granule of the dog adrenal medulla.[2] By implication, it would appear that both an amine pump and chromaffin storage granules are required for the successful accumulation of mIBG. As tumors may be expected to demonstrate heterogeneity for these characteristics, it is reasonable to speculate that a variation in the tumor uptake of mIBG may be found.

Evidence from the scintigraphy of neuroblastoma *in vivo* indicates that in excess of 90% of neuroblastoma deposits accumulate the compound at presentation of the disease. Unfortunately, this characteristic does appear to be modified by chemotherapy as the proportion of tumor sites accumulating mIBG falls at the end of chemotherapy.[17]

A second feature reported from the Amsterdam clinical experience, is a diminishing uptake of mIBG at tumor sites at repeated administration of high-dose mIBG.[17] Whether this reflects selective tissue destruction or other factors remains to be established. Unfortunately, this aspect cannot be investigated in the animal model as SK-N-SH xenografts poorly.

B. Behavior of the Conjugate *in Vivo*

A detailed biodistribution study has been undertaken at the Royal Marsden Hospital and the Hospital for Sick Children, London, in 17 children with stage III/IV neuroblastoma.[16] The major features are a very rapid initial clearance of the vascular compartment. At 60 min a mean of only 4.4% of the injected dose remains in blood. This loss is not explained by renal loss or liver uptake of isotope which accounts for 10% and between 0.5 to 13%, respectively.

These results have been confirmed in a direct tissue resection study on 12 nonhuman primates (marmosets). The data strongly suggest that loss is to a "second space". The radiation dose calculated from the patient series estimated whole body dose from ^{131} I mIBG as of the order of 1.3 rad/mCi (Range 0.9 to 1.8 rad/mCi) and a liver dose of 5.3 rad/mCi (Range 1 to 16 rad/mCi).

These estimates are substantially higher than those derived from tracer work in adults. Moreover, a large variation in dose estimates to liver was observed between patients. Both the magnitude of dose delivery to liver, and its variability, were greater than that observed for patients receiving ^{131}I MAb. Possible explanations of these unexpected observations are measurement errors, or they may reflect a genuine physiological difference in this group of patients. For example, as all children had undergone nephrotoxic chemotherapy, a variation in renal function might result in a shift to hepatic metabolism of the compound.

Clearly the issues are complex. To investigate the problem in the uncompromised host, a comparative study of mIBG and UJ13A has been undertaken in marmosets. Preliminary data suggest that on a mCi/mCi basis, whole body dose is 3.5 times as great from antibody as from mIBG. The indication is that liver dosage is also substantially increased from UJ13A. These data suggest that a systematic study of factors influencing liver uptake should be undertaken.

C. Clinical Experience with High Dose ^{131}I mIBG

A number of centers, notably Amsterdam, Frankfurt, Villejuif, Heidelberg, and Tubingen have gained experience with high-dose mIBG. All have tended to explore the therapeutic effect of the compound in relapsed or chemoresistant disease. Considerable variation in the scheduling and dosage of the compound has been attempted, and so it is difficult to make comparisons between centers.

One approach from Frankfurt is to attempt to standardize for individual differences in metabolizing and clearing the conjugate.[17] With the aim of delivering a whole body of 100 rad and to limit liver dose to 400 rad, the clearance of an initial infusion of mIBG is measured and then "topped" up with a second dose of ^{131}I/mIBG within a few days. Estimated tumor dose delivery in 14 patients has varied between 400 to 26,000 rad. Clinical response in this group of poor risk patients has been two complete responses, five partial responses, and seven nonresponders.

Another large series of 18 patients from Amsterdam, have received a total of 62 doses of between 27 to 200 mCi of ^{131}I/mIBG.[18] The results have been an initial complete response in two patients, sustained for 3 and 9 months and three partial responses (defined as greater than a 50% reduction in tumor volume). Significant marrow toxicity (either as isolated thrombocytopenia and pancytopenia) was seen in 11 patients, and in patients who had previously undergone a unilateral adrenalectomy, adrenal insufficiency was documented.

Troublesome isolated thrombocytopenia or pancytopenia has been the experience of many groups. It remains to be established whether this is largely the result of excess marrow dose due to tumor infiltrates or from other factors.

The few responses documented, although not sustained, are encouraging evidence for the use of mIBG as a targeting agent in neuroblastoma. The compound has several advantages over MAb. First, it is a biologically more robust molecule provided the instructions of the manufacturer are followed. The high specific activity of mIBG does undergo degradation following radiolabeling, but this is retarded by storing the conjugate frozen until use. Antibodies are susceptible to degradation and loss of immunological activity during the process of radiolabeling.

The clinical data appear to support the pilot study in primates in that a larger dose of mIBG can be administered before marrow toxicity supervenes. This probably reflects differences both in whole body dosage and in the variation in rates of loss of isotope from the vascular compartment. Whether the rapid extravascular loss of mIBG will prove to facilitate tumor uptake remains to be established.

V. CONCLUSION

The early clinical trials are sufficiently encouraging to suggest that targeted therapy in neuroblastoma using mIBG is within reach. Further work on the MAb is required to define whether this can be an equally useful approach in neuroblastoma. However, it should be emphasized that considerable potential for manipulation of monoclonals exist, including site specific labeling, alternative radionuclides, the use of fragments, and the prospect of human and other murine monoclonals. At our current level of technology, MAb looks encouraging in the treatment of diffuse disease, in a closed compartment. It is likely that the combination of modified antibody and an appropriate clinical scenario may make targeted radiotherapy in a variety of tumor systems feasible.

REFERENCES

1. **Buch, J., Bruchett, G., and Girgert, R.,** Specific uptake of 123-I meta-iodobenzylguanidine in the neuroblastoma cell line SK-N-SH, *Cancer Res.*, 45, 6366, 1985.
2. **Wieland, D., Wu, J., Brown, L., Manger, T., Swanson, D., and Bierwaltes, W.,** Radiolabelled adrenergic neuro blocking agents: adrenomedullary imaging with (131)-iodobenzylguanidine, *J. Nucl. Med.*, 21, 349, 1980.
3. **Shapiro, B., Copp, J., Sisson, J., Eyre, P., Wallis, J., and Bierwaltes, W.,** Iodine-131 meta-iodobenzylguanidine for the locating of suspected phaeochromocytoma: experience in 400 cases, *J. Nucl. Med.*, 26, 576, 1985.
4. **Cheung, N., Landmeier, B., Neely, J., Nelson, D., Abramowsky, C., Ellery, S., Adams, R., and Miraldi, F.,** Complete tumour ablation with 131-I radiolabelled disialoganglioside GD2 — specific monoclonal antibody against human neuroblastoma xenografted in nude mice, *J. Natl. Cancer Inst.*, 77(3), 739, 1986.
5. **Allan, P., Garson, J., Harper, E., Asser, U., Coakham, H., Brownell, B., and Kemshead, J.,** Biological characterisation and clinical application of a monoclonal antibody recognising an antigen restricted to neuroectodermal tissues, *Int. J. Cancer,* 31, 591, 1983.
6. **Goldman, A., Vivian, G., Gordon, I., Pritchard, J., and Kemshead, J.,** Immunolocalisation of neuroblastoma using radiolabelled monoclonal antibody UJ13A, *J. Paediatr.*, 105, 252, 1984.
7. **Jones, D., Goldman, A., Gordon, I., Pritchard, J., Gregory, B., and Kemshead, J.,** Therapeutic application of a radiolabelled monoclonal antibody in nude mice xenografted with human neuroblastoma: tumouricidal effects and distribution studies, *Int. J. Cancer,* 35, 715, 1986.
8. **Jones, D., Lashford, L., Dicks-Mireaux, C., and Kemshead, J.,** Comparison of pharmacokinetics of radiolabelled monoclonal antibody UJ13A in patients and animal models, *Natl. Cancer Inst. Monog.*, 3, 125, 1987.
9. **Dixon, F., Talmage, D., Maurer, D., and Deizchmiller, M.,** The half-life of homologous gamma globulin in several species. *J. Exp. Med.*, 96, 313, 1952.
10. **Dillman, R., Shawler, D., Dillman, J., Clutter, M., Wormsley, S., Markman, M., and Frisman, D.,** Monoclonal antibody therapy of cutaneous T cell lymphoma (CTCL), *Blood,* 62, 212, 1983.
11. **Schroff, R., Foon, K., Beatty, S., Oldham, R., and Morgan, R.,** Human anti-murine immunoglobulin responses in patients receiving monoclonal antibody therapy, *Cancer Res.*, 45, 879, 1985.
12. **Lashford, L., Jones, D., Pritchard, J., Gordon, I., Breatnach, F., and Kemshead, J.,** Therapeutic application of radiolabelled monoclonal antibody UJ13A in children with disseminated neuroblastoma, *Natl. Cancer Inst.* Monog., 3, 53, 1987.
13. **Lashford, L., Jones, D., Evans, K., Gordon, I., Pritchard, J., and Kemshead, J.,** The biodistribution of the monoclonal antibody UJ13A in children with neuroblastoma — implications for targeted radiation therapy, submitted. 1987.
14. **Mach, J., Chatal, J., Lumboroso, J., Bucheggar, F., Forni, M., Ripschard, J., Berche, C., Douillard, J., Carrel, S., Herlyn, M., Steplewski, Z., and Koprowski, H.,** Tumour localisation in patients by radiolabelled monoclonal antibodies against colon carcinoma, *Cancer Res.*, 43, 5593, 1983.
15. **Lashford, L., Davis, A., Richardson, R., Bullimore, J., Eckert, H., Coakham, H., and Kemshead, J.,** A pilot study of 131-I monoclonal antibodies in the therapy of leptomeningeal tumour, *Cancer,* in press, 1987.
16. **Lashford, L., Moyes, J., Oh, R., Fielding, S., Mellers, S., Gordon, I., Evans, K., and Kemshead, J.,** The biodistribution and pharmacokinetics of m-IBG in childhood neuroblastoma, submitted, 1987.
17. Reported at Conference ''mIBG in Therapy, Diagnosis, and Monitoring of Neuroblastoma'', Rome, September 22-23, 1986.
18. **Hoefnagel, C. and Voute, P.,** Radionuclide therapy of neural crest tumours, Nucleaire Geneeskunde oud en niew. Pauwels, E. K. J., Ed., 1986.

Chapter 7

MONOCLONAL ANTIBODIES AS AGENTS TO PURGE TUMOR CELLS FROM BONE MARROW: LABORATORY AND CLINICAL EXPERIENCES

Adrian P. Gee

TABLE OF CONTENTS

I. INTRODUCTION

In recent years, there has been a dramatic increase in the use of bone marrow transplantation for the treatment of a variety of diseases, particularly refractory cancer.[1] The feasibility of transplanting marrow for hematological reconstitution was first demonstrated in the early 1950s,[2] and to date, more than 11,000 patients have been treated. About three quarters of these procedures have been carried out since 1983.[1] In the treatment of malignant diseases, bone marrow transplantation has been used extensively as rescue, following marrow-ablative high dose therapy for refractory leukemia, lymphoma, and certain solid tumors. An impediment to its more extensive application has been the scarcity of suitable tissue-matched normal marrow donors. Within the immediate family of a patient, the probability of finding a match is one in four, although in practice, this chance is closer to one in three,[3] since patients usually have multiple siblings. The probability of finding a donor in the general population is correspondingly smaller,[4] even if the HLA-typing information was readily available. Two approaches are being used to circumvent this scarcity. The first is the use of mismatched marrow.[3,5]

Transplantation of even HLA-matched bone marrow often produces severe graft vs. host disease in the recipient;[6] the use of mismatched marrow further increases the severity of this reaction, sometimes to a fatal degree.[7] Graft vs. host disease is mediated by immunocompetent T lymphocytes in the donor's marrow,[8,9] and can be ablated or reduced by depletion of these cells *in vitro* prior to marrow infusion.[10,13] Recent evidence suggests, however, that clinically manageable graft vs. host disease may be beneficial in combating residual disease in leukemia patients.[12,14,15] This indicates that complete elimination of mature T lymphocytes from mismatched marrow may be undesirable. This is further supported by the finding that there is a higher incidence of graft failure in patients receiving highly T cell-depleted marrow,[13,16] suggesting that the presence of functional T cells may also be important in establishment of the graft. Current laboratory and clinical investigations should allow us to develop methods for the selective depletion of T lymphocyte subpopulations,[17-21] to permit both full engraftment of the marrow, and the development of a potentially beneficial graft vs. leukemia response, in the absence of severe graft vs. host disease.

II. AUTOLOGOUS TRANSPLANTATION WITH PURGED BONE MARROW

A second solution to the problem of transplanting a patient without a suitable matched donor is to use autologous marrow.[22] In this procedure, bone marrow is harvested from a patient whose disease is in clinical remission, and stored, either frozen in liquid nitrogen,[23] at 4°C,[24,25] or ambient temperature[26] (for much shorter periods). If the patient relapses and requires high-dose therapy, he can be rescued using his own stored marrow. This technique ensures that every suitable patient has a donor, i.e., him or herself, and obviates the potential for development of graft vs. host disease (but also any beneficial effects of a graft vs. residual disease response). To date, more than 2,000 patients have received autologous transplants, and early clinical data on the success of this approach has been presented at three international meetings,[27] and extensively reviewed.[22,28-30]

A source of major concern when using autologous marrow for transplantation is the possibility that it may contain viable tumor cells that would be returned to the patient at reinfusion, and could initiate disease relapse. Although this is a particular problem in the hematological malignancies, it is also true for various solid tumors that metastasize to the bone marrow.[31] It has been estimated, for example, that 30 to 40% of patients with Ewing's sarcoma or neuroblastoma have bone marrow involvement.[32] Although the bone marrow for autologous transplantation is collected during clinical remission, it is clear that our ability to detect infiltration of the marrow by tumor is severely limited, with the result that many "remission" marrows may actually contain appreciable numbers of tumor cells.[33]

The limit of detection of cancer cells in bone marrow smears by conventional histology is about one cell in 100 to 1000 normal cells, or 1% to 0.1%. The sensitivity can be increased to 0.01% to 0.1% using indirect immunofluorescence with panels of tumor-directed monoclonal antibodies,[34] and the use of microcomputer-based digital imaging of the fluorescent cells should produce a further increase in the sensitivity of this approach.[35] If we assume, however, that for most laboratories, the limit of detection is about 0.1%, and that 10^{10} nucleated cells are reinfused during an average pediatric transplant, this means that up to 10 million tumor cells could be returned to a patient in a conventionally "tumor-free" remission bone marrow. The validity of this risk is supported by a recent study demonstrating the presence of leukemia cells in the marrow of patients who were clinically disease-free (by conventional criteria), using a sensitive tumor colony-forming assay.[33] In addition, one of these marrows had been used for autologous transplantation. While it is not possible to estimate what proportion of these tumor cells would be clonogenic *in vivo*, it is clear that in animal systems, infusion of as few as ten malignant cells can produce lethal disease in all of the recipients.[36] Extrapolation from animal models for acute myelogenous leukemia, has suggested that the ED_{50} for the human disease is probably 1,000 to 10,000 cells.[37] This level of infiltration would be exceptionally difficult, if not impossible, to detect in a bone marrow harvest by most of the currently available techniques.

In the human situation, it is also not possible to determine whether the clonogenic potential of tumor cells infiltrating the marrow has been decreased by therapy that the patient received prior to marrow harvest.[38] If this was the case, then the incidence of disease relapse in patients receiving marrow harvested during second or subsequent remission should be lower than in those transplanted with first remission marrow (with the rather large assumption that the high-dose therapy *in vivo* is equally effective in both groups). Unfortunately, at this time, there is too much variability between treatment regimens and patient selection procedures, to make any meaningful comparison of this type. In general, however, clinical results using unmanipulated autologous bone marrow harvested in second or later remission, have been poorer rather than better.[39-41]

The risks associated with reinfusing viable tumor in autologous transplantation, and the absence of definitive information from controlled clinical trials to support the use of untreated marrow, have prompted the development of procedures for eliminating, or "purging", tumor cells *in vitro* prior to marrow reinfusion. Provided that these techniques do not adversely affect engraftment potential, and are capable of effective levels of tumor cell depletion, it would seem preferable to use purged marrows in those patients in whom there is a risk of bone marrow involvement.

The procedures that are being developed for purging tumor can also be adapted for the elimination of T lymphocytes from marrow that is to be used for allogeneic transplantation.[13,17,18,21,42] These approaches can be broadly classified into two groups: (1) *in situ* destruction methods, in which the cell is destroyed within the marrow; and (2) removal techniques, in which the tumor cells are physically separated from the normal marrow cells. In both groups, methods have been developed which exploit the exquisite specificity of monoclonal antibodies to identify the tumor cells, and to target the elimination technique selectively towards these cells. When used in this context, these antibodies need not be directed against "tumor-specific" antigens, it is sufficient that they identify an antigen that is present on the target tumor cell, but is not shared by hematopoietic marrow cells. Many reagents of this type have been described, and have been used for purging of acute lymphoblastic and myelogenous leukemia,[43-47] non-Hodgkin's lymphoma,[48,49] breast carcinoma,[50,51] neuroblastoma,[52,53] and other malignancies.[54-56] It is clear that the efficiency of any antibody-mediated purging procedure can be enhanced significantly by combining antibodies into disease-related panels, and the importance of this concept will be discussed later. It is, however, outside the scope and intent of this article to describe the composition and selection of particular antibody panels.[45,57] The reader is referred to several excellent review articles for this information.[58-62]

III. MARROW PURGING TECHNIQUES

A. *In Situ* Purging Methods

In situ purging techniques generally rely upon the addition of a toxic or lytic agent to the marrow. The specificity of this agent towards tumor cells is either preexisting, in the case of cytotoxic drugs, or conferred by targeting, using tumor-directed antibodies. A variety of unconjugated cytotoxic drugs have been evaluated for purging, but most interest has focused on cyclophosphamide derivatives, and in particular 4-hydroperoxycyclophosphamide and mafosamide.[63,64] Although preclinical reports described enormous variability in the relative specificity of these derivatives towards tumor cells,[65,66] it has now been demonstrated that marrow chemo-purged using these agents is capable of achieving full hematopoietic reconstitution.[67,68] It is still too early, however, to evaluate the clinical effectiveness of this approach. The availability of new cyclophosphamide derivatives,[69] and other agents, both in combination,[70] and in the presence of drugs that exert a protective effect on normal marrow cells,[71] is likely to result in the more widespread use of this type of purging, particularly as a valuable adjunct to monoclonal antibody-mediated techniques.

Attempts have been made to increase the specificity of chemo-purging by using agents that can be activated to their toxic form after they have been efficiently targeted to the tumor cells. This technique has been described by Sieber and his colleagues.[72,73] Merocyanin is an agent that is preferentially incorporated into the lipid bilayer of neuroblastoma and leukemia cells,[74] and can then be activated by exposure to light. Alternatively, specificity can be conferred on a drug by linking it to a tumor-directed antibody. Conjugates of this type have been prepared using daunomycin,[75] methotrexate,[76] and chlorambucil.[77] In common with the use of other antibody-targeted toxic agents, it is important to ensure that the conjugated drug retains its activity, is efficiently translocated to its point of action within the cell, or on the cell membrane, and is not released in an unconjugated, nonspecifically toxic form.

Antibody-mediated delivery has also been described for a variety of plant-derived toxins,[78,79] including abrin and amanitin. The majority of studies have focused on ricin — a potent toxic lectin from the castor bean (*Ricinis communis*).[80] The ricin molecule consists of a short, toxic, polypeptide A chain, disulfide-linked to a longer B chain, which is the source of lectin activity.[81] The specific sugar for ricin lectin is lactose, which is present on many normal cells, including those in bone marrow. Antibody-conjugated intact ricin must, therefore, be prevented from binding to nontumor cells through the B chain, by carrying out the reaction in buffers containing lactose to block the lectin activity.[82] Alternatively, conjugates can be prepared using only the toxic A chain;[83] however, these have usually been found to be less effective,[84,85] since the B chain aids in translocation, and conjugation of the A chain can sterically hinder binding of the antibody to the cell.[86] The efficiency of cell killing can be increased, however, by the addition of lysosomotropic agents, e.g., ammonium chloride[87] during incubation. Intact ricin has been conjugated to anti-cALLa[88] and anti-T cell antibodies,[89] and used clinically for depletion of normal or malignant T cells from bone marrow.[82,89] Conditions must be carefully controlled to ensure effective specific toxicity within an acceptable *in vitro* treatment time.[82,87] The high toxicity of ricin probably compensates for the low level of conjugate binding to cells that express only small amounts of the target antigen. This is supported by recent studies in which no correlation could be demonstrated between the number of antigen-binding sites on the cells and the efficiency of toxin killing.[90] Conversely, the high toxicity also necessitates special precautions during conjugate preparation. For effective purging a variety of conjugates must be prepared, using monoclonal antibodies with different target antigen specificities, to ensure elimination of all tumor cells of a particular histological type from marrows of patients with a range of immunophenotypes. Another potential problem is the release of active toxin from cells, resulting in "innocent bystander killing" of normal marrow cells. This may be a particular difficulty when toxin-purged cryopreserved marrow is thawed for reinfusion.

Many of the problems associated with high potency toxin can be avoided by the use of an antibody-targeted agent that exists in a nontoxic precursor form, and can be activated only when bound to the target cell. Complement is a physiological agent of this type. The complement system consists of a series of more than 20 serum proteins that circulate in an inactive form. The system can be activated by a change in the level of the regulating components by, for example, certain bacteria (the alternative pathway), or via the classical pathway, by binding of the initial components to the Fc region of a cell-bound antibody molecule (or molecules, in the case of IgG antibody).[91] Activation of the complement system results in the generation of a membrane attack complex, which produces a characteristic lesion on the target cell membrane and colloid osmotic lysis of the cell. The use of the classical pathway for tumor cell purging has a number of distinct advantages over immunotoxins.[30,57] It retains and exploits the specificity of monoclonal antibodies to identify the target cells and direct the cytotoxic mechanism. However, the procedure is technically simpler since it is not necessary to prepare conjugates of each antibody that is to be used for purging. A very wide variety of monoclonal antibodies can, therefore, be incorporated into the purging panel, and added directly to the marrow without any form of conjugation procedure. The complement is bound and activated only by those cells to which the monoclonal antibody is bound, and there is no risk of innocent bystander killing. The only limitation to the choice of antibodies is that they belong to a complement-fixing isotype and subclass e.g., usually IgM and IgG_{2a}.

In some cases, an exogenous complement source has not been added to the marrow after antibody treatment.[92] Tumor cell elimination has been achieved either by antibody-dependent cellular cytotoxicity, or via residual complement components present in the treated cell suspension or in the recipient. More frequently, xenogeneic complement is added after antibody treatment, the most common source being baby rabbit serum. This choice is based on (1) the efficiency of rabbit complement for lysis of human cells,[93] (2) the good reactivity between murine antibodies and rabbit complement,[94] and (3) the low direct toxicity of neonatal sera towards nonantibody-sensitized cells. It has proved possible to produce monoclonal antibodies that will fix human complement efficiently, and these can be used for marrow purging.[95,96] For most monoclonals, however, the selection of suitable xenogeneic complement sources has been a major difficulty associated with using this approach. It has usually necessitated screening a large number of different batches of serum to find one in which antibody-mediated toxicity is high, in the absence of direct toxic effects[97] towards nonantibody-sensitized cells.

The lytic efficiency of a complement source has generally been measured as the CH50,[91] that is, the reciprocal of the dilution of serum that is required to lyse 50% of a fixed number of sheep erythrocytes, optimally sensitized with antibody. Red cells have routinely been used as the target cell of choice in complement research, due to their high sensitivity to this form of cytolysis. Previous studies, however, indicate that the lytic efficiency of complement towards nucleated tumor cells varies widely,[98] and may not be directly related to its potency as measured on erythrocytes. In the context of marrow purging, it would be preferable to establish a complement potency unit based on the dilution of complement required to kill 50% of an appropriate tumor cell target,[57] e.g., a tissue culture cell line of the same histological type. The use of this more relevant measure does not, in itself, do anything to increase the availability of suitable complement sources. This problem can be resolved by absorption of direct toxic effects using human erythrocytes, although this often reduces the lytic efficiency of the serum. An alternative approach may be to manipulate the composition of the complement source, by supplementing the components that are present at limiting concentrations.[57] This would allow preparation of high titer, large volume, standardized batches of complement, without significant direct toxicity.

Probably the major difficulty associated with the use of complement, in combination with monoclonal antibodies, for bone marrow purging, is elimination of tumor cells that express small amounts of the target antigen.[57,99] The majority of monoclonal antibodies that have been produced are of the IgG isotype. Activation of the classical pathway by IgG antibody is critically dependent on the membrane distribution of the target antigen, since two molecules must be bound to the cell surface in close proximity, in order to activate the first component of the complement cascade.[100] This conformation will be increasingly difficult to achieve as the amount of target antigen on the cell surface decreases. It would, therefore, be predicted that low antigen density tumor cells would be particularly resistant to complement-mediated elimination. This has proved to be the case. We[99] and others[101,102] have demonstrated that low antigen leukemia and lymphoma cells can be isolated by their ability to survive treatment with monoclonal antibody and complement. It is reasonable to believe that similar low antigen-expressing tumor cells are present in patients,[103] and may, in fact, be selected for, by the therapy that the patient has previously received.[104,105] This should strongly caution against the clinical use of any purging protocol that employs a single monoclonal antibody,[44,106] and although use of panels of antibodies should reduce the risk of the escape of low antigen expressing cells, it is still possible that some tumor cells are multiple low expressors, and could resist most forms of antibody-mediated elimination. As more sensitive techniques are used to detect and characterize residual, unpurged tumor cells,[33,101,107,108] the magnitude of this limitation to the use of complement will become more evident.

It is of interest that many centers originally using single antibodies for marrow cleaning, have successively added extra antibodies,[109] and/or supplementary purging techniques[110-112] to their protocols. This could be explained entirely by the ability of low antigen density tumor cells to evade their earlier purging strategies. It is possible that antigen expression on the target cell population could be enhanced by treatment of the marrow with drugs,[113] enzymes,[114] metabolic inhibitors,[113] and interferon.[115,116] These agents should, however, be used with extreme caution, since they may expose cryptic cross-reacting antigens on normal cells and adversely affect engraftment potential of the marrow. Our studies indicate that the efficiency of antibody-mediated purging can be increased by the use of a magnetic system, rather than complement, to eliminate the cells,[117] since this technique is not as highly dependent on the distribution of target antigen. Alternatively, if complement is to be retained as the primary means of elimination, then it is preferable to use IgM monoclonal antibodies. Since a single cell-bound IgM molecule is capable of triggering the complement cascade,[118] target antigen density is less critical when the antibodies of this isotype are used. It is important to appreciate, however, that efficient binding and activation of the first component of the complement system does not, in itself, ensure efficient lysis of the cell.

Several studies have indicated that multiple complement treatments are required to achieve maximal purging efficiency.[101,119] This may be due to changes in expression of target antigen during treatment *in vitro*, although the incubation conditions generally used would not always support this explanation. Alternatively, we have described the existance of an anticomplementary factor associated with normal human marrow cells.[120] This acts by accelerating the decay of an unstable, cell-bound complement intermediate, and its effects are maximal within 30 min at 37°C. The factor would, therefore, exert its action only during the first incubation of the marrow with complement. This would partly explain the requirement for multiple treatments. While it is technically possible to perform multiple purges, this inevitably increases the amount of marrow manipulation *in vitro*, with a corresponding increase in the risk of microbial contamination, and nonspecific stem cell damage and loss. This should obviously be avoided, particularly when working with an autologous marrow, with its potentially fragile engraftment potential[121] and limited availability.

In spite of these limitations, complement has been extensively used for clinical purging. Two of the largest published studies are from the groups in Minnesota and Boston, both of which have treated patients with acute lymphoblastic leukemia. At last report[110] (December 1986), 51 patients had been entered in the Minnesota study in which a panel of anti-CD24, CD9, and CD10 monoclonal antibodies was used. All patients were in remission at the time of transplant, but two different conditioning regimens were used. The engraftment time of purged marrow was shorter (24 days) in patients receiving purged autologous marrow than in those having allogeneic transplants (31 days). Overall the relapse rate in the autologous patients was 76% (vs. 55% in allogeneic patients), and the relapses occurred earlier (a median of 147 days vs. 557 days post transplant). This was taken as an indication that the purging procedure was not completely effective, and it has now been supplemented with chemo-purging using a cyclophosphamide derivative. As of September 1985, 34 patients had been entered in the Boston study.[109] Fourteen of these were purged using an anti-CD10 monoclonal antibody alone. One patient was treated with an anti-GP26 IgM monoclonal, and the remainder were purged using a combination of the two antibodies. This combination was capable of a four log depletion in preclinical experiments. Ten patients relapsed with cALLa-positive blasts in the marrow, mostly within 10 months of transplant. Twelve were in unmaintained complete remission at a median of 22 months post-transplant, and an equal number had died in remission. Three of six patients had inversions i.e., were currently in remissions that had lasted longer than their first remission. The engraftment times, relapse rate, and lethal toxicity were all greater in these patients than in a group receiving allogeneic bone marrow. In a recent study of purging in acute myelogenous leukemia,[47] two antibodies (an IgM and an IgG_{2a} that bind to mature myeloid cells, but not CFU-GM) have been used to treat 16 patients in first or second remission or at first relapse. Six patients have relapsed and there have been three toxic deaths; the survivors are presently at between 1 and 7 months post-transplant. As the results from other large studies (e.g., the European CAMPATH experience)[95] are published, it should be possible to determine whether there is a consistent pattern of early relapse, suggesting purging failure. This can only be properly decided, however, in a comparative study using purged and nonpurged marrow.[28]

B. Physical Separation Techniques

An alternative to the *in situ* destruction of infiltrating tumor cells is their separation from the marrow. These techniques rely either on inherent physical differences between the normal marrow cells and the target tumor cells, or on the use of procedures that artificially create this difference.

Inherent differences in the size and/or density of malignant and normal cells have been exploited for the removal of leukemia and neuroblastoma cells from bone marrow.[122-124] The former have been separated by centrifugation on albumin gradients, and the latter by centrifugal elutriation. In both cases, the efficiency of depletion (about 95%) is insufficient to allow either procedure to be used alone for clinical purging. The future of these techniques is more likely to be for bulk depletion of tumor from heavily infiltrated marrow, prior to the use of a more efficient method.

A more promising approach is to use a procedure that can enhance or create a difference between tumor and normal marrow cells, that can then be exploited in the separation technique. Again, the most efficient method for achieving this is to use monoclonal antibodies to identify the target cell population. By linking the antibody to a particle, the effective density of the tumor cell can be increased for easier physical separation. Immunogold, colloidal gold linked to antibody,[125] has been used for cell separation; however, the increase in target cell mass that results, is insufficient to obtain the separation efficiency that would be required clincially. This can be achieved by the use of paramagnetic particles.[52,126,127] Cells coated with these particles can be rapidly and effectively separated from the mixture by passage of the treated marrow through a magnetic field. This approach has several advantages over *in situ* tumor cell destruction using complement. It does not require antibodies of a particular isotype or subclass. It is also unaffected by humoral factors, such as the anticomplementary factor associated with normal marrow cells and, in our studies, it is not as critically dependent on the density of target antigen on the tumor cells. We have found that low antigen-expressing, complement-resistant cells can be eliminated by the immunomagnetic procedure.[128] It is still possible, in the model system that we have used (tissue culture leukemia cell lines seeded into peripheral blood or normal bone marrow), to detect a very small number of cells that are apparently resistant to both approaches. It remains to be determined whether a multiply resistant subpopulation of this type would be sufficient in number, and clonogenic potential, to pose a significant threat of relapse if reinfused into a patient.

Two types of magnetic particles are currently being tested, colloids[126,129] and microspheres.[52,130] The colloidal system, originally described by Poynton et al.[131] presently consists of a colloidal suspension of 30 to 40 nm particles that are treated with avidin,[129] and react with biotinylated monoclonal antibody or lectin, coupled to the target cell. The magnetic affinity colloid must be prepared on the day of use and "passivated" by treatment with dichromate. Cell separation is accomplished in a closed system using internal screens magnetized by externally placed samarium cobalt permanent magnets. Using this technique, 1 to 2 logarithm depletions of T cells have been achieved using anti-CD3, CD4, CD8, and CD11 monoclonal antibodies. Addition of a biotinylated T cell-directed agglutinin to the system increased this efficiency to 4 to 5 logarithms. This was believed to be due to lectin-mediated removal of T cells that did not bind any of the monoclonals in the panel. In preliminary studies using patient-derived leukemic cells, 2 logarithms of tumor cell depletion could be achieved with monoclonal antibodies.

The microsphere technique originated with the development by Ugelstad of a procedure for the preparation of paramagnetic beads with absolutely uniform physical properties[130] (Figure 1). These particles, produced by the polymerization of styrene divinylbenzene, contain magnetite dispersed throughout their volume, and are treated to make their surface hydrophilic, allowing for coupling of proteins, such as antibodies, by passive adsorption.[132-134] Alternatively, they can be chemically modified to permit covalent coupling of antibody by tosylation. For marrow purging, 3.5 and 4.5 μm diameter beads have been used in modifications of a procedure originally developed by Kemshead and his colleagues.[52]

Laboratory studies have repeatedly shown that efficient target cell separation cannot be achieved by directly adsorbing the tumor-directed IgG monoclonal antibodies to the microspheres, due presumably to steric hindrance effects.[128,135] A spacer arm, consisting of polyclonal, high-affinity, sheep or goat anti-mouse immunoglobulin antibody, must first be adsorbed, or covalently coupled to the beads, which are then admixed with the monoclonal antibody-sensitized target cells.[52] (Figure 2) A single treatment using this approach (indirect magnetic separation)[136] is more efficient (greater than 5 logarithm depletion) than the one step procedure, in which antiimmunoglobulin-coated beads are preincubated with the monoclonals, washed, and added directly to the untreated nucleated marrow cells (direct magnetic separation). This difference relates both to heterogeneity of expression of target antigen by tumor cells, and the radically different reaction kinetics in the two systems.[137,138] It is not clear how variations in target antigens can be addressed when using the direct technique. In the indirect procedure it is possible to saturate every binding site for each monoclonal, by adding a large excess of fluid-phase antibody. Binding is maximal within 30 min, and unbound antibody is removed by extensive washing. In contrast, in the direct system, the only way to ensure saturation is to add a tremendous excess of precoated beads. To allow

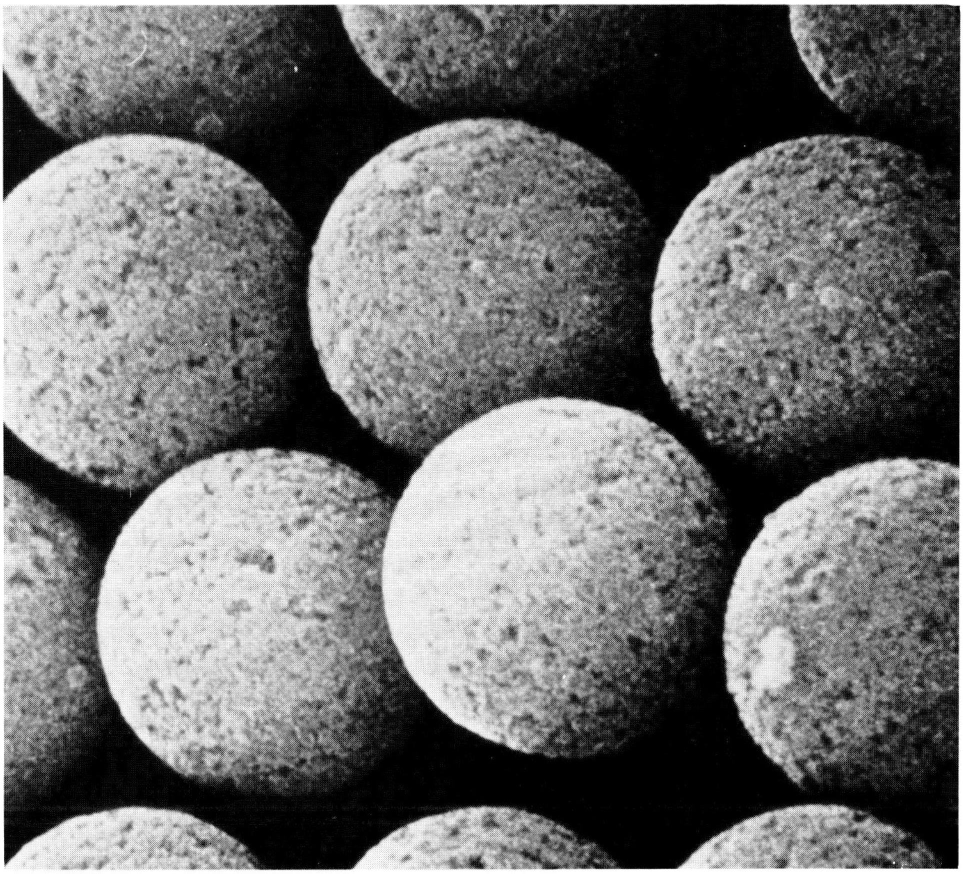

FIGURE 1. Uniform M450 polystyrene microspheres. (Courtesy of Dynal A.S., Oslo, Norway.)

for immunophenotypic differences, it is preferable to prepare batches of microspheres coated with only one monoclonal from the panel, and adjust the proportion of each bead type to the immunophenotype of individual patients. Combined with the change in the kinetics of the bead-target cell interaction seen in direct separations, these disadvantages outweigh the longer treatment time required when using the indirect procedure. In contrast, the direct and indirect systems have been shown to be equally effective for depleting cells that are more homogeneous in their antigen expression, for example T lymphocytes.[117,139] If the direct procedure is chosen, it is possible to use beads with IgM monoclonal antibodies adsorbed directly to their surface, without an antiimmunoglobulin spacer arm.

The Kemshead immunomagnetic purging technique has been used by several groups,[52,140,141] including ourselves,[121] primarily in the treatment of a pediatric cancer, neuroblastoma. The results from these studies are currently accumulating, and it is too early to determine whether the use of purged bone marrow has conferred any clinical advantage on these patients. To date, more than 110 neuroblastoma patients have been transplanted with immunomagnetically purged marrow.[142] The technique has also been adapted for use in acute lymphoblastic leukemia[136-138] and lymphoma.[48,49] The only complication that may relate directly to the procedure is delayed or nonengraftment that has been reported in a small number (less than 10%) of the patients.[121,143] It is not clear whether this is due to the manipulation of the marrow *in vitro*, or the generally poorer quality of the marrow that must be used for autologous transplantation. We have been able to relate engraftment times in our patients directly to

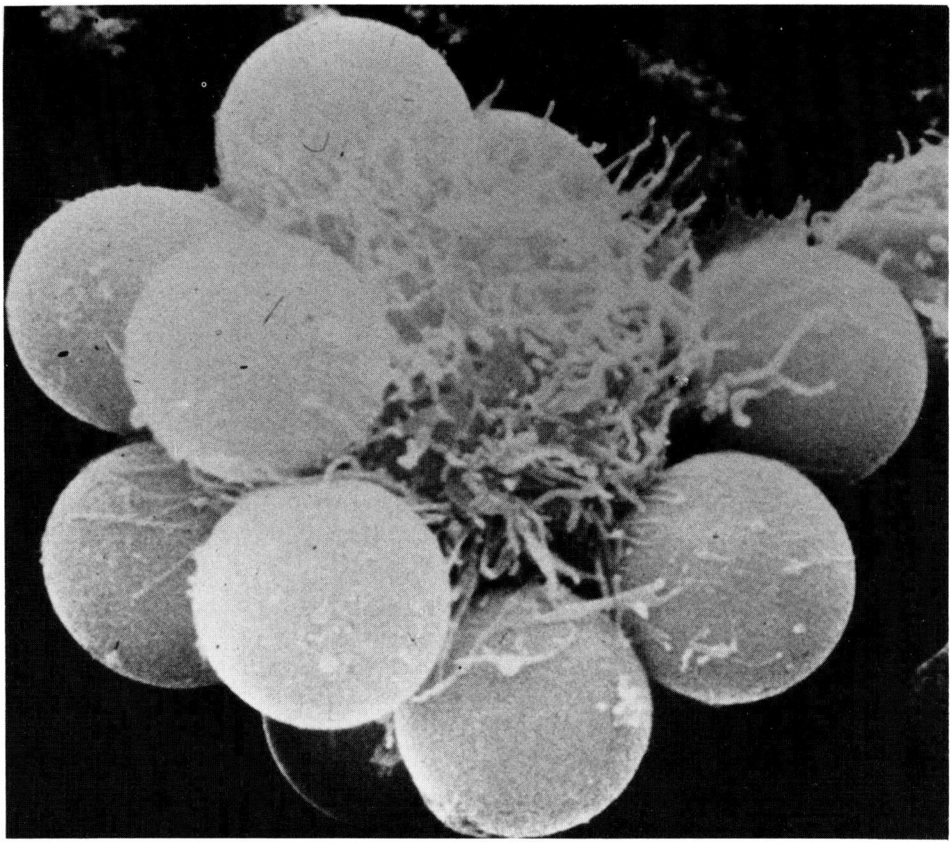

FIGURE 2. M450 microspheres targeted to tumor cells. (Courtesy of Dynal A.S., Oslo, Norway.)

the amount of therapy that they received prior to marrow harvesting.[121] Studies by Favrot[143] have described the appearance of increased numbers of CD8-positive cells in their patients with engraftment problems, and, in two cases, they were able to correct this situation clinically by the *in vivo* administration of anti-CD8 monoclonal antibody.[143]

Several groups have described an advantage in repeated magnetic treatments to increase separation efficiency.[48,49,53,144] This has not been a universal finding,[136-138,142] and this difference probably relates to major variations in the model systems, the panels of monoclonal antibodies, and the methods used for detecting residual target cells. It is likely that repeated purging treatments using any technique, will achieve an increase in the level of depletion. It is not clear, however, that the advantage of removing a very small additional number of tumor cells by a second application of the same purging technique, is not counteracted by the potential for damage to the engraftment potential of an already fragile marrow. If multiple purges are shown to be uniformly advantageous, it would seem preferable to use complimentary techniques e.g., immunomagnetic and chemo-purging, rather than either two identical treatments, or two methods that share similar limitations e.g., two antibody-mediated techniques.

In the design of a purging protocol, it should also be remembered that each of the steps in the procedure may profoundly affect the efficiency of overall tumor cell elimination. For example, enrichment of nucleated marrow cells by Hetastarch-mediated erythrocyte sedimentation can also selectively remove some neuroblastoma cells.[145] Nonspecific cell losses (averaging 50% in immunomagnetic purging for neuroblastoma,[52,135] and slightly higher for acute lymphoblastic leukemia),[146] can also be minimized by careful control of the hematocrit and packed cell volume during marrow processing. The experimental and clinical results of immunomagnetic purging are at least as good as those obtained using other monoclonal antibody-mediated methods. The system does not rely on the use of potent toxins and is less subject to factors that may limit the efficiency of other techniques.

IV. GENERAL CONSIDERATIONS

It remains to be determined whether the level of tumor cell depletion achievable by any of these procedures is sufficient to significantly reduce the chance of bone marrow relapse in the recipients. Our inability to measure the absolute efficiency of any purging procedure is the single greatest obstacle to determining the superiority of a particular technique. The difficulties that hamper the detection of occult tumor in remission bone marrow from patients are amplified when the aim is to determine whether the number of these cells has been further depleted by an *in vitro* manipulation. Model systems permit some degree of quantitation, since known number of target cells, from cell lines, or isolated from patients, can be seeded into the marrow at levels that can be more easily monitored. In addition, it is possible to prelabel these cells with fluorochrome to assist in their detection.[108] Unless a continuous-flow or automated counting technique[35] is used to detect residual cells, however, multiple small samples must be analyzed and a considerable sampling error, in the form of a multiplication factor, is introduced when calculating the total number of tumor cells remaining in the treated sample. For example, a single cell detected in a hemacytometer may represent between one cell and 10,000 residual cells per milliliter, and large numbers of replicate counts must be taken to obtain a more accurate estimate. In our experience, the most sensitive techniques for determining purging efficiency are tumor cell colony assays.[107,144] While these methods differ widely, they generally involve culturing the treated samples under conditions that favor the selective growth of malignant cells e.g., an hypoxic atmosphere. We [138] and others[48] have used the Courtenay system in which samples of purged marrow are cultured in semisolid agar with rat erythrocyte feeder cells, in an atmosphere of 5% carbon dioxide, 5% oxygen, and 90% nitrogen for three weeks, and have been able to detect fewer than ten residual leukemic cells per culture. The plating efficiency of tissue culture leukemia lines in this assay approaches 50%, and a similar system has been described for the detection of occult tumor cells in patient marrow samples, where it has proved to be highly efficient.[33] These techniques can usually be easily adapted for limiting dilution analysis for added sensitivity.[147] While colony assays measure the clonogenic capability of nonpurged tumor cells, this may not accurately reflect the proliferative capacity of these cells *in vivo*. It is, therefore, advisable to use a combination of techniques (fluorochrome prelabeling, indirect immunofluorescent post-labeling, and colony-forming assays) to measure purging efficiency in any model system.

Many early studies described animal models for the development of marrow purging techniques using antibody and complement[148-151] or immunotoxins.[83,152] While these are able to provide indications of optimal treatment conditions, and of the relative efficiencies of different approaches, they are of limited value for establishing the conditions for clinical purging. Unfortunately, neither model nor animal systems effectively simulates the clinical situation. Bone marrow is much more heterogeneous in its cellular content and properties than peripheral blood, and conditions that are optimized in a model system using either small marrow samples or peripheral blood to simulate bulk marrow, usually cannot be reliably transferred directly for use with the volumes of marrow that must be handled during clinical purging. Aggregation and gelation, accelerated by DNA release,[101,128] can be real problems in some marrows, particularly those that have been traumatized during harvesting or handling. These difficulties can usually be minimized by keeping the marrow cold during manipulation and by gentle treatment. We have avoided the addition of DNAase to prevent the possibility of an anaphylactic reaction if reinfused into a sensitive patient.

Another limitation in the development of marrow cleaning protocols is the lack of a reliable *in vitro* method to predict the engraftment potential of treated bone marrow. Various committed hematopoietic cells can be assayed using colony-forming assays, but the general consensus is that these tests are of limited predictive value in the clinical situation.[153,154] It is possible that some of the newer long-term marrow culture systems[155-157] may provide this information. Until then, colony assays can only really be used as an indication of the viability of treated bone marrow.

V. SUMMARY

Ultimately, the only real test of any purging technique can be to evaluate it in the patients for whom it was designed. Marrow purging studies are presently at the Phase I stage, in which the aim is to show that bone marrow treated *in vitro* is capable of producing full hematological engraftment, without unacceptable toxic side effects, when reinfused. Although the patterns and rates of disease relapse in these patients may indicate whether recurrence is due to failure of the high dose therapy, or of marrow purging, definitive proof can only be obtained by carefully designed, controlled clinical trials that compare allogeneic and purged and unpurged autologous transplantation.[28] It has been calculated that 135 patients would be required in each arm of a study to determine the efficacy of using purged bone marrow for first remission patients, assuming that the *ex vivo* procedure is effective in 50% of cases. For second remission patients, this number increases to 235 in each arm. If, however, a uniformly effective purging technique is developed, these numbers decline to 31 and 55, respectively.[28] While these numbers appear daunting for any single institution, it has been shown that marrow can be transported from distant institutions to a central facility for *in vitro* treatment, and returned cryopreserved for reinfusion.[117,121,135] This makes multicenter cooperative studies of this sort feasible, and several American trials are currently in the planning stages. As we prepare for these studies, we must continually refine both the techniques that we use for bone marrow cleaning and the methods to assess the efficacy of these techniques, bearing in mind that this technology will also be of potential value to patients receiving T cell-depleted, mismatched marrow. The ability to separate subpopulations of cells from bone marrow can only increase our understanding of transplantation and hematopietic reconstitution, both of which will ultimately benefit the patient.

ACKNOWLEDGMENTS

The author's work described in this article was carried out at the University of Florida and supported in part by grants from the Pardee Foundation, Midland, Michigan, the American Cancer Society (CH-33), the Florida Affiliate of the American Cancer Society (F86UF-3), the Leukemia Society of America, and Stop Children's Cancer, Florida.

REFERENCES*

1. **Gale, R. P.,** Analysis of bone marrow transplantation data in man, *Bone Marrow Transplant.*, 1, 3, 1986.
2. **Bortin, M. M.,** A compendium of reported human bone marrow transplants, *Transplantation*, 9, 571, 1970.

* See Note Added in Proof, at end of Reference list.

3. **O'Reilly, R. J.**, Allogeneic bone marrow transplantation: current status and future directions, *Blood,* 62, 941, 1983.
4. **Hansen, J. A., Clift, R. A., Thomas, E. D., Buckner, C. D., Storb, R., and Giblett, E. R.**, Transplantation of marrow from an unrelated donor to a patient with acute leukemia, *N. Engl. J. Med.*, 303, 565, 1980.
5. **Reisner, Y., Kapoor, N., Kirkpatrick, D., Pollack, M. S., Dupont, B., Good, R. A., and O'Reilly, R. J.**, Transplantation for acute leukemia with HLA-A and B nonidentical parental marrow cells fractionated with soybean agglutinin and sheep red cells, *Lancet,* 2, 327, 1981.
6. **Thomas, E. D., Storb, R., Clift, R. A., Fefer, A., Johnson, F. L., Neiman, P. E., Lerner, K. C., Glucksberg, H., and Buckner, C. D.**, Bone marrow transplantation, *N. Engl. J. Med.*, 292, 895, 1975.
7. **Buckley, R. H.**, Reconstitution: grafting of bone marrow and thymuses, in *Progress in Immunology,* Amos, B., Ed., Academic Press, New York, 1971, 1061.
8. **Yunis, E. J., Good, R. A., Smith, J., and Stutman, O.**, Protection of lethally irradiated mice by spleen cells from neonatally thymectomized mice, *Proc. Natl. Acad. Sci. U.S.A.*, 71, 2544, 1974.
9. **Lum, L. G., Orcutt-Thordarson, N., Seigneuret, M. C., and Storb, R.**, The regulation of Ig synthesis after marrow transplantation IV. T4 and T8 subset functions in patients with chronic graft-versus-host disease, *J. Immunol.*, 82, 113, 1982.
10. **Slocombe, G. W., Newland, A. C., Yeatman, N. W. J., Macey, M., Jones, H. M., and Knott, L.**, Allogeneic bone marrow transplantation for adult leukemia with soy bean lectin fractionated marrow, *Bone Marrow Transplant.*, 1, 31, 1986.
11. **Prentice, H. G., Blacklock, H. A., Janossy, G., Bradstock, K. F., Skeggs, D., Goldstein, G., and Hoffbrand, A. V.**, Use of the anti-T cell monclonal antibody OKT3 for prevention of acute graft versus host disease in allogeneic histocompatible bone marrow transplantation for acute leukemia, *Lancet,* 1, 1266, 1982.
12. **Apperley, J. F., Jones, L., Hale, G., Waldmann, H., Hows, J., Rombos, Y., Tsatalas, C., Marcus, R. E., Goolden, A. W. G., Gordon-Smith, E. C., Catovsky, D., Galton, D. A. G., and Goldman, J. M.**, Bone marrow transplantation for patients with chronic myeloid leukaemia: T cell depletion with Campath-1 reduces the incidence of graft-versus-host disease but may increase the risk of leukaemic relapse, *Bone Marrow Transplant.*, 1, 53, 1986.
13. **O'Reilly, R. J., Collins, N. H., Kernan, N., Brochstein, J., Kirkpatrick, D., Siena, S., Keever, C., Jordan, B., Shank, B., Wolf, L., Dupont, B., and Reisner, Y.**, Transplantation of marrow depleted of T cells by soybean lectin agglutination and E rosette depletion. Major histocompatibility complex related graft resistance in leukemic transplant recipients, *Transplant. Proc.*, 17, 455, 1985.
14. **Weiden, P. L., Sullivan, K. M., Fluornoy, N., Storb, R., and Thomas, E. D.**, Antileukemic effect of chronic graft versus host disease, *N. Eng. J. Med.*, 304, 1529, 1981.
15. **Bacigalupo, A., Van Lint, M. T., Frassoni, F., and Marmont, A.**, Graft versus leukemia effect following allogeneic bone marrow transplantation, *Br. J. Hemato.*, 61, 749, 1985.
16. **Liu Yin, J. A., Gordon-Smith, E. C., Hows, J. M., Goldman, J., and Chipping, P.**, Bone marrow transplants from unrelated donors, *Exp. Hematol.*, 12 (Suppl. 15), 40, 1984.
17. **De Witte, T., Raymakers, R., Plas, A., Koekman, E., Wessels, H., and Haanen, C.**, Bone marrow repopulation capacity after transplantation of lymphocyte depleted allogeneic bone marrow using counterflow centrifugation, *Transplantation,* 37, 151, 1984.
18. **Gee, A. P., Sleasman, J., Lee, C., Ugelstad, J., and Barrett, D. J.**, T-lymphocyte depletion of bone marrow using monoclonal antibodies and magnetic microspheres, *Exp. Hematol.*, 6, 544, 1986.
19. **Vallera, D. A., Ash, R. C., Zanjani, E. D., LeBien, T. W., Beverly, P. C. L., Neville, D. M., and Youle, R. J.**, Anti-T cell reagents for human bone marrow transplantation: ricin linked to three monoclonal antibodies, *Science,* 222, 512, 1983.
20. **Filipovich, A. H., Vallera, D. A., Youle, R. J., Neville, D. M., and Kersey, J. H.**, *Ex vivo* T cell depletion with immunotoxins in allogeneic bone marrow transplantation: the pilot clinical study for prevention of graft versus host disease, *Transplant. Proc.*, 17, 442, 1985.
21. **Blazar, B. R., Quinones, R. R., Heinitz, K. J., Sevenich, E. A., and Filipovich, A. H.**, Comparison of three techniques for the *ex vivo* elimination of T cells from human bone marrow, *Exp. Hematol.*, 13, 123, 1985.
22. **Kaizer, H. and Chow, H. S.**, Autologous bone marrow transplantation (ABMT) in the treatment of cancer, *Cancer Invest.*, 2, 203, 1984.
23. **Gorin, N. C.**, Collection, manipulation and freezing of haemopoietic stem cells. *Clin. Haematol.*, 15, 19, 1986.
24. **Burnett, A. K., Tansey, P., Watkins, R., Alcorn, M., Maharaj, D., Singer, C. R., McKinnon, S., McDonald, G. A., and Robertson, A. G.**, Transplantation of unpurged autologous marrow in acute myeloid leukemia in first remission, *Lancet,* 2, 1068, 1984.
25. **Takahashi, M. and Singer, J. W.**, Effects of marrow storage at 4°C on the subsequent generation of long term marrow cultures, *Exp. Hematol.*, 13, 691, 1985.

26. **Wells, J. R. and Cline, M. J.,** Preservation of granulopoietic precursors in non frozen stored human bone marrow, *Transplantation,* 22, 568, 1976.
27. **Dicke, K. A., Spitzer, G., and Zander, A. R.,** Autologous Bone Marrow Transplantation: Proceedings of the First International Symposium. University of Texas M. D. Anderson Hospital and Tumor Institute at Houston, Texas, 1985.
28. **Appelbaum, F. R. and Buckner, C. D.,** Overview of the clinical relevance of autologous bone marrow transplantation, *Clin. Hematol.,* 15, 1, 1986.
29. **Dicke, K. A. and Spitzer, G. S.,** Evaluation of the use of high dose cytoreduction with autologous marrow rescue in various malignancies, *Transplantation,* 41, 4, 1986.
30. **Graham-Pole, J. and Gee, A. P.,** Cancer treatment using autologous bone marrow infusions, *J. Fla. Med. Assoc.,* 71, 336, 1984.
31. **Pinkerton, R., Philip, T., Bouffet, E., Lashford, L., and Kemshead, J. T.,** Autologous bone marrow transplantation in paediatric solid tumors, *Clin. Haematol.,* 15, 187, 1986.
32. **Anner, R. M. and Trewinko, B.,** Frequency and significance of bone marrow involvement by metastatic solid tumor, *Cancer,* 38, 1344, 1977.
33. **Estrov, Z., Grunberger, T., Dube, I. D., Wang, Y-P., and Freedman, M. H.,** Detection of residual acute lymphoblastic leukemia cells in cultures of bone marrow obtained during remission, *N. Engl. J. Med.,* 315, 538, 1986.
34. **Kemshead, J. T. and Pritchard, J.,** Neuroblastoma: recent developments and current challenges. *Cancer Surv.,* 3, 691, 1987.
35. **Reynolds,, C. P.,** Microcomputer-based digital imaging for detection of infrequent cells, presented at 3rd Int. Symp. Autologous Bone Marrow Transplantation, Houston, December 4 to 5, 1986.
36. **Bast, R. C. and Ritz, J. C.,** Application of monoclonal antibodies to autologous bone marrow transplantation, in *Biological Response in Cancer,* Vol. 12, Plenum Press, New York, 1984, 185.
37. **Hagenbeek, A. and Martens, A. C.,** Reinfusion of leukemic cells with the autologous marrow graft: preclinical studies on lodging and regrowth of leukemia, *Leuk. Res.,* 9, 1389, 1985.
38. **Burnett, A. K. and McKinnon, S.,** Autologous bone marrow transplantation in first remission using nonpurged marrow, in *Minimal Residual Disease in Acute Leukemia,* Hagenbeek, A., and Lowenberg, B., Eds., Martinus Nijhoff, Dordrecht, The Netherlands, 1986, 211.
39. **Gorin, N. C.,** Autologous bone marrow transplantation for acute leukemia in Europe, *Exp. Hematol.,* 12 (Suppl. 15), 123, 1984.
40. **Stewart, P., Buckner, C. D., Bensinger, W., Appelbaum, F., Fefer, A., Clift, R., Storb, R., Sanders, J., Meyers, J., and Hill, R.,** Autologous marrow transplantation in patients with acute nonlymphocytic leukemia in first remission, *Exp. Hematol.,* 13, 267, 1985.
41. **O'Reilly, R. J.,** New promise for autologous transplants in leukemia, *N. Engl. J. Med.,* 315, 186, 1986.
42. **Vartdal, F., Qvalheim, G., Lea, T. E., Bosnes, V., Gaudernack, G., Ugelstad, J., and Albrechtsen, D.,** Depletion of T lymphocytes from human bone marrow. Use of magnetic monosized polymer microspheres coated with T lymphocyte-specific monoclonal antibodies, *Transplantation,* 43, 366, 1987.
43. **Ramsay, N. K. C., LeBien, T. W., Nesbit, M., McGlave, D., Weisdorf, D., Hurd, D., Kenyon, A., and Kersey, J.,** Autologous bone marrow transplantation for acute lymphoblastic leukemia following marrow treatment with BA-1, BA-2, BA-3 and rabbit complement, *Exp. Hematol.,* 12, 461, 1984.
44. **Ritz, J., Sallan, S. E., Bast, R. C., Lipton, J. M., Clavell, L. A., Feeney, M., Hercend, T., Nathan, D. G., and Schlossman, S. F.,** Autologous bone marrow transplantation in CALLA-positive acute lymphoblastic leukemia after *in vitro* treatment with J5 monoclonal antibody and complement, *Lancet,* 2, 60, 1982.
45. **LeBacq-Verheyden, A. M., Humblet, Y., Neirynck, A., Ravoet, A., and Symann, M.,** Four rat cytotoxic monoclonal antibodies for the *in vitro* treatment of bone marrow autografts in non-T, non-B acute lymphoblastic leukemia, in *Autologous Bone Marrow Transplantation,* Dicke, K. A., Spitzer, G., and Zander, A. R., Eds., University of Texas M. D. Anderson Hospital and Tumor Institute, Houston, 1985, 419.
46. **Howell, A. L. and Ball, E. D.,** Monoclonal antibody mediated cytotoxicity of human myeloid leukemia cells: an *in vitro* model for estimating efficiency and optimal conditions for cytolysis, *Blood,* 66, 649, 1985.
47. **Ball, E. D.,** Acute myeloid leukemia/monoclonal antibody purging, presented at 3rd Int. Symp. Autologous Bone Marrow Transplantation, Houston, December 3 to 5, 1986.
48. **Kvalheim, G., Fodstad, O., Pihl, A., Nustad, K., Pharo, A., Ugelstad, J., and Funderud, S.,** Elimination of B lymphoma cells from human bone marrow, I. The use of monodisperse magnetic particles with attached monoclonal antibodies, *Cancer Res.,* 47, 846, 1987.
49. **Favrot, M. C., Philip, I., Philip, T., Pinkerton, R., LeBacq, K., Forster, P., Adeline, P., and Dore, J. F.,** Bone marrow purging procedure in Burkitt lymphoma with monoclonal antibodies and complement, *Br. J. Hematol.,* in press, 1986.
50. **Buckman, R., McIlhinney, R. A. J., Shepherd, V., Patel, S., Coombes, R. C., and Neville, A. M.** Elimination of carcinoma cells from human bone marrow, *Lancet,* 2, 1428, 1982.

51. **Kries, M. S., Vriesendorp, H. P., Gordon, L. I., Kucuk, O., Rosen, S. T., Fey, T. A., McDonough, C., and Prachand, S.**, Autologous bone marrow transplantation in metastatic breast cancer, *Exper. Hematol.* 11 (Suppl. 14), 128, 1983.
52. **Treleaven, J. G., Gibson, F. M., Ugelstad, J., Rembaum, A., Philip, T., Caine, G. D., and Kemshead, J. T.**, Removal of neuroblastoma cells from bone marrow with monoclonal antibodies conjugated to magnetic microspheres, *Lancet,* 1, 70, 1984.
53. **Reynolds, C. P., Seeger, R. C., Vo, D. D., Black, A. T., Wells, J., and Ugelstad, J.**, Model system for removing neuroblastoma cells from bone marrow using monoclonal antibodies and magnetic immunobeads, *Cancer Res.*, 46, 5882, 1986.
54. **Stahel, R. A., Mabry, M., Sabbath, K., Speak, J. A., and Bernal, S. D.**, Selective cytotoxicity of murine monoclonal antibody LAM2 against human small-cell carcinoma in the presence of human complement: possible use for *in vitro* elimination of tumor cells from bone marrow, *Int. J. Cancer,* 35, 587, 1985.
55. **Bernal, S. D., Mabry, M., Stahel, R. A., Griffin, J. D., and Speak, J. A.**, Selective cytotoxicity of SM-1 monoclonal antibody towards small cell carcinoma of the lung, *Cancer Res.* 45, 1026, 1985.
56. **Okabe, T., Kaizu, T., Ozawa, K., Urabe, A., and Takaku, F.**, Elimination of small cell lung cancer cells *in vitro* from human bone marrow by a monoclonal antibody, *Cancer Res.*, 45, 1930, 1985.
57. **Boyle, M. D. P. and Gee, A. P.**, Low antigen density tumor cells — an obstacle to effective autologous bone marrow purging, *Cancer Invest.*, 5, 113, 1987.
58. **Macintyre, E. A.**, The use of monoclonal antibodies for purging autologous bone marrow in the lymphoid malignancies, Clin. Haematol., 15, 249, 1986.
59. **Jansen, J., Falkenburg, J. H. F., Stepan, D. E., and LeBien, T. W.**, Removal of neoplastic cells from autologous bone marrow grafts with monoclonal antibodies, Semin. Hematol., 21, 164, 1984.
60. **Ritz, J., Bast, R. C., Takvorian, T., and Sallan, S. E.**, Clinical applications of monoclonal antibodies in acute leukemia, N.Y. *Ann. Acad. Sci.*, 428, 308, 1984.
61. Human Leucocyte Differentiation Antigens Detected by Monoclonal Antibodies, Proc. 3rd Int. Workshop on Human Leucocyte Differentiation Antigens, Oxford, September 21 to 26, 1986.
62. **Matthay, K. K.**, Monoclonal antibodies in the diagnosis and treatment of childhood diseases, *Adv. Pediatr.*, 32, 101, 1985.
63. **Santos, G. W., Sharkis, S. J., and Colvin, O. M.**, Elimination of acute myelogenous leukemia cells from marrow and tumor suspensions in the rat with 4-hydroperoxycyclophosphamide, *Blood,* 55, 521, 1980.
64. **Herve, P., Tamayo, E., and Peters, A.**, Autologous stem cell grafting in acute myeloid leukemia, technical approach of marrow incubation *in vitro* with pharmacological agents (prerequisite for clinical applications), *Br. J. Haematol.*, 53, 683, 1983.
65. **Kluin-Nelemans, J. C., Martens, A. C. M., Hagenbeek, A., and Lowenberg, B.**, *In vitro* sensitivity of human leukemic clonogenic cells and normal hematopoietic progenitors to Asta Z-7557 is not different, *Exp. Hematol.*, 11 (Suppl. 14), 9, 1983.
66. **Gorin, N. C., Douay, L., and Najman, A.**, Study of the *in vitro* sensitivity of human leukemic cells and normal hematopoietic progenitors to 4-hydroperoxycyclophosphamide (4HC): the interest for the preparation of antileukemic autologous bone marrow transplantation, *Exp. Hematol.*, 10 (Suppl. 13), 14, 1982.
67. **Yeager, A. M., Kaizer, H., Santos, G. W., Saral, R., Colvin, O. M., Stuart, R. K., Braine, H. G., Burke, P. J., Ambinder, R. F., Burns, W. H., Fuller, D. J., Dacis, J. M., Karp, J. E., Stratford May, W., Rowley, S. D., Sensenbrenner, L. L., Vogelsang, G. B., and Wingard, J. R.**, Autologous bone marrow transplantation in patients with acute nonlymphocytic leukemia, using *ex vivo* marrow treatment with 4-hydroperoxycyclophosphamide, *N. Eng. J. Med.*, 315, 142, 1986.
68. **Gorin, N. C.**, Acute myeloid and acute lymphoblastic leukemia/chemopurging, presented at 3rd Int. Symp. Autologous Bone Marrow Transplantation, Houston, December 4 to 5, 1986.
69. **Beran, M.**, Aldophosphamide a new cyclophosphamide derivative for *in vitro* chemotherapy of leukemia, presented at 3rd Int. Symp. Autologous Bone Marrow Transplantation, Houston, December 4 to 5, 1986.
70. **Spitzer, G.**, Chemopurging methods, presented at 3rd Int. Symp. Autologous Bone Marrow Transplantation, Houston, December 4 to 5, 1986.
71. **Janowska, A.**, Biochemical modulation for selected toxicity against leukemic cells, presented at 3rd Int. Symp. Autologous Bone Marrow Transplantation, Houston, December 4 to 5, 1986.
72. **Sieber, F., Rao, S., Rowley, S. D., and Sieber-Blum, M.**, Dye-mediated photolysis of human neuroblastoma cells for autologous bone marrow transplantation, *Blood,* 68, 32, 1986.
73. **Sieber, F. and Sieber-Blum, M.**, Dye-mediated photosensitization of murine neuroblastoma cells, *Cancer Res.*, 46, 2072, 1986.
74. **Porcellini, A.**, Photodynamic purging, presented at 3rd Int. Symp. Autologous Bone Marrow Transplantation, Houston, December 4 to 5, 1986.
75. **Arnon, R. and Sela, M.**, *In vitro* and *in vivo* efficacy of conjugates of daunomycin with anti-tumour antibodies, *Immunol. Rev.*, 62, 5, 1982.

76. **Calendi, E., Constanzi, G., Idiveri, F., Lotti, G., and Zini, C.,** Histo-immunologic specificity of an anti-lymphoid tissue sarcoma gammaglobulin bound to methotrexate, *Bull. Chem. Pharmacol.*, 108, 25, 1969.
77. **De Weger, R. A., Dullens, H. J. F., and Den Otter, W.,** Eradication of murine lymphoma and melanoma cells by chlorambucil antibody complexes, *Immunol. Rev.*, 62, 29, 1982.
78. **Moller, G., Ed.,** Antibody Carriers of Drugs and Toxins in Tumor Therapy, *Immunol. Rev.*, 62, 1982.
79. **Ramakrishnan, S., Uckun, F. M., and Houston, L. L.,** Anti-T cell immunotoxins containing pokeweed anti-viral protein: potential purging agents for human autologous bone marrow transplantation, *J. Immunol.*, 135, 3616, 1985.
80. **Olsnes, S. and Pihl, A.,** Abrin, ricin and their associated agglutinins, in *Receptors and Recognition*, Cuatrecasas, P., Ed., Chapman and Hall, London, 1976, 129.
81. **Olsnes, S., Refsnes, K., and Pihl, A.,** Mechanisms of action of the toxic lectins abrin and ricin, *Nature*, 249, 627, 1974.
82. **Leonard, J. E., Taetle, R., To, D., and Rhyner, K.,** Preclinical studies on the use of selective antibody-ricin conjugates in autologous bone marrow transplantation, *Blood*, 65, 1149, 1985.
83. **Thorpe, P. E., Mason, D. W., Brown, A. N. F., Simmonds, S. J., Ross, W. C. J., Cumber, A. J., and Forrester, J. A.,** Selective killing of malignant cells in a leukemic rat bone marrow using an antibody ricin conjugate, *Nature*, 297, 594, 1982.
84. **Vallera, D. A., Youle, R. J., Neville, D. M., Soderling, C. C. B., and Kersey, J. H.,** Monoclonal antibody toxin conjugates for experimental graft-versus-host disease prophylaxis. Reagents selectively reactive with T cells and not murine stem cells, *Transplantation*, 36, 73, 1983.
85. **Weiss, L., Morecki, S., Vitteta, E. S., and Slavin, S.,** Suppression and elimination of BCL_1 leukemia by allogeneic bone marrow transplantation, *J. Immunol.*, 130, 2452, 1983.
86. **Jansen, F. K., Blythman, H. E., and Carriere, D.,** Replacement of the B chain of ricin with specific conventional or monoclonal antibodies, in *Receptor-mediated Binding and Internalization of Toxins and Hormones*, Middlebrook, J. L., and Kohn, D., Eds., Academic Press, Orlando, 1981, 351.
87. **Casellas, P., Bourrie, B. J. P., Gros, P., and Jansen, F. K.,** Kinetics of cytotoxicity induced by immunotoxin: enhancement by lysosomotropic amines and carboxylic ionophores, *J. Biol. Chem.*, 257, 9359, 1984.
88. **Herrman, R., Pelham, J., Meyer, B., Davis, R., Raphael, C., Kraft, N., and Atkins, R.,** An immunotoxin for immunologic manipulation of marrow *ex vivo* in autologous transplantation for acute lymphoblastic leukemia, *Transplant. Proc.*, 18, 278, 1986.
89. **Vallera, D. A., Ash, R. C., Zanjani, E. D., Kersey, J. H., LeBien, T. W., Beverly, P. C., Neville, D. M., and Youle, R. J.,** Anti-T cell reagents for human bone marrow transplantation. Ricin linked to three monoclonal antibodies, *Science*, 222, 512, 1983.
90. **Laurent, G.,** Chemopurging — immunotoxins, presented at 3rd Int. Symp. Autologous Bone Marrow Transplantation, Houston, December 4 to 5, 1986.
91. **Gee, A. P.,** Molecular titration of the components of the classical complement pathway, *Methods Enzymol.*, 93, 339, 1983.
92. **Netzel, B., Haas, R. J., Rodt, H., Kolb, H. J., and Thierfelder, S.,** Immunological conditioning of bone marrow for autotransplantation in childhood acute lymphoblastic leukemia, *Lancet*, 1, 1330, 1980.
93. **Ohanian, S. H., Yamazaki, M., Schlager, S. I., and Faibisch, M.,** Cell growth dependent variation in the sensitivity of human and mouse tumor cells to complement-mediated killing, *Cancer Res.*, 43, 491, 1983.
94. **Spiegelberg, H. L.,** Biological activities of immunoglobulins of different classes and subclasses, *Adv. Immunol.*, 19, 259, 1974.
95. **Hale, G., Swirsky, D., Waldmann, H., and Chan, L. C.,** Reactivity of rat monoclonal antibody CAMPATH-1 with human leukemia cells and its possible application for autologous bone marrow transplantation, *Br. J. Haematol.*, 60, 41, 1985.
96. **Clark, M., Cobold, S., Hale, G., and Waldmann, H.,** Advantages of rat monoclonal antibodies, *Immunol. Today*, 4, 100, 1983.
97. **Buckman, R., Shepherd, V., Coombers, R. C., McIlhinney, R. A. J., Patel, S., and Neville, A. M.,** Elimination of carcinoma cells from human bone marrow, *Lancet*, 2, 1428, 1982.
98. **Ohanian, S. H. and Schlager, S. I.,** Humoral immune killing of nucleated cells, I. Mechanisms of complement-mediated attack and target cell defense, CRC *Crit. Rev. Immunol.*, 1, 165, 1981.
99. **Gee, A. P., Bruce, K. M., Van Hilten, J., Siden, E. J., Braylan, R. C., Bauer, P. C., and Boyle, M. D. P.,** Selective loss of expression of a tumor-associated antigen on a human leukemia cell line induced by treatment with monoclonal antibody and complement, *J. Natl. Cancer Inst.*, 78, 29, 1987.
100. **Borsos, T.,** Immunoglobulin classes and complement-fixing activity, *Prog. Immunol.*, 1, 842, 1971.
101. **LeBien, T. W., Stepan, D. E., Bartholomew, R. M., Strong, R. C., and Anderson, J. M.,** Utilization of a colony assay to assess the variables influencing elimination of leukemic cells from human bone marrow, *Blood*, 65, 945, 1985.

102. **Fabritiis, P. D., Bregni, M., Lipton, J., Reynolds, C., Nadler, L., Ritz, J., and Bast, R. C.,** Antigenic heterogeneity among Burkitt's lymphoma cells surviving treatment with monoclonal antibody and complement, *Leuk. Res.,* 10, 35, 1986.
103. **Grob, J. P., Campana, D., Timms, A., Janossy, G., and Prentice, H. G.,** Purging in autologous bone marrow transplantation: importance of antigen density on leukemic blasts for the efficiency of complement-mediated cytolysis, Proc. 2nd Int. Symp. on the Detection and Treatment of Residual Disease in Acute Leukemia, Rotterdam, 84 (Abstr.), 1985.
104. **Shapiro, S. J., Leibson, P. J., Loken, M. R., and Schreiber, H.,** Changes in susceptibility to cytotoxic antibody among tumor cells surviving exposure to chemotherapeutic agents, *Cancer Res.,* 42, 2622, 1982.
105. **Taupier, M. A., Kerney, J. F., Leibson, P. J., Loken, M. R., and Schreiber, H.,** Nonrandom escape of tumor cells from immune lysis due to intraclonal fluctuations in antigen expression, *Cancer Res.,* 43, 4050, 1983.
106. **Saarinen, U. M., Coccia, P. F., Gerson, S. L., Pelley, R., and Chung, N-K. V.,** Eradication of neuroblastoma cells *in vitro* by monoclonal antibody and human complement: method for purging autologous bone marrow, *Cancer Res.,* 45, 5969, 1985.
107. **Courtenay, V. D. and Mills, J.,** An *in vitro* assay for human tumors grown in immune suppressed mice and treated *in vivo* with cytotoxic agents, *Br. J. Cancer,* 37, 261, 1978.
108. **Reynolds, C. P., Black, A. T., and Woody, J. N.,** Sensitive method for detecting viable cells seeded into bone marrow, *Cancer Res.,* 46, 5878, 1986.
109. **Takvorian, T.,** Monoclonal antibody purged autologous bone marrow transplantation for relapsed non-T acute lymphoblastic leukemia, presented at 2nd Int. Symp. on the Detection and Treatment of Minimal Residual Disease in Acute Leukemia, Rotterdam, 1985.
110. **Ramsay, N. K.,** Acute lymphoblastic leukemia/monoclonal antibody purging, presented at 3rd Int. Symp. Autologous Bone Marrow Transplantation, Houston, December 4 to 5, 1986.
111. **Bast, R. C.,** Elimination of T lymphoma cells, presented at 3rd Int. Symp. Autologous Bone Marrow Transplantation, Houston, December 4 to 5, 1986.
112. **Uckun, F. M., Ramakrishnan, S., and Houston, L. L.,** *Ex vivo* elimination of neoplastic T-cells from human marrow using an anti-Mr 41,000 protein immunotoxin: potentiation by Asta Z7557, *Blut,* 50, 19, 1985.
113. **Schlager, S. I., Boyle, M. D. P., Ohanian, S. H., and Borsos, T.,** Effect of inhibiting DNA, RNA and protein synthesis of tumor cells on their susceptibility to killing by antibody and complement, *Cancer Res.,* 37, 1432, 1977.
114. **Boyle, M. D. P., Ohanian, S. H., and Borsos, T.,** Effect of protease treatment on the sensitivity of tumor cells to antibody-GPC killing, *Clin. Immunol. Immunopathol.,* 10, 84, 1978.
115. **Giacomini, P., Aguzzi, A. S., Pestka, S., Fisher, P. B., and Ferrone, S.,** Modulation by recombinant DNA leucocyte (alpha) and fibroblast (beta) interferons of the expression and shedding of HLA- and tumor-associated antigens by melanoma cells, *J. Immunol.,* 133, 1649, 1984.
116. **Liaso, S. K., Kwong, P. C., Khosravi, M., and Dent, P. B.,** Enhanced expression of melanoma-associated antigens and beta 2 microglobulin on cultured human melanoma cells by interferon, *J. Natl. Cancer Inst.,* 68, 19, 1982.
117. **Gee, A. P., Barrett, D. J., Lee, C., Bruce, K., Janssen, W., Ugelstad, J., Kemshead, J., and Gross, S.,** Use of magnetic microspheres and monoclonal antibodies for purging bone marrow in autologous and haplotype-mismatched transplantation, *J. Cell. Biochem.,* Suppl. 10D, 255, 1986.
118. **Borsos, T. and Rapp, H. J.,** Hemolytic titration based on fixation and activation of the first component of complement: evidence that one molecule of hemolysin suffices to sensitize an erythrocyte, *J. Immunol.,* 95, 559, 1965.
119. **Bast, R. C., Ritz, J., Lipton, J. M., Feeney, M., Sallan, S. E., Nathan, D. G., and Schlossman, S. F.,** Elimination of leukemic cells from human bone marrow using monoclonal antibody and complment, *Cancer Res.,* 43, 1389, 1983.
120. **Gee, A. P., Bruce, K. M., Morris, T. D., and Boyle, M. D. P.,** Evidence for an anti-complementary factor associated with human bone marrow cells, *J. Natl. Cancer Inst.,* 75, 441, 1985.
121. **Gee, A. P., Graham-Pole, J., Lee, C., Bruce, K., Pick, T., Harvey, W., Worthington-White, D., Hintz, M., Janssen, W., and Gross, S.,** Transplantation for neuroblastoma using immunomagnetically-purged autologous bone marrow — factors influencing engraftment, presented at 3rd Int. Symp. Autologous Bone Marrow Transplantation, Houston, December 4 to 5 1986.
122. **Dicke, K. A., McCredie, K. B., Spitzer G., Zander, A., Peters, L., Verma, D. S., Stewart, D., Keating, M., and Stevens, F. F.,** Autologous bone marrow transplantation in patients with adult acute leukemia in relapse, *Transplantation,* 26, 269, 1978.
123. **Rubin, P., Wheeler, K. T., Keng, P. C., Gregory, P. K., and Croizot, H.,** The separation of a mixture of bone marrow stem cells from tumor cells: an essential step for autologous bone marrow transplantation, *Int. J. Radiat. Oncol. Biol. Phys.,* 7, 1405, 1981.

124. **Figdor, C. G., Voute, P. A., De Kraker, J., Vernie, L. N., and Bent, W. S.,** Physical cell separation of neuroblastoma cells from bone marrow, in *Advances in Neuroblastoma Research,* Evans, A. E., D'Angio, G. J., and Seeger, R. C., Eds., Alan R. Liss, New York, 1985, 471.
125. **Vellekoop, L., Reading, C. L., and Chandran, M.,** Cell separation on the basis of immunogold-coupled monoclonal antibodies, *Blood,* 60 (Suppl. 1) (Abstr.), 174a, 1982.
126. **Poynton, C. H., Reading, C. L., and Dicke, K. A.,** Colloidal immunomagnetic fluids for cell separation, in *Autologous Bone Marrow Transplantation,* Dicke, K. A., Spitzer, G., and Zander, A. R., Eds., The University of Texas M. D. Anderson Hospital and Tumor Institute at Houston, Texas, 1985, 433.
127. **Reynolds, C. P., Seeger, R. C., Vo, D. D., Ugelstad, J., and Wells, J.,** Purging of bone marrow with immunomagentic beads: studies with neuroblastoma as a model system, in *Autologous Bone Marrow Transplantation,* Dicke, K. A., Spitzer, G. and Zander, A. R., Eds., The University of Texas M. D. Anderson Hospital and Tumor Institute at Houston, Texas, 1985, 439.
128. **Gee, A. P.,** unpublished observations, 1986.
129. **Reading, C. L.,** Leukemia purging/detection of minimal residual disease — monoclonal antibody purging methods, presented at 3rd Int. Symp. Autologous Bone Marrow Transplantation, Houston, Texas, December 4 to 5, 1986.
130. **Ugelstad, J., Soderberg, L., Berge, A., and Hergstrom, J.,** Monodisperse polymer particles — a step forward for chromatography, *Nature,* 303, 96, 1983.
131. **Poynton, C. H., Dicke, K. A., Culbert, S., Frankel, L. S., Jagganath, S., and Reading, C. L.,** Immunomagnetic removal of CALLA positive cells from human bone marrow, *Lancet,* 1, 524, 1983.
132. **Ugelstad, J., Kaggerud, K. H., Hansen, F. K., and Berge, A.,** Absorption of low molecular weight compounds in aqueous dispersions of polymer-oligomer particles: a two step swelling process of polymer particles giving an enormous increase in absorption capacity, *Makromol. Chem.,* 180, 737, 1979.
133. **Ugelstad, J., Mork, P. C., Kaggerud, K. H., Ellingsen, T., and Berge, A.,** Swelling of oligomer particles. New methods of preparation of emulsions and polymer dispersions, *Adv. Colloid Interface Sci.,* 13, 1010, 1980.
134. **Ugelstad, J., Mork, P. C., Berge, A., Ellingsen, T., and Khan, A. A.,** Effects of additives on the formation of monomer emulsions and polymer dispersions, in *Emulsion Polymerization,* Purma, I., Ed., Academic Press, New York, 1982.
135. **Kemshead, J. T.,** personal communication, 1985.
136. **Gee, A. P., Bruce, K., Lee, C., Bauer, P. C., Janssen, W., and Gross, S.,** Depletion of cALLa-positive leukemia cells from bone marrow using monoclonal antibodies and magnetic microspheres, *Proc. Am. Assoc. Cancer Res.,* 27, 367, 1986.
137. **Gee, A. P., Gross, S., Lee, C., Bruce, K., Ugelstad, J., Kemshead, J. T., and Barrett, D. J.,** Immunomagnetic removal of cell subpopulations from bone marrow that is to be used for autologous transplantation, presented at 6th Int. Congr. Immunol., Toronto, July 6 to 11, 1986.
138. **Gee, A. P., Lee, C., Bruce, K., Janssen, W., Graham-Pole, J., and Gross, S.,** High efficiency immunomagnetic depletion of cALLa-positive leukemia cells from bone marrow, in Proc. 3rd Natl. Leuk. Soc. Am. Symp., Leukemia, (Abstr.) 1, 275, 1987.
139. **Gaudernack, G., Leivestad, T., Ugelstad, J., and Thorsby, E.,** Isolation of pure functionally active CD8+ T cells: positive selection with monoclonal antibodies directly conjugated to monosized magnetic microspheres, *J. Immunol., Methods,* 90, 179, 1986.
140. **Philip, T., Bernard, J. L., Zucker, J. M., Pinkerton, R., Lutz, P., Bordigoni, P., Plouvier, E., Robert, A., Carton, R., Phillipe, N., Philip, I., and Favrot, M.,** High dose chemoradiotherapy with bone marrow transplantation as consolidation treatment in neuroblastoma: an unselected group of stage IV patients over one year of age, manuscript in preparation, 1986.
141. **Seeger, R. C., Wells, J., Lenarsky, C., Feig, S. A., Selch, M., Moss, T. J., Ugelstad, J., and Reynolds, C. P.,** Bone marrow transplantation for poor prognosis neuroblastoma, *J. Cell. Biochem.,* Suppl. 10D, 215, 1986.
142. **Kemshead, J. T.,** personal communication, 1986.
143. **Favrot, M.,** Purging in neuroblastoma, presented at 3rd Int. Symp. Autologous Bone Marrow Transplantation, Houston, December 4 to 5, 1986.
144. **Favrot, M. C., Philip, I., Combaret, V., Frappaz, D., Pinkerton, R., Ugelstad, J., Portoukalian, J., Dore, J. F., and Philip, T.,** Experimental evaluation of an immunomagnetic bone marrow procedure using the Burkitt lymphoma model, *J. Immunol. Methods,* 1986, In press.
145. **Seeger, R. C.,** Purging in neuroblastoma, presented at 3rd Int. Symp. Autologous Bone Marrow Transplantation, Houston, December 4 to 5, 1986.
146. **Kemshead, J. T., Treleaven, J., Heath, L., O'Meara, A., Gee, A., and Ugelstad, J.,** Monoclonal antibodies and magnetic microspheres for the depletion of leukaemic cells from bone marrow harvested for autologous transplantation, *Bone Marrow Transpl.,* 2, 133, 1987.
147. **Lefkovits, I. and Waldmann, H.,** Limiting dilution analysis of cells of the immune system, *Immunol. Today,* 5, 265, 1984.

148. **Thierfelder, S., Rodt, H., and Netzel, B.,** Transplantation of syngeneic bone marrow incubated with leukocyte antibodies, I. Suppression of lymphatic leukemia of syngeneic donor mice, *Transplantation,* 23, 459, 1977.
149. **Trigg, M. E. and Poplack, D. G.,** Transplantation of leukemic bone marrow treated with cytotoxic antileukemic antibodies and complement, *Science,* 217, 259, 1982.
150. **Economou, J. S., Shin, H. S., Kaizer, H., Santos, G. W., and Schron, D. S.,** Bone marrow transplantation in cancer therapy: inactivation by antibody and complement of tumor cells in mouse syngeneic marrow transplants, *Proc. Soc. Exp. Biol. Med.,* 158, 449, 1978.
151. **Feeney, M., Knapp, R. C., Greenberger, J. S., and Bast, R. C.,** Elimination of leukemic cells from rat bone marrow using antibody and complement, *Cancer Res.,* 41, 3331, 1981.
152. **Krolick, K. A., Uhr, J. W., and Vitteta, E. S.,** Selective killing of leukaemia cells by antibody-toxin conjugates: implications for autologous bone marrow transplantation, *Nature,* 295, 604, 1982.
153. **Douay, L., Gorin, N. C., Mary, J. Y., Lemaire, E., Lopez, M., Najman, A., Stachowiak, J., Giarratana, M. C., Baillou, C., Salmon, C., and Duhamel, G.,** Recovery of CFU- GM from cryopreserved marrow and *in vivo* evaluation after autologous bone marrow transplantation are predictive of engraftment, *Exp. Hematol.,* 14, 358, 1986.
154. **Knight, W. A., Roodman, G., and Clarke, G. M.,** Correlation of colony forming units — granulocyte, erythrocyte, megakaryocyte, macrophage "CFU-GEMM" with marrow recovery following autologous bone marrow transplantation "ABMT", *Proc. Am. Assoc. Cancer Res.,* 24, 163, 1983.
155. **Dexter, R. M., Allen, T. D., and Lajtha, L. G.,** Conditions controlling the proliferation of hemopoietic stem cells, *in vitro, J. Cell. Physiol.,* 91, 335, 1979.
156. **Gordon, M. Y., Hibbin, J. A., Kerney, L. U., Gordon-Smith, E. C., and Goldman, J. M.,** Colony formation by primitive hemopoietic progenitors in cocultures of bone marrow cells and stromal cells, *Br. J. Haematol.,* 60, 129, 1985.
157. **Gordon, M. Y., Hibbin, J. A., Dowding, C., Gordon-Smith, E. C., and Goldman, J. M.,** Separation of human blast progenitors from granulocytic, erythroid, megakaryocytic and mixed colony forming cells by "panning" on cultured marrow derived stromal layers, *Exp. Hematol.,* 13, 937, 1985.

NOTE ADDED IN PROOF

References which refer to presentations at the Third International Symposium on Autologous Bone Marrow Transplantation have now been published in *Autologous Bone Marrow Transplantation, Proceedings of the Third International Symposium,* Dicke, K. A., Spitzer, G., and Jagannath, S., Eds., University of Texas M.D. Anderson Hospital and Tumor Institute at Houston, 1987.

Chapter 8

MOLECULAR APPROACHES TOWARDS THE ISOLATION OF PEDIATRIC CANCER PREDISPOSITION GENES

John K. Cowell

TABLE OF CONTENTS

I. INTRODUCTION

The majority of human cancers appear to occur sporadically within the population, but it is becoming more apparent that, in a few cases, genetic determinants are involved. In polyposis coli, medullary carcinoma of the thyroid, and neurofibromatosis, the inheritance of a predisposition to malignancy is well established[1] although the location and the identity of these predisposing genes is unknown. Familial clustering of some breast cancer cases suggests a genetic basis for this disease, though the complexities of the pedigrees prevent the emergence of a clear pattern. Our ability to isolate and characterize the genetic defects in conditions such as these will, undoubtedly, increase our understanding of the initial stages of neoplasia and offer an opportunity for the prenatal prediction of those at risk. The analysis of two particular childhood cancers, Wilms' tumor and retinoblastoma, has been particularly important since the location of the predisposition loci are known and, in retinoblastoma, the means for effective prenatal diagnosis are now available.

In this article the events leading to the identification of the predisposition loci, their genetic and molecular analysis, and how this information can be used in prenatal diagnosis and management of pediatric cancers will be reviewed. All of the techniques discussed here are also proving powerful tools in the analysis of other human disease processes.

II. GENE TRACKING

The principle of following disease phenotypes through families is known as "gene tracking" and requires that the location of the disease locus is known. The distance between two given genetic loci can be defined in two ways; actual physical distance and relative recombination distance. As its name implies, "physical distance" can be defined as the number of basepairs (bp), or thousands of basepairs — kilobases (kb) — between the two loci. The recombination distance is determined by the frequency with which genetic recombination occurs between given loci. In general, the farther the two loci are apart, the greater the chance of recombination. However, within the genome, there are some areas which show proportionately more recombination events and others which show fewer events than might be expected considering the physical distance between the two loci, a phenomenon illustrated by the long arm of the X chromosome.[2] This concept is important when discussing gene tracking strategies since too frequent recombination between marker and disease loci makes prenatal prediction unreliable.

Successful gene tracking depends on being able to distinguish between chromsomes derived from both parents. This distinction is made using natural variations — polymorphisms — at individual genetic loci, due either to different electrophoretic mobilities of the gene product,[3] or to natural variations in DNA sequences around the locus of interest. Whatever the tracking system, if the chromosome region derived from the affected transmitting parent can be unequivocally identified, the inheritance of that gene can be followed. As the use of DNA polymorphisms is the most versatile[4] system, this will be considered in more detail below.

A. Restriction Fragment Length Polymorphisms

Restriction enzymes cleave DNA at specific recognition sequences usually composed of 4 base pairs (bp), such as the one recognized by the enzyme Sau 3A, AGTC, or 6 bp, such as GAATTC, recognized by Eco R1. Less frequently, restriction enzyme sites involve larger numbers of bases and these special enzymes will be discussed in more detail later.

When total genomic DNA is "cut" with a particular enzyme, a heterogeneous population of characteristic restriction fragments is produced. Each fragment has a fixed length, the restriction fragment length (RFL). Agarose gels can be used to separate these fragments

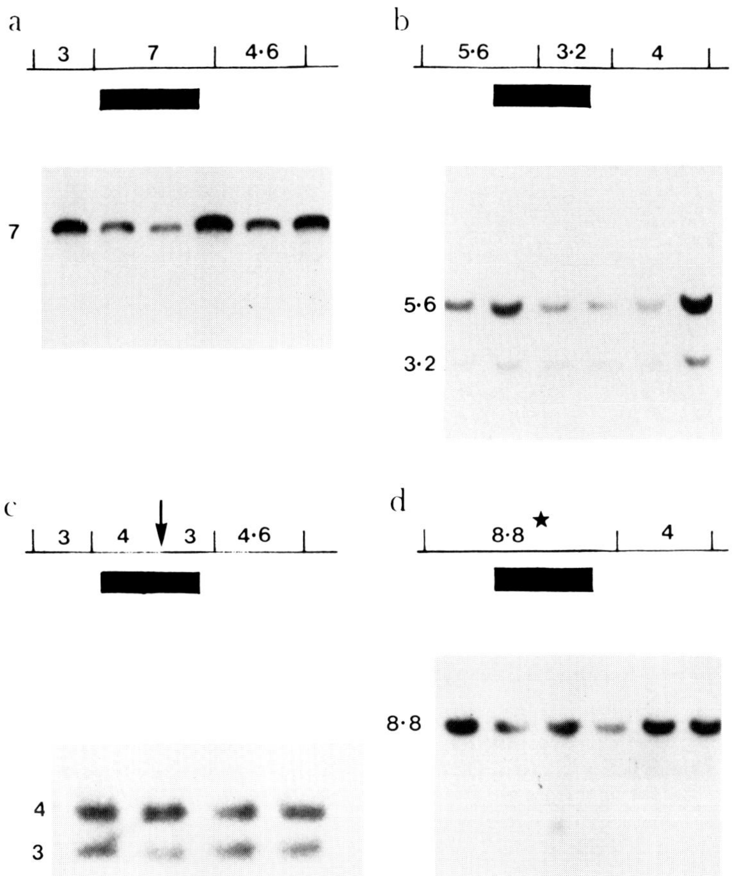

FIGURE 1. Diagrammatical interpretation of the production of restriction band patterns on an autoradiograph. A linear genomic sequence is represented by a continuous line on which specific restriction enzyme sites have been marked by vertical lines. The distance between the adjacent sites is indicated by a number and is in kilobases. Homology between the probe (solid box) and a single restriction fragment 7 kb long produces a single band on the autoradiograph (a). If the enzyme used to digest the genomic DNA has a restriction site within the region of homology (b), then two bands are produced on the autoradiograph. If this internal site (indicated by the arrow) is lost, then a single band is produced with the sum length of the two original bands (d). Alternatively, if a restriction site is generated (indicated by the arrow) within the region of homology with the probe (compare a and c), then two smaller bands are produced (c). All of these changes have occurred within the region of homology with the probe. (From *Cancer Surv.*, 3, 573, 1985. With permission of L. M. Franks, Executive Editor.)

according to size. Using standard techniques, developed by Southern[5] and Rigby et. al.,[6] radioactive DNA probes can be used to hybridize with, i.e., "recognize", homologous sequences within the heterogenous population. This homology is manifested as a band (or set of bands) on an autoradiograph at one or more specific locations determined by the size of the fragment being recognized (Figure 1). If there is no sequence variation between individuals in the region of the chromosome recognized by the probe, a consistent band pattern is produced at the same position on the gel. However, any variation in DNA sequence that affects a given restriction site, such that an existing one is removed or a new one is created, will generate variations in the band pattern observed. Since the bands produced are polymorphic, the variation is referred to as a restriction fragment length polymorphism (RFLP). This principle is illustrated in Figure 2. If an individual is heterozygous for the polymorphic variants, then both of the individual homologous chromosomes can be identified (see Figure 2). Differences in DNA sequence at the same locus are allelic and the bands produced on the autoradiograph are conveniently referred to as alleles.

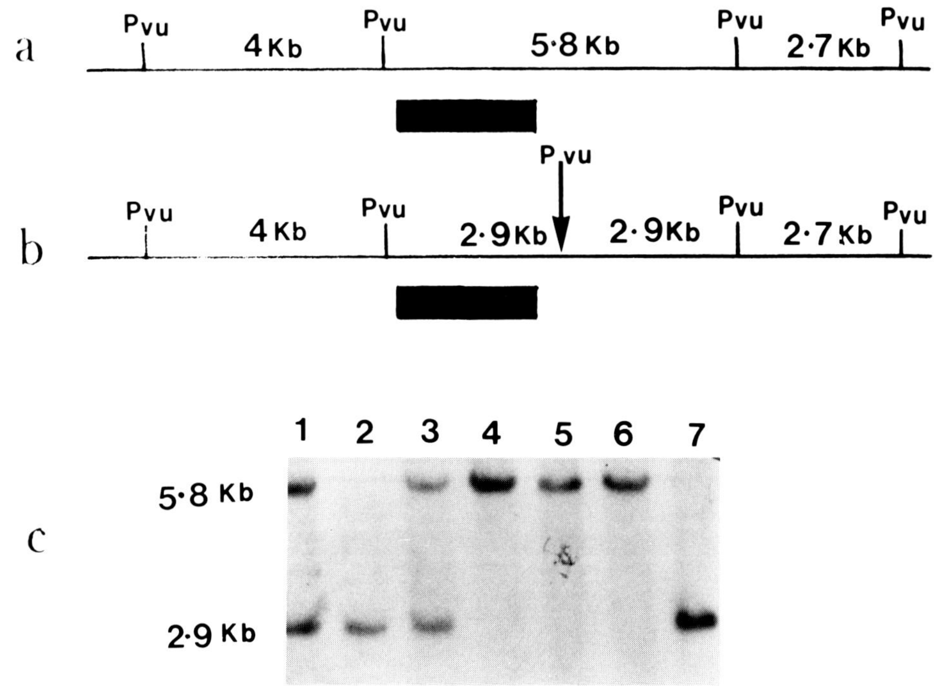

FIGURE 2. A restriction fragment length polymorphism identified in total genomic human DNA digested with the restriction enzyme Pvu I. The probe (indicated by the filled box) recognizes a 5.8 kb restriction fragment (a) and produces the corresponding band on the autoradiograph (c). The generation of a new Pvu I site (indicated by the arrow) within this 5.8 kb fragment produces two fragments 2.9 kb long. The probe now only has homology with a single 2.9 kb fragment and produces the correspondingly smaller band on the autoradiograph (c). Homozygotes for the 5.8 kb band (lanes 4, 5, and 6) in (c) have a single band in the appropriate position as do homozygotes for the 2.9 kb band (lines 2 and 7). Heterozygotes have both bands (lanes 1 and 3). (From *Cancer Surv.*, 3, 573, 1985. With permission of L. M. Franks, author.)

B. Linkage

RFLPs are useful only if they show tight linkage to the disease locus. The degree of linkage can be determined by an analysis of the segregation of the disease and marker loci in families. Loose linkage can be useful in preliminary studies by identifying the part of the genome containing the disease locus. If the two loci recombine too freely, however, prenatal diagnosis is unreliable. The more closely linked the two loci, the more confident the prenatal prediction. For example, if the frequency of recombination between two loci is 10%, then the prediction may be wrong one time in ten, whereas, if the frequency of recombination is only 1%, then, theoretically, errors are reduced to only one in 100. The estimate of the linkage distance between the two loci, however, is a mathematical consideration dependent upon variables, such as the number of meioses and recombination events included in the calculation. The results of the analysis are presented as a ''lod score'': the log of the odds that the two loci are not linked. In practice a lod score of 3 (1000:1 chance) is taken to indicate linkage. Gene tracking achieves maximum accuracy if there are zero recombinations between the disease and marker loci. This is achieved if the probe is the gene itself. This principle has been well illustrated in both thalassemia and phenylketonuria where defects in the β-globin gene and phenylalanine-hydroxylase gene, respectively, are responsible for the two diseases. In each case, the gene producing the disease has been cloned and used in prenatal diagnosis.[7,8] This approach cannot yet be used to detect individuals at risk to cancer predisposition syndromes since, with the possible exception of retinoblastoma (see later), the nature and location of the responsible genetic defect is unknown.

Unless there is a specific DNA defect that causes a consistent band change, the isolation

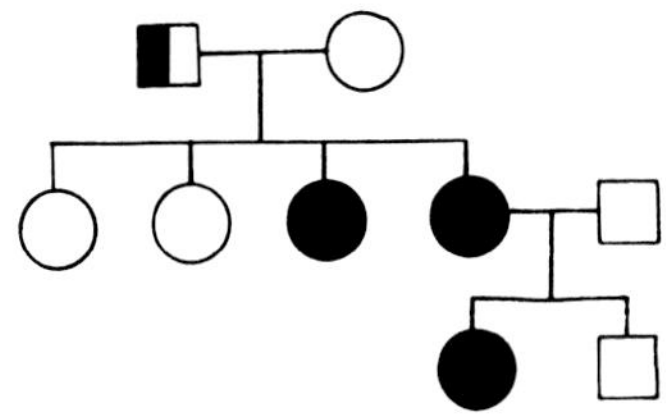

FIGURE 3. Segregation of the retinoblastoma phenotype in a pedigree from a family showing dominant inheritance of the Rb gene. (□) Male, (○) female, (◧) unilaterally affected male,(●) bilaterally affected female.

of the gene itself does not necessarily indicate that prenatal diagnosis will be available for all families. This has been shown in hemophilia A[9] where, even though the factor VIII gene responsible for the phenotype is available, it must still be used in combination with neighboring anonymous DNA probes for maximum effectiveness in counseling.

In the absence of gene probes, the problems of recombination can be further overcome by using flanking DNA markers, i.e., those on either side of the disease locus. In this case, individual recombination events can be observed and incorporated in the counseling and risk assessment. Only in cases where there are double recombination events between both markers and the disease locus will this approach be ineffective. In practice, if both flanking markers are closely linked, the chance of two adjacent recombination events is very small.

III. RETINOBLASTOMA

Retinoblastoma (Rb) is an intraocular eye tumor affecting young children. Most cases are diagnosed before the age of 5 and the disease rarely occurs after the age of 11. If tumors remain within the confines of the eye, Rb has the best prognosis of all childhood cancers; if the tumor escapes the orbit, it has the worst prognosis. Metastasis usually occurs down the optic nerve to the brain and central nervous system.

The incidence of Rb in the Western World is about 1:20,000 live births, although in some Third World countries it is reportedly higher.[10] In these cases, it is difficult to determine whether the relatively high incidence is related to incomplete ascertainment of other types of cancer or to interpopulation variation in the incidence of genetic predisposition.

The majority of Rb are apparently sporadic, but a significant proportion are hereditary and demonstrate autosomal dominant inheritance with high penetrance (Figure 3). Hereditary cases are usually bilateral, multifocal, and have an earlier age of onset compared with the sporadic cases which tend to be unifocal and unilateral.[11] These observations led Knudson[12] to postulate a "two-hit" hypothesis for the development of Rb and other hereditary cancers. Knudson assumed that Rb behaves as a recessive trait at the cellular level and that expression of the malignant phenotype requires mutation of both normal counterparts of the gene. Without a second "hit", all retinal cells would be expected to produce tumors which is clearly not the case. Sporadic appearance of a tumor results from at least two post-zygotic mutations. The chances of two such random events is very low and accounts for the unilateral, unifocal nature of sporadic tumors. In the hereditary cases, however, the "first hit" is inherited. Since the chances of one additional event occurring are relatively high, more cells will be affected and tumors will develop earlier in life. The mean age of onset of the hereditary tumors is 10 months compared with 18 months for the sporadic cases.

The proportion of patients with hereditary Rb varies from study to study. Vogel[11] estimated that hereditary, bilateral tumors constituted 40% of the total. In a study of over 1100 cases in the U.K.,[13] approximately 50% were bilateral. From a subset of these cases, 23% showed a family history.[14] It is not always possible to demonstrate unequivocally that bilateral cases

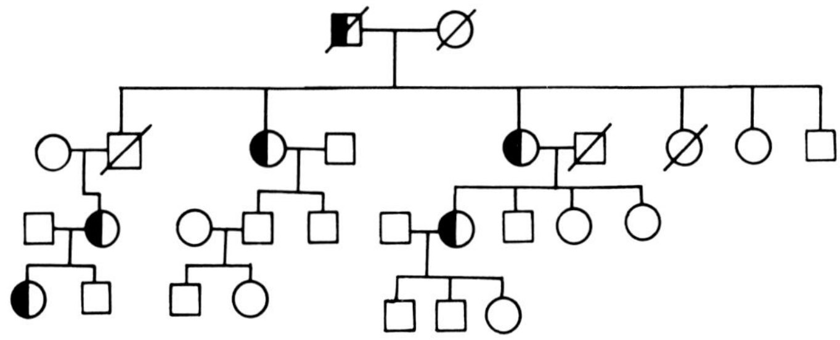

FIGURE 4. Segregation of the retinoblastoma phenotype in a family where there are only unilaterally affected individuals. (□) Male, (○) female, (⧄, ∅) deceased, (◧, ◑) unilaterally affected.

are hereditary since these patients, aware of the risks, usually have small families often without affected children. However, we noted that in 15% of families, the initial transmitting individual was unilaterally affected (Figure 4). These observations have a direct bearing on the relative risks given to individuals seeking genetic counseling. In practice, the hereditary nature of Rb means that all siblings and children of Rb patients are screened regularly during the first few years of life. These examinations take the form of ophthalmoscopy under anesthetic. The 90% success rate in treatment of Rb may have influenced the increased frequency of hereditary cases seen in our series. Early diagnosis means that conservative treatment with laser beam, cryosurgical procedures, or cobalt plaque implantation, is possible. These procedures selectively destroy the tumor without significantly affecting surrounding tissue. Therefore, depending on where the tumor occurs on the retina, it may be possible to save the individual's sight. More advanced tumors require more drastic treatment, such as external beam irradiation, to which Rb has been shown to be particularly sensitive. The most drastic treatment is to remove the eye.

A. Chromosome Analysis

The dominant Mendelian inheritance of Rb strongly implies a single gene effect. The first clues to the location of the gene came from cytogenetic studies in a small group of patients with Rb, who also often had other congenital abnormalities including mental retardation which suggested a constitutional deletion on one of the D-group chromosomes. Subsequent G-banding analysis implicated chromosome 13. Compiling the data from several reports[11] suggested a subregion of band 13q14 was always deleted (Figure 5). The principle of this analysis is shown in Figure 6. Several reports have reached conflicting conclusions concerning the exact location of the Rb locus. From high resolution cytogenetic analysis of a tiny deletion, Yunis and Ramsay[15] suggested that region 13q14.2 was the most likely candidate, whereas, Sparkes et al.[16] and Ward et al.[17] favored 13q14.1. Subband deletions in several of our own patients involve only half of band 13q14, but it has not been possible to determine whether these deletions are proximal or distal. A patient with normal ESD levels but a deletion of 13q14-q31 shows a breakpoint which appears to be in the distal half of q14.[18] These observations would suggest a more distal location of the Rb gene in 13q14.2-q14.3.

The frequency of deletion cases in the population is only about 4%.[14] Evidence indicating the same locus in the hereditary nondeletion form of the disease came from linkage studies using the esterase-D gene (ESD) which has also been mapped to chromosome 13.[19] Sparkes et al.[20] showed that patients with heterozygous 13q14 deletions had levels of the enzyme in red blood cells which were approximately 50% that of normal. Reduced activity was associated with the smallest deletions, placing the ESD gene very close to the Rb locus. The ESD enzyme has been shown to have two electrophoretic variants, type 1 and type 2.[21] Using this polymorphism, Sparkes et al.[22] were able to show close linkage between hereditary

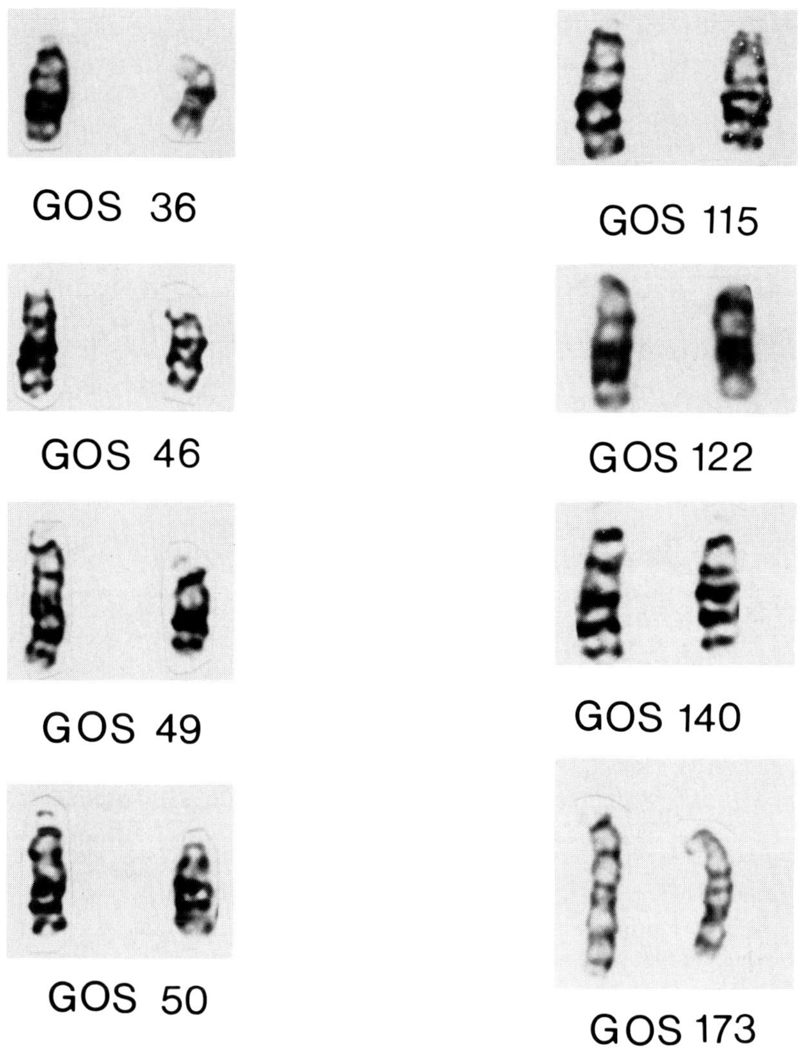

FIGURE 5. Chromosome 13 pairs from eight retinoblastoma patients. The normal homologue is presented on the left in all cases and the deleted chromosome on the right.

Rb and ESD, confirming the localization of the hereditary, nondeletion form of the disease to 13q14.

Abnormalities of chromosome 13 are also implicated in sporadic tumors. Direct chromosome analysis of tumor cells has shown considerable variability. Balaban-Malenbaum et al.[23] reported deletions of 13q14 in 5/6 tumors but this finding was not confirmed by others.[24,25] In an extensive analysis, Squire et al.[26] showed rearrangement of chromosome 13 in only 3 of 27 tumors. In contrast, aneuploidy for chromosome arms 6p and 1q were observed in 15/27 and 21/27, respectively. The involvement of iso-6p had also been reported previously.[25,27] This abnormality was originally thought to be iso-17q, but somatic cell hybrid studies confirmed the involvement of chromosome 6.[27]

Banding of tumor cell chromosomes is often poor and the possibility of subtle changes in 13q14 cannot always be excluded. Analysis of tumor/normal pairs with polymorphic DNA sequences is likely to provide a better indication of the reorganization of the genetic material on chromosome 13.

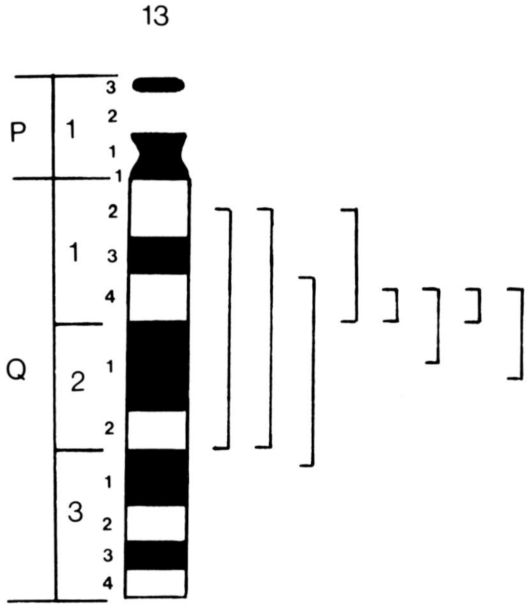

FIGURE 6. Diagrammatical representation of the extent of the eight chromosome deletions presented in Figure 5; the minimum region of overlap is only a subregion of band 13q14.

B. Homozygosity Studies

If Knudson's prediction[12] is correct, precursor tumor cells should be homozygous for the mutant gene. The mutation refers to any disruption of the gene, including deletion and rearrangement, resulting in loss or distortion of function. Several groups have compared the chromosomes from the tumor cells with those in normal tissues in the same individual. Cavenee et al.[28] and Dryja et al.[29] showed that patients heterozygous for chromosome 13 specific probes in normal tissues became homozygous at these loci in the tumors so demonstrating the loss of one allele in the tumor cells. Was this due to the generation of hemizygosity, homozygosity, deletion, or some other mechanism? In some cases chromosome analysis of the tumor cells showed that two copies of chromosome 13 were still present. Dosage studies on the bands produced on the autoradiographs in other tumors also suggested that two copies of chromosome 13 were retained. Thus, simple loss of one copy of chromosome 13 was excluded. Nondisjunction of the chromosome carrying the mutant Rb allele and loss of the corresponding normal chromosome seemed the more likely explanation (Figure 7). Alternatively, homozygosity over large regions of the chromosome, generated as a result of mitotic recombination, may have occurred (see Figure 7). Evidence for this mechanism has been presented recently by Cavenee et al.[30] Furthermore, Cavenee et al.[30] were able to show that, when nondisjunction did occur, it was the chromosome which was inherited from the affected parent which was retained in the tumor. Similarly, using the ESD protein polymorphism, Godbout et al.[31] were able to demonstrate generation of homozygosity in Rb tumors.

C. Chromosome Translocations

Genetic predisposition to Rb can also result from chromosome rearrangements[32-34] such as translocations, inversions, and insertions. The chromosome rearrangement is usually carried in a "balanced" form by the parent who is unaffected; inheritance of the unbalanced form confers the predisposition because of a net loss of material from q14. Figure 8 shows an apparently balanced chromosome translocation from an Rb patient. The ESD levels from

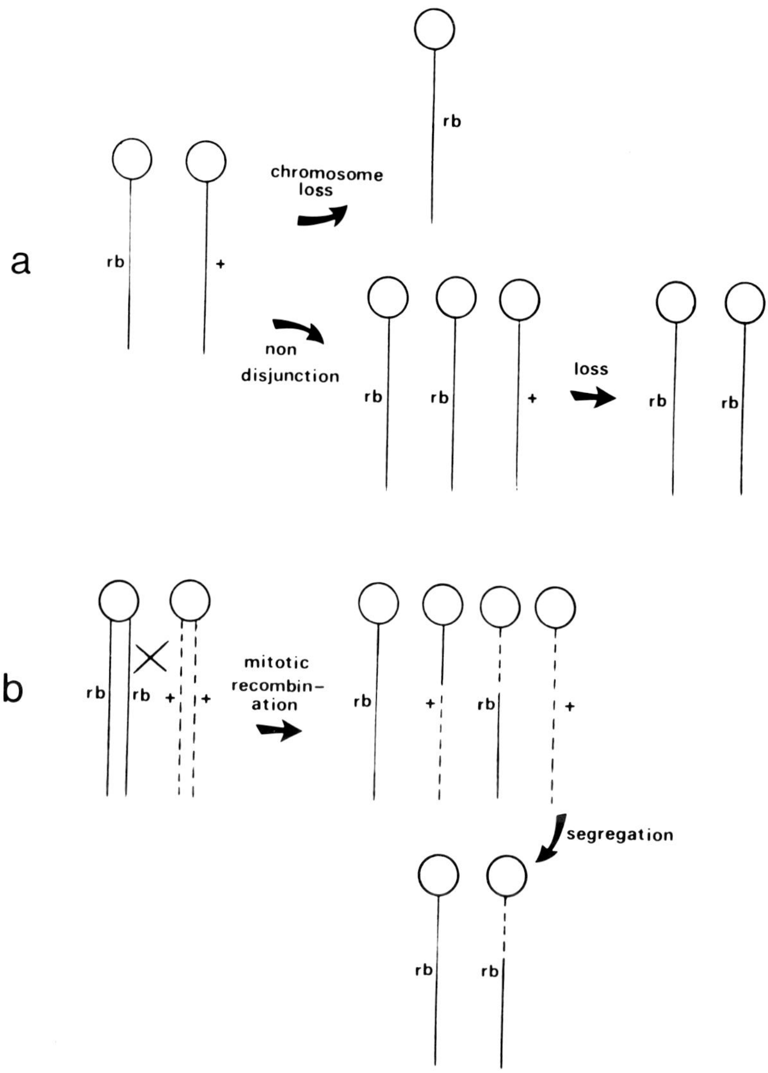

FIGURE 7. Mechanisms for the generation of homozygosity in retinoblastoma cells. Cells which are heterozygous for the predisposing "rb" allele (a) can either lose the normal chromosome altogether, thereby becoming hemizygous for "rb" or, as a result of nondisjunction, could acquire a second copy of the "rb"-bearing chromosome. Loss of the chromosome with the normal (+) allele in these cells results in homozygosity for "rb". Mitotic recombination (b) can reorganize the "rb" alleles such that, with appropriate segregation, individual cells can become homozygous for "rb" without any chromosome loss.

red blood cells from this patient were normal suggesting that the breakpoint in this case has occurred within the coding sequence of the Rb gene or its control elements. In two other cases, the translocation has involved the relocation of 13q14 onto the X chromosome.[35,36] The apparent random inactivation of the derivative chromosome responsible for tumor development represents a functional, rather than a physical, deletion of the Rb locus.

D. N-myc Expression

Analysis of chromosome translocations has failed to implicate the involvement of any oncogene in the genesis of Rb although dosage studies in tumors have shown an elevated level of the N-myc oncogene in one case associated with double minute chromosomes.[26]

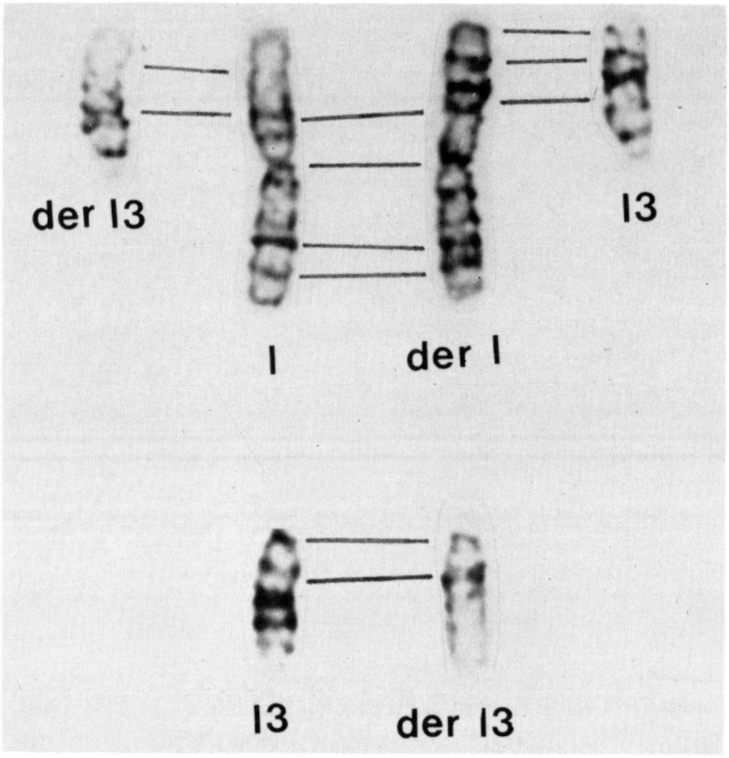

FIGURE 8. Partial trypsin-Giemsa banded karyotype from a patient with retinoblastoma who carried a constitutional chromosome translocation involving chromosomes 1 and 13. The breakpoint on chromosome 13 is at band q14, the site of the retinoblastoma predisposition locus.

One cell line, Y79, contains a homogeneously staining chromosome region.[37,38] Both these chromosome abnormalities have been shown to represent the cytological manifestation of gene amplification.[39] Squire et al.[26] were able to analyze chromosomes in tumors from different foci in the same patient, but failed to reveal a consistent pattern of chromosome abnormality suggesting that most of these changes probably represent events associated with progression, rather than with initiation of the tumor. Squire et al.[40] confirmed this suggestion with the analysis of N-myc expression in normal and tumor tissue. Only tumors showing genomic amplification of N-myc had elevated mRNA levels. N-myc expression was present in normal adult tissues, including brain and retina, and N-myc mRNA levels in retinoblastoma cells were the same as those seen in normal fetal tissue. Thus N-myc expression in tumors probably reflects the origin of the cells rather than indicating a role in oncogenic transformation.

E. Mental Retardation

The close linkage between ESD and Rb has been used for the identification of 13q14 deletions in the Rb population.[14] ESD levels can be measured quickly in lysates of red blood cells and individuals with deletions show 50% normal levels. In a preliminary survey, we analyzed samples from 200 patients[14] and detected eight deletions. This study has now been extended to over 400 patients from whom 16 deletions have been identified, a frequency of 4%. Of the patients detected with reduced enzyme levels, 6/14 had not previously been diagnosed. In at least one case,[41] chromosome analysis had been undertaken and pronounced "normal". With only one exception, the newly detected chromosome deletions were very small, and none of the five patients had mental retardation or other congenital abnormalities. Although larger deletions are almost always accompanied by mental retardation, one of our patients with a deletion of 13q12-14 showed only minor developmental delay. Other patients, with the same deletion, had severe mental retardation. It is possible that the exceptional patient is a tissue mosaic. Mental retardation in Rb patients, however, is not always accompanied by a chromosome deletion. In our series, for example, three mentally retarded patients with normal ESD levels were identified. None has a chromosome deletion. Quantitative determination of ESD levels has proved to be an excellent screening method for detection of chromosome deletions. It is not, however, infallible. We have identified one patient[18] with mental retardation and a series of other congenital abnormalities but normal ESD levels. Chromsome analysis revealed a substantial deletion of 13q14-31. Because the ESD level is not affected, it has been concluded that the breakpoint in this case must have occurred between the ESD and Rb loci.

F. Prenatal Diagnosis

1. Chromosome Deletions

Children of patients with 13q-deletions are at risk for inheritance of the abnormality and, hence, for tumor development. Rb patients with large chromosome deletions usually have a variety of other congenital abnormalities, including severe mental retardation, which tend to exclude them from the mating pool. However, patients with small deletions, though predisposed to Rb, often have apparently normal development and reproductive ability. Since ESD quantitation in cord blood samples are comparable with those in mature adults, it is possible to offer prenatal diagnosis to almost all deletion patients. The exceptions are those rare cases where the ESD gene in not involved. This procedure offers a much quicker alternative to standard amniotic cell chromosome analysis. Chromosome deletions can also be detected in this way in cultured chorionic villus (CV) cells.[42] Thus, even allowing the 4 to 5 weeks needed for culture of CV samples, the results can be available after 12 to 13 weeks of pregnancy, significantly sooner than the 18 to 20 weeks that must elapse before cord blood samples can be safely taken.

The first four small deletion patients identified in our series had a negative family history of 13q- associated Rb. The most recent patient diagnosed as a deletion carrier also apparently had sporadic disease with a unilateral tumor and a negative family history. ESD analysis of the parents showed the father had normal levels, but the mother only had 50% normal ESD activity. In both mother and patient, chromosome analysis revealed a small deletion in 13q14. Detailed ophthalmological analysis of the mother showed no retinal abnormality. This family represents the first recognized instance of transmission of a small chromosome deletion and also the first example of a chromosome deletion carrier without detectable tumor development. Dryja et al.[29] have suggested that deletion carriers may only develop unilateral, unifocal disease because the deletion also predisposes to the expression of other recessive lethal genes in the same region. Thus, potential tumor precursor cells are removed from the dividing population of cells in the embryonic retina. The mother in this family might represent the extreme form of this hypothesis with no "transformed" cells surviving development. Alternatively, she could have been a tissue mosaic with the hemopoietic and germ lines carrying the deletion but not retinal cells. Finally, it might be that the deletion in the mother does not include the Rb locus but predisposes to an additional adjacent deletion in the son. The isolation of the Rb gene should allow clarification of this issue.

2. Linkage to ESD

Sparkes et al.[22] demonstrated linkage between ESD and Rb. Although the frequency of the type 2 allele in the U.S. was only 0.1, from a survey of 35 families, three large pedigrees were identified where the transmitting carriers of the Rb gene were heterozygous at the ESD

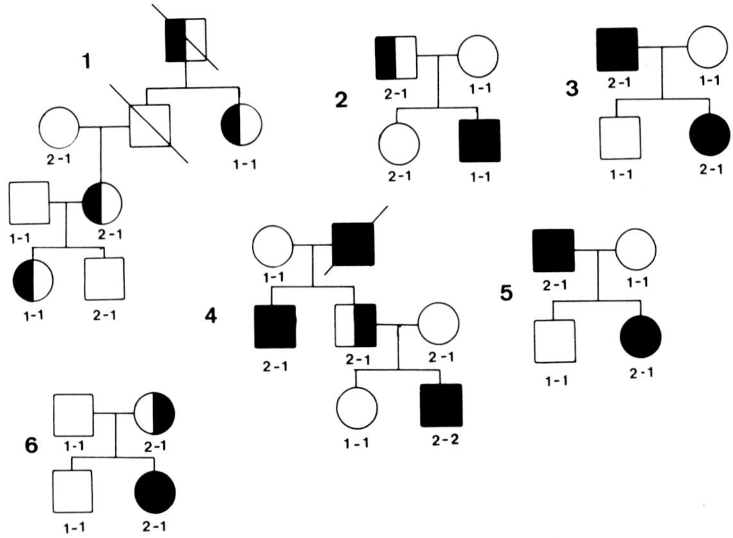

FIGURE 9. Co-segregation of the Rb gene with particular polymorphic variants of the ESD genes in six families. (□) Male, (○) female, (◪, ∅) deceased, (●) bilaterally affected, (◑) unilaterally affected.

locus. No recombination was observed in 12 phase-known meioses, giving a lod score of 3.5. Subsequently, Mukai et al.[43] and Halloran et al.[44] presented two other families in which there was no recombination between ESD and Rb. Recently,[42] we have presented data from 50 families which, with no recombination in 13 meioses (Figure 9), give an additional lod score of 2.61. A cumulative lod score of 13.69 has now been obtained. Thus, the maximum real recombination rate is 6% with 95% confidence limits and 10% with 99% confidence limits. A major drawback to the widespread use of this polymorphism for prenatal diagnosis, however, is the low frequency (0.116 in the U.K.) of the 2-allele.[45] With a heterozygote frequency of 0.172, one in seven families were informative for the polymorphism.[42]

The close linkage between the ESD gene and Rb prompted several groups to clone the ESD gene sequence.[46,47] Clones of 1.1 and 1.4 kb were isolated which spanned a genomic sequence between 25 to 40 kb. Only one RFLP has been identified to date, in digests using the Apa I enzyme. The frequency of the rare allele in this case is 0.2, giving a heterozygote frequency of 32% which means that more families will be informative for prenatal diagnosis than with the ESD protein polymorphism.

Vogel[11] presented evidence that the Rb gene was only 80 to 90% penetrant, an observation that affects the prediction of the risk to offspring of Rb patients. In our series of 70 families, only one example of incomplete penetrance was observed. In a second family the apparent lack of penetrance was accounted for by the identification, in the transmitting parent, of a retinoma indicating the presence of the Rb gene. Connelly et al.[48] reported an unusual family where the penetrance was only 70% with three unaffected individual carriers clearly identifiable and without evidence of retinomas. Recently, a similar family has been identified in the U.K.[49] and is illustrated in Figure 10.

G. 13q14 Probes

Several groups have attempted to isolate chromosome region 13q14-specific probes to identify the Rb gene. Using somatic cell hybrids containing human chromosome 13 as well as other individual human chromosomes, Cavenee et al.[50] and Dryja et al.[29] isolated a series of human probes from DNA libraries constructed in bacteriophage lambda. Chromosome 13-specific probes were identified using somatic cell hybrid panels. Subregional localization

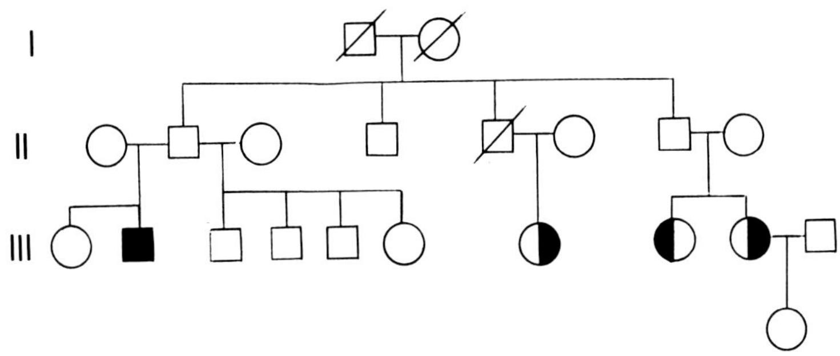

FIGURE 10. A family pedigree demonstrating incomplete penetrance of the Rb predisposition gene. Unaffected individuals in generation II clearly transmit the predisposition to their offspring. Details of this pedigree presented by kind consent of Professor P. Harper. (□) Male, (○) female, (⍁, ∅) deceased, (■) bilaterally affected male, (◑) unilaterally affected female.

was achieved either using somatic cell hybrids containing different overlapping deletions[50] or by *in situ* hybridization.[51] Lalande et al.[52] constructed a chromosome 13 specific library from flow sorted chromosomes. Individual unique sequences were identified and mapped along chromosome 13.[53] One of these probes, H3-8, demonstrated homozygous deletion in 2/37 retinoblastomas,[54] suggesting that this DNA sequence is close to the Rb locus. Chromosome walking in phage libraries from this probe[54] generated an adjacent sequence which showed a high degree of sequence conservancy between species, suggesting it was localized within a coding region. Using this probe, Friend et al.[55] identified an mRNA sequence which was 4.7 kb long. A cDNA clone was subsequently isolated from a fetal retinal cell line which was immortalized using adenovirus 12. This cDNA sequence, 4.7R, recognizes a genomic sequence approximately 200 kb long. The 4.7R probe was apparently not present in fetal retina or retinoblastoma cells, but was present in a wide variety of other tumor types. Histopathology of retinoblastomas is variable, but individual cells can resemble immature photoreceptors seen in embryonic retina. Although pseudorosettes are sometimes formed, the general appearance is consistent with the suggestion that the tumors represent an arrested stage of development.

Gallie and colleagues have demonstrated that the H3-8 sequence is present at all stages of fetal retinal development and also in adult retina.[56] Analysis of 50 Rb tumors demonstrated either homozygous deletions or rearrangements of the gene sequence in 30%.[55] Many of the deletions extended beyond the chromosome region identified by the 4.7 gene, but in one case was interstitial. These data make this gene a strong candidate for the Rb gene although its ubiquity is surprising, since it might be expected that the Rb gene would be expressed only at certain stages of development. In a recent study by Gallie and colleagues,[56] rearrangement of H3-8 was not detected in any Rb cells analyzed and showed normal levels of expression in 5/8 tumors.

H. Osteosarcoma

Survivors of the inherited form of Rb have a 200 times greater than average risk for developing a second tumor,[57] the most common being osteosarcoma (OS).[59] This does not appear to be the case in the nonhereditary form of the tumor. Radiation treatment of Rb undoubtedly contributes to the high incidence of osteosarcomas, with many tumors arising within the irradiated field, but more than one third of OS in Rb patients occur in unirradiated bones. Another interesting second neoplasm in patients with inherited Rb is pinealoma.[58] Since the pinea is considered a vestigial photoreceptor, this condition has been referred to as "trilateral retinoblastoma".

Cells from Rb patients may be more prone than normal cells to radiation induced mutation.

Several groups have tried to investigate this possibility. Sister chromatid exchange (SCE) has been used as an index of fragility in cells from Rb patients. Whereas Wechselbaum et al.[60] claimed increased SCE frequencies in fibroblasts, others[61] could not repeat this observation. Recently, Sanford and colleagues have shown chromosome fragility in all Rb patients compared with normal controls.[62] In their experiments, lymphocytes were subjected to radiation but only in the more sensitive G2 period of the cell cycle. This stage specificity may account for the variability seen by others. Interestingly, the same sensitivity was shown in cells from Wilms' tumor patients.[62]

The high incidence of OS in Rb patients suggests that the same genetic locus could be responsible for the predisposition to both tumors. In this respect, Gilman et al.[63] reported an interesting family with OS. There was an associated 13;14 Robertsonian translocation in one parent but no tumor. Two of the daughters developed OS and showed an inversion within the Robertsonian translocation with breakpoints in 13q12 and 14q11, possibly implicating region 13q12 in OS development. Hansen et al.[64] investigated OS tumors both from retinoblastoma patients and sporadic cases with chromosome 13 specific DNA probes. They demonstrated homozygosity for the 13pter-q21 region in one patient who had previously had bilateral retinoblastoma and also in a sporadic case of OS. Many loci on other chromosomes were also analyzed but shown to be unaffected demonstrating the specificity of the genetic reorganization. The presumptive Rb gene[55] was also investigated in OS and in two cases reorganization of the gene was found. Similar results have also been reported by Dryja et al.[65]

IV WILMS' TUMOR

Wilms' tumor is a pediatric kidney tumor which affects about 1 in 10,000 children in the U.K. and accounts for 6% of all childhood cancers. Knudson and Strong[66] estimated that 38% of all Wilms' tumors are inherited in an autosomal dominant pattern with reduced penetrance, but familial and bilateral tumors are much less common than in Rb. For example, of the first 300 cases in the first U.K. Childhood Cancer Study Group trial, none were familial and only 4% were bilateral.[67] It is clear that, if this tumor can be described as hereditary, the penetrance must be low. Analysis of chromosome deletion patients (see below) shows that there is only a 50% chance of tumor formation in the presence of a predisposing deletion[68] which also indicates reduced penetrance of the gene. Several examples of familial Wilms' tumor have been reported.[69,70] In the U.K., the mean age of onset of the bilateral cases is 30 months compared with 42 months for the unilateral cases supporting a two-hit hypothesis.

A. The WAGR Phenotype

Analysis of the Wilms' tumor registers in the U.S. shows a high frequency, 1/73, of coincident aniridia (absence of irises) referred to as the aniridia-Wilms' association (AWTA).[71] Careful examination of these patients has revealed a more complex phenotype with mental retardation and/ or genitourinary abnormalities also evident in many cases. Patients with the so-called AGR-triad[72] — for aniridia, gonadal abnormalities, and mental retardation — have been shown to have a 50% chance of developing Wilms' tumor[68] — the so called WAGR phenotype. Chromosome analysis has shown, almost without exception,[73] that these patients have a constitutional deletion from the short arm of chromosome 11. Variable lengths of region 11p13 are involved (Figure 11) strongly implicating this region as the site of the Wilms' predisposition locus.[68,74,75] The larger deletions tend to be associated with the full phenotypic triad, while patients with smaller deletions usually only have aniridia and Wilms' tumor. Some of these patients had previously been described as having no deletion, but careful karyotypic studies revealed an abnormality. The deletion of 11p13 was shown in

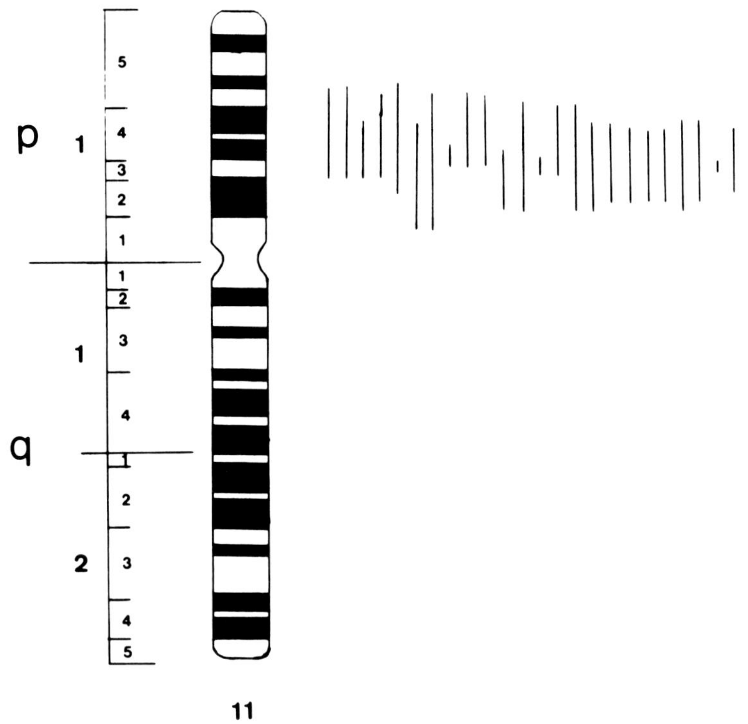

FIGURE 11. Schematic representation of the variability in the size of deletions on 11p in patients with the WAGR phenotype. Each vertical line represents the extent of an individual deletion.

one family to be transmitted from an individual who carried a balanced translocation with insertion of the 11p13 region into the long arm of chromosome 2.[76] The inheritance of the unbalanced form of this rearrangement led to the WAGR phenotype. Hittner et al.[77] reported a case of transmission of a deletion from a patient who carried an insertion of 11p13-p14 in the long arm of chromosome 11. They reasoned that the deletion was generated through recombination between the normal and rearranged homologues. Wilms' tumor is rarely hereditary, but in cases such as these, where the predisposing rearrangement can be identified, prenatal diagnosis would be possible. Similarly, the inheritance of small 11p13 deletions which do not affect reproductive ability, can be detected.

Wilms' tumor is not the only malignancy associated with 11p deletion and the AGR triad. Andersen et al.[78] reported one AGR patient, a girl, who developed bilateral gonadoblastoma at 21 months. Particularly interesting is that both the kidneys and gonads are of mesodermal origin and derive from embryologically adjacent structure involving the mesonephros. These observations imply that genes in 11p13 must act pleiotrophically, and affect development of a number of different tissues (see later).

B. The 11p Gene Map

The gene for catalase was the first to be mapped to the 11p13 region.[79] Patients with larger 11p13 deletions have only 50% normal catalase activity in their cells. We have identified a Wilms'-aniridia patient with a sub-band deletion of chromosome 11p13 and two copies of the catalase gene. *In situ* hybridization suggests that the catalase gene is in the proximal part of 11p13.[80] If so, the Wilms' gene (Wg) and aniridia gene (Ag) must be in the distal half of 11p13 (Figure 12). The relative orientation of these two genes can be inferred from the report of a deletion in a patient with Wilms' tumor and mental retardation

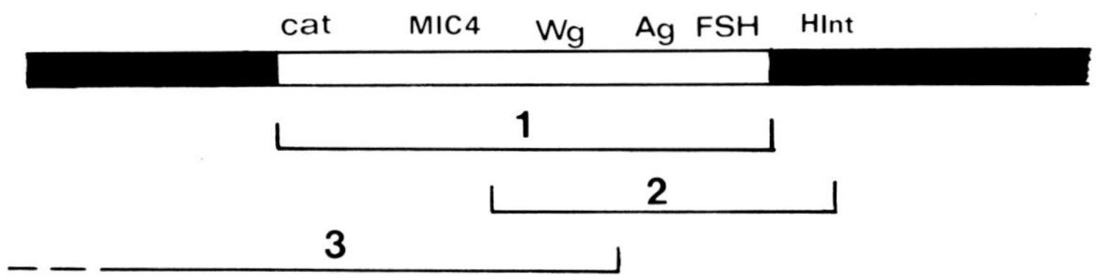

FIGURE 12. The relative gene order in region 11p13. Deletion 1 was from a patient with the WAGR syndrome who showed deletion of one copy of the catalase gene. Deletion 2 was from a patient with Wilms' tumor (Wg) and aniridia (Ag) but who had two copies of the catalase gene. Deletion 3 was from a patient with reduced catalase activity, Wilms' tumor, but no aniridia.[81]

but no aniridia.[81] In this case, the breakpoints were in 11p11 and 11p13. Thus, Ag appears to be distal to Wg. Several other genes have now been located to 11p13 including a cell surface marker, MIC4, and the gene for the beta-subunit of follicle stimulating hormone (FSH).[82] A locus representing the integration site of the hepatitis B virus[83] was shown to be close, but distal, to the FSH gene.[82] The relative order of these genes on 11p is given in Figure 12. It can be seen that the Wg locus is flanked by the CAT and FSH genes.

C. Chromosome Analysis of Wilms' Tumors

Several distinct cytogenetic analyses of Wilms' tumors have been presented and indicate that, although abnormalities involving 11p are observed, they are not universal. Kaneko et al.[84] reported an instance where an 11p deletion was the only chromosome abnormality. This patient had a normal constitutional karyotype. In two other tumors, both copies of chromosome 11 were normal but translocations involved chromosomes 1 and 16.[85] Kondo et al.[86] demonstrated 11p abnormalities in 1/9 Wilms' tumors whereas Douglass et al.[87] showed 6/14 carried abnormalities.

In this study, simple deletions and deletions produced as a result of complex chromosome translocations were identified. Slater et al.[88] showed aberrations of 11p in 3/11 Wilms' tumors studied and, in a later review,[89] reported that 11p deletions were the most common abnormality, present in 13/38. The next most commonly involved region was 1q, although abnormalities of this chromosome arm are very common in tumor cells.[90] Chromosome 16 was also frequently involved in rearrangements. It appears, therefore, that 11p is often involved in structural chromosome rearrangements but frequently within a background of other chromosome abnormalities. It is difficult to determine, therefore, which, if any, of these abnormalities are causal in tumorigenesis or consequences of it.

Nephroblastomatosis — nodular renal blastema — is a histologically benign lesion frequently associated with Wilms' tumor[91,92] and is considered to be a premalignant condition. Heidemann et al.[93] reported a child who presented with bilateral nephromegaly and eventually developed Wilms' tumor. Chromosome analysis of nodular renal blastema taken from this patient demonstrated a deletion of 11p11-p14.2. The sample analyzed was taken from an area remote from the tumor and histological examination revealed no recognizable tumor components. These observations lend further support to the view that deletion from the 11p13 region is an important predisposing event in the development of Wilms' tumor.

Chromosome analysis of Wilms' tumors has been used to aid assessment of the relative aggression of the tumor. With current treatment regimes, over 80% of Wilms' patients with favorable histology and stage I-III disease are long-term survivors. However, in advanced stage disease and in tumors with unfavorable histologic subtypes, the prognosis is less favorable.[94] Douglass et al.[95] analyzed 48 Wilms' tumors by FACS and demonstrated that the majority of tumors with favorable histology had diploid or hyperdiploid DNA content. By contrast, 90% (9/10) of the anaplastic tumors had a DNA content in the tetraploid and hypertetraploid range. Of the seven near-tetraploid tumors analyzed karyotypically, all showed major structural and numerical chromosome abnormalities compared with 15 nonanaplastic tumors.

It appears, therefore, that a highly abnormal karyotype is associated with a more aggressive course of the disease. If these studies can be confirmed, this type of analysis could provide useful confirmation of pathological subtypes.

D. Homozygosity

Demonstration of the generation of homozygosity in the tumors of retinoblastoma patients who were constitutionally heterozygous for the same DNA ''markers'' was followed closely by the same observation in Wilms' tumors. Using 11p distal probes, several groups showed that, in a proportion of tumors, homozygosity was generated.[96-98] The mechanism was shown not to be due to simple chromosome loss, but to nondisjunction or, in one case[99] mitotic recombination. Analysis of tumor material from one of our own patients with an 11p13-p15 deletion showed that the tumor had retained a copy of the catalase gene, excluding the possibility that a large homozygous deletion had been generated in these cells.

E. Beckwith-Wiedemann Syndrome

Beckwith-Wiedemann syndrome is a condition involving somatic overgrowth.[100,101] In a few cases, it is also associated with a chromosome abnormality involving the distal tip of chromosome 11.[102,103] One of the features of this condition is that individuals often develop specific rare pediatric tumors, most frequently Wilms' tumors, but also hepatoblastomas, rhabdomyosarcomas, adrenal adenocarcinomas, and non-Burkitt's lymphoma. In some patients, combinations of these tumors have been reported, suggesting a common etiological event arising as a result of a mutation at the same locus. Koufos et al.[104] analyzed three hepatoblastomas and showed that in two, homozygosity for chromosome 11 markers developed, while in a third tumor, heterozygosity was retained. There were similar findings in two rhabdomyosarcomas. Markers from other chromosomes were the same in tumor and normal tissues showing that loss of alleles was restricted to chromosome 11. Recently Haas et al.[102] reported a patient with BWS who developed nephroblastoma and carried a constitutional chromosome deletion of region 11p11.1-p11.2. These studies suggest a common pathogenicity mechanism by these clinically associated tumor types. It is not clear whether the locus involved is the same or constitutes a complex of several genes in the same region of the chromosome. It does appear, however, that these genes contribute to the normal differentiation of the tissues involved.

F. Isolation of 11p DNA Sequences

Histopathology of WT is variable, but is normally characterized by undifferentiated blastemal cells similar to those seen in the developing kidney. Grobstein[105] showed that differentiation of the kidney mesenchyme was triggered by a factor produced by the ureter bud. Possibly, disruption of this induction system could allow continuous proliferation of blastemal cells which overcome the growth limitations imposed by differentiation. The implication that specific genes in region 11p13 are involved with the predisposition to WT and other rare embryonic tumors has prompted several groups to look for genes in 11p13 showing abnormal expression of the type described for retinoblastoma. Several approaches being used will be discussed below, but all depend on the isolation of DNA sequences from within the 11p13 region. One option would be to use existing 11p13 markers to attempt chromosome walking towards the Wilms' locus. Chromosome walking is the sequential isolation of clones which are normally adjacent within the genome (Figure 13). Walking is relatively time consuming and requires the isolation of the end regions of each clone in order to achieve the maximum step. These procedures can be carried out in either lambda or cosmid vectors.

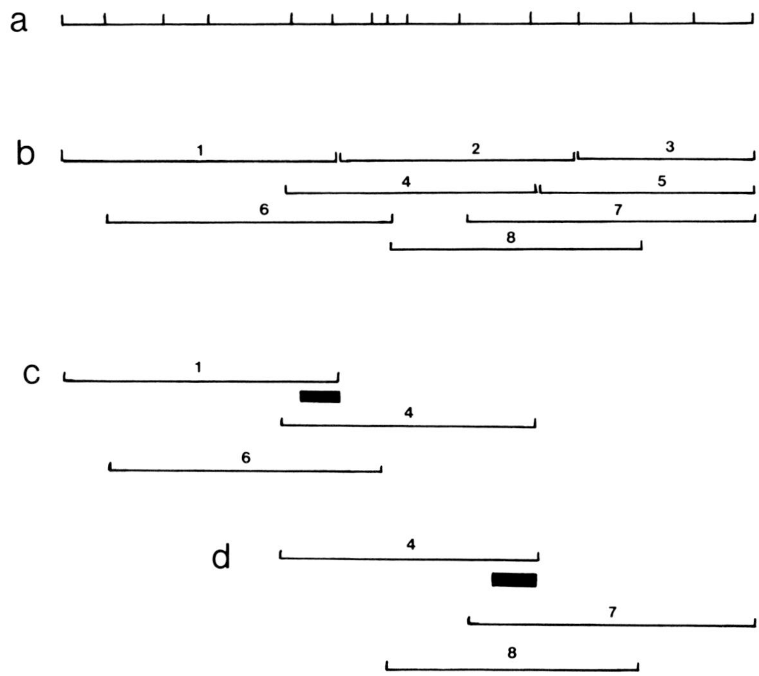

FIGURE 13. Principle of chromosome walking. (a) shows a length of DNA with vertical strokes representing cleavage sites for a particular restriction enzyme. Partial digestion with a restriction enzyme produces a variety of overlapping fragments, examples of which are shown in (b). Starting from fragment 1, the end region is isolated following restriction enzyme digest analysis and used as a probe (■) to find other fragments with the same sequence. In this example, fragments 4 and 6 have partial sequence homology. Fragment 4 represents a piece of DNA with only one short region in common with clone 1, whereas fragment 6 is virtually the same as fragment 1 and would extend the walk only a short distance. Therefore, clone 4 is used to extend the walk. If the distalmost region of clone 4 is now isolated and used in a similar way to probe for homologous sequences, clones 7 and 8 will be recognized but clone 7 used to extend the walk because of its lesser overlap with clone 4.

The isolation of a single overlapping clone constitutes a ''step'' and a series of steps constitutes a ''walk''. Such strategies for walking long distances in the human genome are not practical for a variety of reasons.[106] Cosmid walking offers the best opportunity for covering large distances and the development of new vectors such as the one described by Little and Cross[107] might make walking slightly quicker. Into their cosmid vector, LORIC,[107] the SP6 and T7 promotors have recently been introduced.[108] This allows rapid generation of radioactive RNA probes directly from the end regions of the clone which can be used in the next walking step (see Figure 13).

It is conceivable, although unlikely, that these walking strategies can be used to cover the distance from catalase or FSH to the Wilms' locus (see Figure 12). The large physical distance between even closely linked loci, however, is a major problem. The human haploid genome contains 3×10^9 bp of which, for example, chromosome 11 constitutes 2.4%, i.e., 7.8×10^7 bp. Chromosome band 11p13 (about 4% of the chromosome) contains 3×10^6 bp or 3000 kb. Using cosmid cloning strategies, 45 kb is the largest amount of DNA that can be cloned. To isolate region 11p13, 70 contiguous cosmids would have to be isolated which represents a formidable task even if the libraries are fully representative.[106].

It is clear that probes which are physically closer to the Wilms' locus are required. Chromosome 11 specific probes can be obtained from DNA libraries prepared from somatic cell hybrids containing chromosome 11 as the only human component or from chromosome 11 isolated by flourescent activated cell sorting (FACS). Random isolation of DNA sequences from a chromosome 11 library holds a 1:25 chance that any clone will be derived from 11p13. In our group, we have created a cosmid library from a cell hybrid containing all but the 11pq23-qter region of chromosome 11. The chances of obtaining 11p13 probes could be increased by starting with, for example, only the short arm of chromosome 11. Some groups have attempted to do this by first fragmenting chromosome 11 by irradiation or using caffeine,[109,110] but in general the damage has been nonspecific and the results confusing. Chromosome 11 can be isolated by FACS using twin beam systems only. One such library has been generated by the Lawrence Livermore laboratories[111] from which 11-specific probes can be isolated and mapped. This library is unlikely to be representative of the whole chromosome[112] but will be an invaluable source of chromosome specific probes.

G. Chromosome-Mediated Gene Transfer

Another approach for the isolation of chromosome region specific probes has been pioneered by Hastie and colleagues. Fragments of chromosome 11 were introduced into suitable mouse cells via chromosome mediated gene transfer techniques.[113] The c-Ha-Ras gene is located on the distal tip of chromosome 11 which, when transfected into suitable host mouse cells, produces foci of transformed cells.[113] Chromosomes from the EJ bladder cell line showing activation of the H-ras oncogene were used, and in several transformants, genes from the 11p13 and 11p15 regions were cotransfected; genes from the intervening 11p14 region, however, appeared to be absent. Clearly, during the transformation process, rearrangement of 11p13 had occurred.[114] Libraries made from these transfectants, however, are proving a valuable source of material from the short arm of chromosome 11.

H. T-cell Chromosome Rearrangements

Chromosome analysis of T-cell leukemia (ALL) demonstrates a fairly consistent translocation between chromosome 11 and 14 with breakpoints in p13 and q11, respectively.[115] Isolation of these derivative chromosomes in somatic cell hybrids demonstrates that the breakpoints are between the constant and variable regions of the gene for the alpha-chain.[116-117] Analysis of the derivative chromosome 11 showed that the breakpoint was distal to the catalase gene but proximal to calcitonin[118] and recently, the FSH gene.[119] This places the breakpoint closer to the Wg locus than other available DNA sequences. It might be expected that chromosome walking experiments starting at the alpha-chain locus would eventually cross the breakpoint into the 11p13 region. Attempts to date have covered 100 kb without achieving this aim.[119] The consistent observation that oncogenes are translocated into the vicinity of highly active genes in leukemic cells[120] might suggest, if this rearrangement has anything to do with the transformation of the T-cells, that such an oncogene is located at 11p13.

V. GENE HUNTING

The identification of the retinoblastoma locus represents perhaps, one of the more fortuitous results in the search for cancer predisposition genes. From relatively few clones, one was found to be actually within a gene with some of the characteristics expected for the Rb gene. Attempts to isolate the Wilms' tumor locus have not yet led to similar success. Recent developments in molecular biology, however, are making it increasingly possible to identify genes from flanking sequences which may be considerable distances away from the gene of interest.

The task of walking into the Wilms' locus would be less daunting if it were possible to cover large distances within the genome, quickly, from an initial clone which may be some

Table 1
RECOGNITION SEQUENCES FOR RARE CUTTING RESTRICTION ENZYMES

Bss H1	CGCGCG	Sac II	CCGCGG
Cla 1	ATCGAT	Sal I	GTCGAC
Nae 1	GCCGGC	Sfi I	GGCCNNNNNGGCC
Nar 1	GGCGCC	Sma I	CCCGGG
Not 1	GCGGCCGC	Sna B1	TACGTA
Nru 1	TCGCGA	Xho 1	CTCGAG
Pvu 1	CGATCG	Xma III	CGGCCG

million bp (megabases; Mbp) away. The technology is now available and is referred to as ''hopping'' and ''jumping''.[121]

A. Pulse-Field Gel Electrophoresis

This ability to cover large distances in the genome depends on the activity of specific restriction enzymes which cut very infrequently in the human genome. Several such enzymes exist and are listed in Table 1. It will be noted that most of them have, within their recognition sequences, the CpG dinucleotide which, because the human genome is AT-rich, occur five times less frequently than would be expected. 99% of human CpG dinucleotides are methylated, a requirement for the action of the majority of restriction enzymes. The enzymes listed in Table 1, however, require unmethylated DNA as a substrate which only occurs in 1% of the genome. Digestion with these rare cutting enzymes generates DNA fragments which are 0.2 to 2 Mbp long. Conventional agarose gel methods, however, are only capable of separating DNA fragments up to 50 kb long. To cope with the larger fragments generated, pulse field gel electrophoresis (PFGE) has been developed. This work was pioneered by Cantor and colleagues[122] working with yeast chromosomes, but the system has since been successfully adapted to separating human DNA. The details of this technique are discussed by van Ommen and Verkerk[123] and Anand.[124]

The first part of the procedure is to prepare very high molecular weight DNA which, following enzyme treatment, will yield DNA fragments up to 2 Mbp long. Conventional techniques shear the DNA into relatively small pieces. This is overcome by embedding the cells in blocks of low melting point agarose. Subsequent extraction procedures and enzyme treatments are carried out directly on these blocks which are then loaded into the running gel. There are several different types of equipment for running these gels, all of which are based on the same principle.[125] The DNA is subjected alternately to two approximately perpendicular electric fields. The electrodes may be placed at 45 degrees to the gel[126] producing an orthogonal field (OFAGE). Carle et al.[125] showed that separation can also be achieved by reversing the polarity in a conventional horizontal gel apparatus, so-called ''inverted field agarose gel electrophoresis'' (IFAGE). A switching mechanism with a net forward movement is used, such that the greater part of the cycle promotes DNA migration in the forward direction. Early problems of uneven migration of the DNA were overcome using switching ramps where the time ratio was kept constant but the overall pulse time was increased during the run. This progressive change in time is controlled by a computed driven mechanism. The reason for the separation achieved is not yet fully understood, but some suggestions are reviewed by van Ommen and Verkerk.[123] The DNA in the gels can be transferred using conventional blotting techniques, which in turn can be screened with radioactive probes, and the particular fragment containing the gene of interest can be identified. If two markers are on the same fragment, they will occupy the same band on the autoradiograph. In this case, the particular band can be excised from the gel and subcloned into an appropriate vector. When the gene is not located in the same fragment, it is necessary to employ jumping strategies to move into the adjacent fragment.

B. Chromosome Jumping

Infrequent cutting enzymes generate large fragments with cohesive ends which can be ligated to suitable vectors with the same cohesive ends (Figure 14). Dilution of the DNA at this stage will promote the generation of large circles linked by vector molecules. Cutting these circles with another enzyme which does not cut internally within the vector, followed by religation, produces clones which contain the end sequences of a very large fragment.[121] In this way, it is possible to jump large distances along the genome. All of these jumps can be tested against suitable somatic cell hybrids to determine the orientation of the jumping and whether the region of interest has been reached. To begin the jumping, the nearest rare cutting site to the starting probe has to be identified which usually requires conventional walking strategies. A combination of IFAGE and jumping should eventually allow the region of a chromosome to be delimited by flanking probes. Once the extremes of the region required have been isolated, contiguous DNA maps can be generated which should contain the gene.

C. HTF Islands

Analysis of the localization of the infrequent cutting sites in the genome shows that they tend to be clustered within small regions (0.5 to 2 kb) of the genome.[127] In addition to the rare cutting enzymes, the 4-base pair recognition sequence from the Hpa II restriction enzyme (CCGG) is also frequently located within these islands. Digestion of the human genome with Hpa II produces tiny fragments,[129] the Hpa II-tiny-fragments (HTF). A clustering of rare cutting sites occurs throughout the genome within the "HTF-islands"[128] which are frequently, but not always, located 5′ to genes.[129] The sequences flanking the HTF islands are usually highly methylated and it has been suggested that these islands, in some way, are responsible for the regulation of gene activity.[129] There are an estimated 30,000 HTF islands in the human genome which is strikingly close to the total estimated number of human genes.[129] The exciting possibility in this area is that, in combination with PFGE and chromosome jumping strategies, "island hopping" and, by implication "gene hopping", may be possible.

VI. SUMMARY

The possibility of isolating specific cancer predisposition genes has become a realistic venture over the past few years. This ability is a direct consequence of the considerable pace with which technology in molecular biology is proceeding. The one-time hope of localizing disease genes within the genome through linkage to "classical" markers has become a reality due mainly to the widespread isolation and use of DNA fragments identifying RFLPs. For retinoblastoma and Wilms' tumor, the identification of specific chromosome abnormalities was undoubtedly important, but for other disease where, despite detailed searches, no such clues have been forthcoming, genetic linkage will inevitably prove the means whereby these genes are mapped. Once their chromosomal position is known, the rapidly evolving technology of pulse-field gel electrophoresis, HTF island hopping, and chromosome walking will eventually become a routine means of isolating the gene responsible. The identification of these genes will allow fundamental questions about mammalian development to be asked and provide insights into the cause of complex diseases such as cancer.

ACKNOWLEDGMENTS

I should like to thank Dr. J. Pritchard for his support throughout this work and for his critical reading of the manuscript.

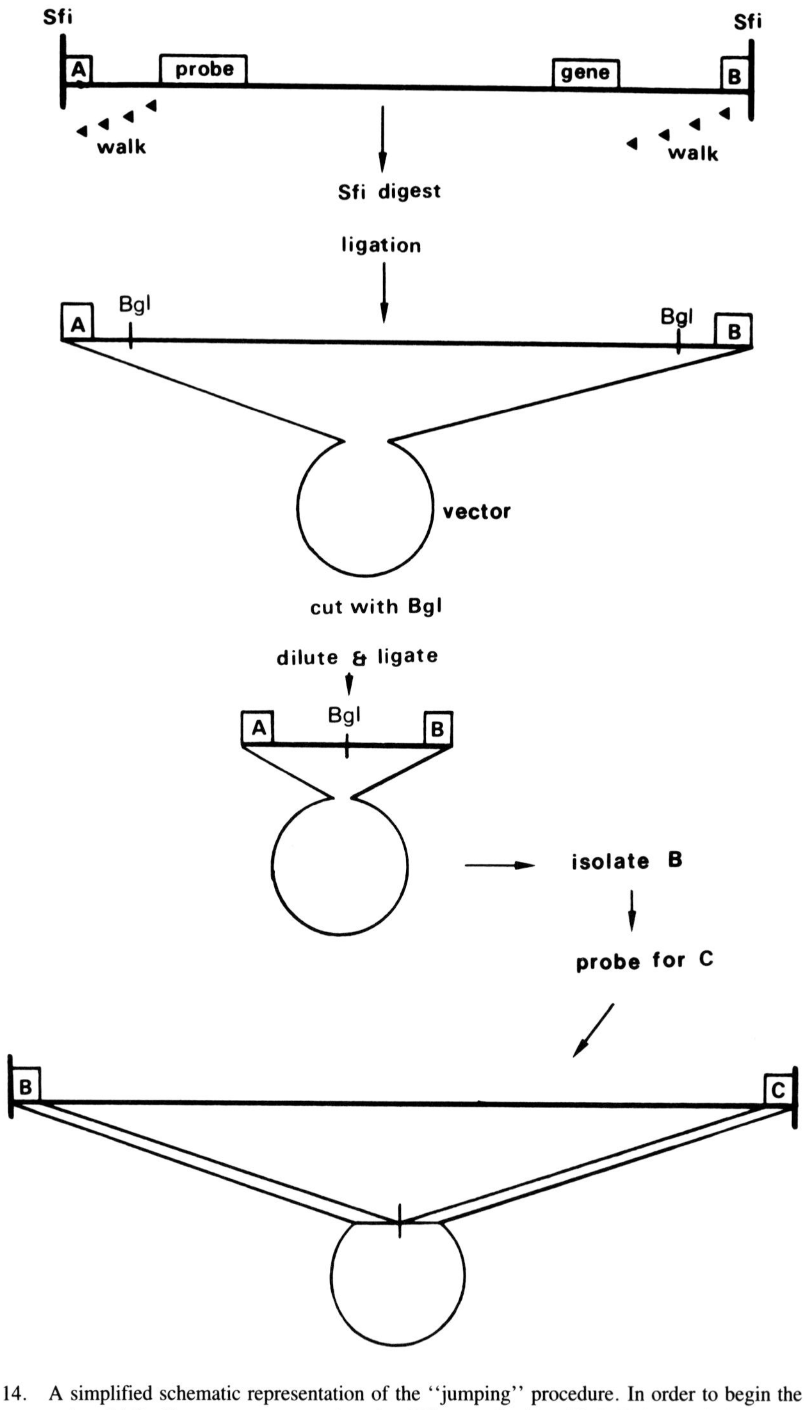

FIGURE 14. A simplified schematic representation of the ''jumping'' procedure. In order to begin the jumping experiment, a region ''A'' adjacent to a rare cutting site (Sfi) must be identified. If the 'probe' is some distance away from ''A'', then chromosome walking must be used to cover the intervening distance. The isolation of the ''gene'' sequence depends on first isolating ''B'', and then walking to the gene. Total genomic DNA is cut with a rare cutting enzyme (Sfi) which generates large (0.2 to 2 Mbp) fragments. Vector molecules are ligated onto the ends of these fragments and, under suitable conditions,[121] large circles of DNA are generated. Cutting these circles with a frequent cutting enzyme (Bgl), which does not have a recognition sequence within the vector, produces smaller fragments, one of which will contain the vector and regions ''A'' and ''B''. Dilution of the DNA at this stage, followed by ligation will generate closed circular plasmids containing the end regions of the Sfi fragment. ''B'' can then be isolated and used either as a start point for walking to the ''gene'', or to initiate another jump in order to isolate ''C''.

REFERENCES

1. **Harnden, D., Morten, J., and Featherstone, T.,** Dominant susceptibility to cancer in man, *Adv. Cancer Res.,* 41, 185, 1984.
2. **Drayna, D., Davies, K. E., Hartley, D., Mandel, J. L., Camerino, G., Williamson, R., and White, R.,** Genetic mapping of the human X chromosome by restriction fragment length polymorphisms, *Proc. Natl. Acad. Sci. U.S.A.,* 81, 2836, 1984.
3. **Harris, H., Hopkinson, D. A., and Robson, E. B.,** The incidence of rare alleles determining electrophoretic variants: data on 43 enzyme loci in man. *Ann. Hum. Genet.,* 37, 237, 1974.
4. **Gusella, J. F.,** DNA polymorphism and human disease, *Ann. Rev. Biochem.,* 55, 831, 1986.
5. **Southern, E.,** Detection of specific sequences among DNA fragments separated by gel electrophoresis, *J. Mol. Biol.,* 98, 503, 1975.
6. **Rigby, P. W., Dieckman, M., Rhodes, C., and Berg, P.,** Labelling deoxyribonucleic acid to high specific activity in vitro by nick translation with DNA polymerase I, *J. Mol. Biol.,* 113, 237, 1977.
7. **Woo, S. L., Lidsky, A. S., Guttler, F., Chandra, T., and Robson, K. J. H.,** Cloned human phenylalanine hydroxylase gene allows prenatal diagnosis and carrier detection of classical phenylketonuria, *Nature,* 306, 151, 1983.
8. **Old, J. M., Heath, C., Fitches, A., Thein, S. L., Weatherall, D. J., Warren, R., Mckensie, C., Rodeck, C. H., Model, B., Petrou, M., and Ward, R. T. H.,** First trimester fetal diagnosis for haemoglobinopathies: Report on 200 cases, *Lancet,* 2, 763, 1986.
9. **Pembrey, M. E.,** personal communication, 1986.
10. **Molyneux, E. M.,** Childhood malignancies in Malawi 1967-1976, *East African Med. J.,* 56, 15, 1979.
11. **Vogel, W.,** The genetics of retinoblastoma, *Hum. Genet.,* 52, 1, 1979.
12. **Knudson, A. G.,** Mutation and cancer: statistical study of retinoblastoma. *Proc. Natl. Acad. Sci. U.S.A,* 68, 820, 1971.
13. **Jay, M.,** manuscript in preparation.
14. **Cowell, J., Rutland, P., Jay, M., and Hungerford, J.,** Deletions of the esterase-D locus from a survey of 200 retinoblastoma patients. *Hum. Genet.,* 72, 164, 1986.
15. **Yunis, J. J. and Ramsay, N.,** Retinoblastoma and subband deletion of chromosome 13. *Am. J. Dis. Child.,* 132, 161, 1978.
16. **Sparkes, R. S., Sparkes, M., Kalina, R. E., Pagon, R. A., Salk, D. J., and Disteche, C. M.,** Separation of the retinoblastoma and esterase-D loci in a patient with sporadic retinoblastoma and del (13)(q14.1-q22.3), *Hum. Genet.,* 68, 258, 1984.
17. **Ward, P., Packman, S., Loughman, W., Sparkes, M., Sparkes, R., McMahon, A., Gregory, T., and Albin, A.,** Location of the retinoblastoma susceptibility gene (s) and the human esterase-D locus, *J. Med. Genet.,* 21, 92, 1984.
18. **Cowell, J. K., Hungerford, J., Rutland, P., and Jay, M.,** A chromosomal breakpoint which separates the esterase-D and retinoblastoma predisposition loci in a patient with del (13) (q14-q31), *Cancer Genet. Cytogenet.,* 27, 27, 1987.
19. **Van Heyningen, V., Bobrow, M., Bodmer, W. F., Gardiner, S. E., Povey, S., and Hopkinson, D. A.,** Chromosome assignment of some human enzyme loci. Mitochondrial malate dehydrogenase to 7, mannosphosphate isomerase and pyruvate kinase to 15, and probably, esterase-D to 13, *Ann. Hum. Genet.,* 38, 295, 1975.
20. **Sparkes, R. S., Sparkes, M. C., Wilson, M. G., Towner, J. W., Benedict, W., Murphree, A. L., and Yunis, J. J.,** Regional assignment of genes for human esterase D and retinoblastoma to chromosome band 13q14, *Science,* 208, 1042, 1980.
21. **Hopkinson, D. A., Mestriner, M. A., Cortner, J., and Harris, H.,** Esterase-D: a new human polymorphism, *Ann. Hum. Genet.,* 37, 119, 1973.
22. **Sparkes, R. S., Murphree, A. L., Lingua, R. W., Sparkes, M. C., Field, L. L., Funderbuck, S., and Benedict, W. F.,** Gene for hereditary retinoblastoma assigned to human chromosome 13 by linkage to esterase-D, *Science,* 217, 971, 1983.
23. **Balaban-Malenbaum, G., Gilbert, F., Nichols, W. W., Hill, R., Shields, J., and Meadows, A. T.,** A deleted chromosome number 13 in human retinoblastoma cells: Relevance to tumorigenesis, *Cancer Genet. Cytogenet.,* 3, 243, 1981.
24. **Gardner, H. A., Gallie, B. L., Knight, L. A., and Phillips, R. A.,** Multiple karyotypic changes in retinoblastoma tumour cells: presence of normal chromosome number 13 in most tumours. *Cancer Genet. Cytogenet.,* 6, 201, 1982.
25. **Kusnetsova, L. E., Prigogina, E. L., Pogosianz, H. E., and Belkina, B. M.,** Similar chromosome abnormalities in several retinoblastomas, *Hum. Genet.,* 61, 201, 1982.
26. **Squire, J., Gallie, B. L., and Phillips, R. A.,** A detailed analysis of chromosomal changes in heritable and non-heritable retinoblastoma, *Hum. Genet.,* 70, 291, 1985.

27. **Squire, J., Phillips, R. A., Boyce, S., Godbout, R., Rodgers, B., and Gallie, B. L.,** Isochromosome 6p, a unique chromosomal abnormality in retinoblastoma: verification by standard staining techniques, new densitometric methods, and somatic cell hybrids, *Hum. Genet.*, 66, 46, 1984.
28. **Cavenee, W. K., Dryja, T. P., Phillips, R. A., Benedict, W. F., Godbout, R., Gallie, B. L., Murphree, A. L., Strong, L. C., and White, R.,** Expression of recessive alleles by chromosomal mechanisms in retinoblastoma, *Nature,* 305, 779, 1983.
29. **Dryja, T. P., Cavenee, W. K., White, R., Rapaport, J. M., Peterson, R., Albert, D. M., and Bruns, G. A.,** Homozygosity of chromosome 13 in retinoblastoma, *N. Engl. J. Med.*, 310, 550, 1984.
30. **Cavenee, W. K., Murphree, A. L., Schull, M. M., Benedict, W. F., Sparkes, R. S., Kock, E., and Nordenskjold, M.,** Prediction of familial predisposition to retinoblastoma, *N. Engl. J. Med.*, 314, 1201, 1986.
31. **Godbout, R., Dryja, T. P., Squire, J., Gallie, B. L., and Phillips, R. A.,** Somatic inactivation of genes on chromosome 13 is a common event in retinoblastoma, *Nature,* 304, 451, 1983.
32. **Turleau, C., De Grouchy, J., Chavin-Colin, F., Despoisses, S., and Leblanc, A.,** Two cases of deletion (13q) retinoblastoma and two cases of partial trisomy due to familial insertion, *Ann. Genet.*, 26, 158, 1983.
33. **Turleau, C., De Grouchy, J., Chavin-Colin, F., Junien, C., Seger, J., Schlienger, P., Leblanc, A., and Haye, C.,** Cytogenetic forms of retinoblastoma: their incidence in a survey of 66 patients, *Cancer Genet. Cytogenet.*, 16, 321, 1985.
34. **Strong, L. C., Riccardi, V. M., Ferrel, R. E., and Sparkes, R. S.,** Familial retinoblastoma and chromosome 13 deletion transmitted via an insertional translocation, *Science,* 213, 1501, 1981.
35. **Cross, H. E., Hansen, R. C., Morrow, G., and Davis, J. R.,** Retinoblastoma in a patient with a 13qXp translocation, *Am. J. Ophthalmol.*, 84, 548, 1977.
36. **Hida, T., Kinoshita, Y., Matsumoto, R., Suzuki, N., and Tanaka, H.,** Bilateral retinoblastoma with 13qXp translocation, *J. Paediatr. Ophthalmol. Strab,* 17, 144, 1980.
37. **Lee, W.-H., Murphree, A. L., and Benedict, W. F.,** Expression and amplification of the N-myc gene in primary retinoblastoma, *Nature,* 309, 458, 1985.
38. **Kohl, N. E., Kanda, N., Schreck, R. R., Bruns, G., Latt, S. A., Gilbert, F., and Alt, F. W.,** Transposition and amplification of oncogene-related sequences in human neuroblastomas, *Cell,* 35, 359, 1983.
39. **Cowell, J. K.,** Double minutes and homogeneously staining regions: gene amplification in mammalian cells, *Ann. Rev. Genet.*, 16, 21, 1982.
40. **Squire, J., Goddard, A. D., Canton, M., Becker, A., Phillips, R. A., and Gallie, B. L.,** Tumour induction by the retinoblastoma mutation is independent of N-myc expression. *Nature,* 322, 555, 1986.
41. **Cowell, J. K., Thompson, E., and Rutland, P.,** The need to screen all retinoblastoma patients for esterase-D activity; detection of submicroscopic deletions, *Arch. Dis. Child.*, 62, 8, 1986.
42. **Cowell, J. K., Jay, M., Rutland, P., and Hungerford, J.,** An assessment of the usefulness of the esterase-D protein polymorphism in the antenatal prediction of retinoblastoma in the United Kingdom, *Br. J. Cancer,* In Press, 1987.
43. **Mukai, S., Rapaport, J. M., Shields, J. A., Augsburger, J. J., and Dryja, T. P.,** Linkage of genes for human esterase-D and hereditary retinoblastoma, *Am. J. Ophthalmol.*, 97, 681, 1984.
44. **Halloran, S. L., Boughman, J. A., Dryja, T. P., Mukai, S., Long, D., Roberts, D., and Craft, A. W.,** Accuracy of the detection of the retinoblastoma gene by esterase-D linkage, *Arch. Ophthalmol.*, 103, 1329, 1985.
45. **Cowell, J., Rutland, P., Jay, M., and Hungerford, J.,** Effect of the esterase-D genotype on its in vitro enzyme activity, *Hum. Genet.*, 74, 298, 1986.
46. **Squire, J., Dryja, T. P., Dunn, J., Goddard, A., Hofmann, T., Musarella, M., Willard, H. F., Becker, A. J., Gallie, B. L., and Phillips, R. A.,** Cloning of the esterase D gene; a polymorphic gene probe closely linked to the retinoblastoma locus on chromosome 13, *Proc. Natl. Acad. Sci. U.S.A.*, 83, 6573, 1986.
47. **Lee, E. H. P. and Lee, W. H.,** Molecular cloning of the human esterase D gene, a genetic marker of retinoblastoma, *Proc. Natl. Acad. Sci. U.S.A.*, 83, 6337, 1986.
48. **Connolly, M. J., Payne, R. H., Johnson, G., Gallie, B. L., Allerdice, P. W., Marshall, W. H., and Lawton, R. D.,** Familial, EsD-linked, retinoblastoma with reduced penetrance and variable expressivity, *Hum. Genet.*, 65, 122, 1983.
49. **Harper, P.,** personal communication, 1986.
50. **Cavenee, W., Leach, R., Mohandas, T., Pearson, P., and White, R.,** Isolation and regional localisation of DNA segments revealing polymorphic loci for human chromosome 13, *Am. J. Hum. Genet.*, 36, 10, 1984.
51. **Dryja, T. P. and Morton, C. C.,** Mapping of seven polymorphic loci on human chromosome 13 by in situ hybridization, *Hum. Genet.*, 71, 192, 1985.

52. **Lalande, M., Dryja, T. P., Schreck, R. R., Shipley, J., Flint, A., and Latt, S. A.**, Isolation of human chromosome 13-specific DNA sequences cloned from flow sorted chromosomes and potentially linked to the retinoblastoma locus, *Cancer Genet. Cytogenet.*, 13, 283, 1984.
53. **Lalande, M., Donlon, T., Petersen, R. A., Liberfarb, R., Manter, S., and Latt, S. A.**, Molecular detection and differentiation of deletions in band 13q14 in human retinoblastoma, *Cancer Genet. Cytogenet.*, 23, 151, 1986.
54. **Dryja, T. P., Rapaport, J. M., Joyce, J. M., and Petersen, R. A.**, Molecular detection of deletions involving band q14 of chromosome 13 in retinoblastomas, *Proc. Natl. Acad. Sci. U.S.A.*, 83, 7391, 1986.
55. **Friend, S. H., Bernards, R., Rogelj, S., Weinberg, R. A., Rapaport, J. M., Albert, D. M., and Dryja, T. P.**, A human DNA segment with properties of the gene that predisposes to retinoblastoma and osteosarcoma, *Nature,* 323, 643, 1986.
56. **Gallie, B. L.**, personal communication, 1986.
57. **Abramson, D. H., Ellesworth, R., and Zimmerman, L.**, Nonocular cancer in retinoblastoma survivors, *Trans. Am. Acad. Ophthalmol. Otolaryngol.*, 81, 454, 1976.
58. **Bader, J. L., Meadows, A. T., Zimmerman, L. E., Rorke, L. B., Voute, P. A., Champion, L. A. A., and Miller, R. W.**, Bilateral retinoblastoma with ectopic intracranial retinoblastoma: trilateral retinoblastoma. *Cancer Genet. Cytogenet.*, 5, 203, 1982.
59. **Draper, G. J., Sanders, B. M., and Kingston, J. E.**, Second primary neoplasms in patients with retinoblastoma, *Br. J. Cancer,* 53, 661, 1986.
60. **Weichselbaum, R. R., Nove, J., and Little, J. B.**, X-ray sensitivity of diploid fibroblasts from patients with hereditary and sporadic retinoblastoma, *Proc. Natl. Acad. Sci. U.S.A.*, 75, 3962, 1978.
61. **Takabayashi, T., Lin, M. C., and Wilson, M. G.**, Sister chromatid exchanges and chromosome aberrations in fibroblasts from patients with retinoblastoma, *Hum. Genet.*, 63, 317, 1983.
62. **Sanford, K. K.**, personal communication, 1986.
63. **Gilman, P. A., Wang, N., Fan, S. F., Reede, J., Khan, A., and Leventhal, B. G.**, Familial osteosarcoma associated with 13;14 chromosomal rearrangement, *Cancer Genet. Cytogenet.*, 17, 123, 1985.
64. **Hansen, M. F., Koufos, A., Gallie, B. L., Phillips, R. A., Fodstad, O., Brogger, A., Gedde-Dahl, T., and Cavenee, W. K.**, Osteosarcoma and retinoblastoma: a shared chromosomal mechanism revealing recessive predisposition, *Proc. Natl. Acad. Sci. U.S.A.*, 82, 6216, 1985.
65. **Dryja, T. P., Rapaport, J. M., Epstein, J., Goorin, A. M., Weichselbaum, R., Koufos, A., and Cavenee, W. K.**, Chromosome 13 homozygosity in osteosarcoma without retinoblastoma, *Am. J. Hum. Genet.*, 38, 59, 1986.
66. **Knudson, A. G. and Strong, L. C.**, Mutation and Cancer: a model for Wilms' tumour of the kidney, *J. Natl. Cancer Inst.*, 40, 313, 1972.
67. **Barnes, J., Morris-Jones, P., and Pritchard, J.**, personal communication, 1987.
68. **Narahara, K., Kikkawa, K., Kimira, S., Kimoto, H., Ogata, M., Kasai, M., and Matsuoka, K.**, Regional mapping of catalase and Wilms' tumour-aniridia, genitourinary abnormalities, and mental retardation triad loci to the chromosome segment 11p1305-p1306, *Hum. Genet.*, 66, 181, 1984.
69. **Cordero, J. F., Li, F. P., Holmes, L. B., and Gerald, P. S.**, Wilms' tumour in five cousins, *Pediatrics,* 66, 716, 1980.
70. **Juberg, R. C., Saint Martin, E. C., and Hundley, J. R.**, Familial occurrence of Wilms' tumour: nephroblastoma in one of monozygotic twins and another sibling. *Am. J. Hum. Genet.*, 27, 155, 1975.
71. **Miller, R. W.**, Association of Wilms' tumour with aniridia, hemihypertrophy and other congenital malformations, *N. Engl. J. Med.*, 270, 922, 1964.
72. **Riccardi, V. M., Sujansky, E., Smith, A. C., and Francke, U.**, Chromosome imbalance in the aniridia-Wilms' tumour association: 11p interstitial deletion, *Pediatrics,* 61, 604, 1978.
73. **Riccardi, V. M., Hittner, H. M., Strong, L. C., Fernback, D. J., Lebo, R., and Ferrell, R. F.**, Wilms' tumour and aniridia/iris dysplasia and apparently normal chromosomes, *J. Pediatr.*, 100, 574, 1982.
74. **Shannon, R. S., Mann, J. R., Harper, E., Harnden, D. G., Morten, J. E. N., and Herbert, A.**, Wilms' tumour and aniridia: clinical and cytogenetic features, *Arch. Dis. Child.*, 57, 685, 1982.
75. **Turleau, C., DeGrouchy, J., Dufier, J. L., Phuc, L. H., Schmelck, P. H., Rappaport, R., Nihoul-Fekete, C., and Diebold, N.**, Aniridia, male pseudohermaphroditism, gonadoblastoma, mental retardation and del 11p13, *Hum. Genet.*, 57, 300, 1981.
76. **Yunis, J. J. and Ramsay, K. C.**, Familial occurrence of the aniridia-Wilms' tumour syndrome with deletion 11p13-14.1, *J. Pediatr.*, 96, 1027, 1980.
77. **Hittner, H. M., Riccardi, V. M., and Francke, U.**, Aniridia caused by a heritable chromosome 11-deletion, *Ophthalmologica,* 86, 1173, 1979.
78. **Andersen, S., Geertingen, P., Larsen, H. W., Mikkelson, M., Parbing, A., Vestermark, S., and Warburg, M.**, Aniridia, cateract and gonadoblastoma in a mentally retarded girl with deletion of chromosome 11, *Ophthalmologica,* 176, 171, 1978.

79. **Junien, C., Turleau, C., DeGrouchy, J., Said, R., Rethore, M. O., Tenconi, R., and Dufier, J. L.,** Regional assignment of catalase(CAT) gene to band 11p13. Association with the aniridia-Wilms' tumour-gonadoblastoma (WAGR) complex, *Ann. Genet.*, 28, 165, 1980.
80. **Junien, C.,** personal communication, 1985.
81. **Turleau, C., DeGrouchy, J., Nihoul-Fekete, C., Dufier, J. L., Chavin-Colin, F., and Junien, C.,** Del 11p13/nephroblastoma without aniridia, *Hum. Genet.*, 67, 455, 1984.
82. **Glaser, T., Lewis, W. H., Bruns, G. A. P., Watkins, P. C., Rogler, C. E., Shows, T. B., Powers, V. E., Willard, H. F., Goguen, J. M., Simola, K. O. J., and Housman, D. E.,** b-subunit of follicle-stimulating hormone is deleted in patients with aniridia and Wilms' tumour, allowing a further definition of the WAGR locus, *Nature,* 321, 882, 1986.
83. **Rogler, C. E., Sherman, M., Su, C. Y., Shafritz, D. A., Summers, J., Shows, T. B., Henderson, A., and Kew, M.,** Deletion in chromosome 11p associated with a Hepatitis B integration site in hepatocellular carcinoma, *Science,* 230, 319, 1985.
84. **Kaneko, Y., Euges, M. C., and Rowley, J. D.,** Interstitial deletion of short arm of chromosome 11 limited to Wilms' tumour cells in a patient without aniridia, *Cancer Res.*, 41, 4577, 1981.
85. **Kaneko, Y., Kondo, K., Rowley, J. D., Moohr, J. W., and Maurer, H. S.,** Further chromosome studies on Wilms' tumour cells of patients without aniridia, *Cancer Genet. Cytogenet.*, 10, 191, 1983.
86. **Kondo, K., Chilcote, R. R., Maurer, H. S., and Rowley, J.,** Chromosome abnormalities in tumour cells from patients with sporadic Wilms' tumour, *Cancer Res.*, 44, 5376, 1984.
87. **Douglass, E. C., Green, A. A., Hayes, F. A., Etcubanas, E., Horowitz, M., and Wilimas, J. A.,** Chromosome 1 abnormalities: a common feature of pediatric solid tumours, *J. Natl. Cancer Inst.*, 75, 51, 1985.
88. **Slater, R. M., De Kraker, J., Voute, P. A., and Delemare, J. F. M.,** A cytogenetic study of Wilms' tumour, *Cancer Genet. Cytogenet.*, 14, 95, 1985.
89. **Slater, R. M.,** The cytogenetics of Wilms' tumour, *Cancer Genet. Cytogenet.*, 19, 37, 1986.
90. **Brito-Babapulle, V. and Atkin, N. B.,** Breakpoints in £1 abnormalities of 218 human neoplasms, *Cancer Genet. Cytogenet.*, 4, 215, 1981.
91. **Machin, G. A.,** Persistent renal blastema (nephroblastomatosis) as a frequent precursor of Wilms' tumour, a pathological and clinical review. I. Nephroblastomatosis in context of embryology and genetics, *Am. J. Pediatr. Hematol. Oncol.*, 2, 165, 1980.
92. **Kulkarni, R., Bailie, M. D., Bernstein, J., and Newton, B.,** Progression of nephroblastomatosis to Wilms' tumour, *J. Pediatr.*, 96, 178, 1980.
93. **Heidemann, R. L., McGravan, L., and Waldstein, G.,** Nephroblastomatosis and deletion 11p, *Am. J. Pediatr. Hematol./Oncol.*, 8, 231, 1986.
94. **Bonadio, J. F., Storer, B., and Norkool, P.,** Anaplastic Wilms' tumour: clinical and pathological studies, *J. Clin. Oncol.*, 47, 2302, 1985.
95. **Douglass, E. C., Look, A. T., Webber, B., Parham, D., Wilimas, J. A., Green, A. A., and Roberson, P. K.,** Hyperdiploidy and chromosomal rearrangements define the anaplastic variant of Wilms' tumour, *J. Clin. Oncol.*, 4, 975, 1986.
96. **Orkin, S. H., Goldman, D. S., and Sallan, S. E.,** Development of homozygosity for chromosome 11p markers in Wilms' tumour, *Nature,* 309, 172, 1984.
97. **Fearon, E. R., Vogelstein, B., and Feinberg, A. P.,** Somatic deletion and duplication of genes on chromosome 11 in Wilms' tumours, *Nature,* 309, 176, 1984.
98. **Koufos, A., Hansen, M. F., Lampkin, B. C., Workman, M. L., Copeland, N. G., Jenkins, N. A., and Cavenee, W. K.,** Loss of alleles at loci on human chromosome 11 during genesis of Wilms' tumour, *Nature,* 309, 170, 1984.
99. **Raizis, A. M., Becroft, D. M., Shaw, R. L., and Reeve, A. E.,** A mitotic recombination in Wilms' tumour occurs between the parathyroid hormone locus and 11p13, *Hum. Genet.*, 70, 344, 1985.
100. **Beckwith, J. B.,** Wilms' tumour and other renal tumours of childhood: a selective review from the National Wilms' tumour study pathology center, *Hum. Pathol.*, 14, 481, 1983.
101. **Wiedemann, H. R.,** Complexe malformatif familial avec hernie ombilicle et macroglossie; un syndrome nouveau? *J. Genet. Hum.*, 13, 223, 1964.
102. **Haas, O. A., Zoubek, A., Grumayer, E. R., and Gadner, H.,** Constitutional interstitial deletion of 11p11 and pericentric inversion of chromosome 9 in a patient with Wiedemann-Beckwith syndrome and hepatoblastoma, *Cancer Genet. Cytogenet.*, 23, 95, 1986.
103. **Pettenati, M. J., Haines, J. L., Higgins, R. R., Wappner, R. S., Palmer, C. G., and Weaver, D. D.,** Wiedemann-Beckwith syndrome: presentation of clinical and cytogenetic data on 22 cases and review of the literature, *Hum. Genet.*, 74, 143, 1986.
104. **Koufos, A., Hansen, M. F., Copeland, N. G., Jenkins, M. A., Lampkin, B. C., and Cavenee, W. K.,** Loss of heterozygosity in 3 embryonal tumours suggests a common pathogenetic mechanism, *Nature,* 316, 330, 1986.

105. **Grobstein, C.,** Morphogenetic interaction between embryonic mouse tissue separated by a membrane filter, *Nature,* 172, 869, 1953.
106. **Little, P. F. R.,** Finding the defective gene, *Nature,* 321, 558, 1986.
107. **Little, P. F. R. and Cross, S. H.,** A cosmid vector that facilitates restriction enzyme mapping, *Proc. Natl. Acad. Sci. U.S.A.,* 82, 3159, 1986.
108. **Cross, S. H. and Little, P. F. R.,** A cosmid vector for systematic walking, *Gene,* in press, 1987.
109. **Gusella, J. F., Keys, C., Varsanyi-Breiner, A., Kao, F., Jones, C., Puck, T. T., and Housman, D.,** Isolation and localisation of DNA segments from specific human chromosomes, *Proc. Natl. Acad. Sci. U.S.A.,* 77, 2829, 1980.
110. **Gusella, J. F., Jones, C., Kao, F., Housman, D., and Puck, T. T.,** Genetic fine structure mapping of chromosome 11 by use of repetitive DNA sequences, *Proc. Natl. Acad. Sci. U.S.A.,* 79, 7804, 1982.
111. **Deaven, L. L. and Van Dilla.,** Construction of human chromosome-specific DNA libraries from flow sorted chromosomes, *Proc. 7th Int. Congr. Human Genetics,* 1, 199, 1986.
112. **Cowell, J. K. and Pritchard, J.,** The molecular genetics of retinoblastoma and Wilms' tumour *Crit. Rev. Oncol. Hematol.,* in press, 1987.
113. **Porteous, D. J., Morten, J. E. N., Cranston, G., Fletcher, J. M., Mitchell, A., Van Heyningen, V., Fantes, J. A., Boyd, P. A., and Hastie, N. D.,** Molecular and physical arrangements of human DNA in HRAS1-selected, chromosome-mediated transfectants, *Mol. Cell. Biol.,* 6, 2223, 1986.
114. **Hastie, N.,** personal communication, 1986.
115. **Williams, D. L., Look, T., Melvin, S. L., Roberson, P. K., Dahl, G., Flake, T., and Stass, S.,** New chromosomal translocations correlate with specific immunophenotypes of childhood acute lymphoblastic leukaemia, *Cell,* 36, 101, 1984.
116. **Lewis, W. H., Goguen, J. M., Powers, V. E., Willard, H. F., and Michalopoulos, E. E.,** Gene order on the short arm of human chromosome 11: regional assignment of the LDH A gene distal to catalase in two translocations, *Hum. Genet.,* 71, 249, 1985.
117. **Erikson, J., Williams, D. L., Finan, J., Nowell, P. C., and Croce, C. M.,** Locus of the a-chain of the T-cell receptor is split by chromosome translocation in T-cell leukemias, *Science,* 229, 784, 1985.
118. **Lewis, W. H., Goguen, J. M., Powers, V. E., Willard, H. F., and Michalopoulos, E. E.,** Gene order on the short arm of human chromosome 11: regional assignment of the LDH A gene distal to catalase in two translocations, *Hum. Genet.,* 71, 249, 1986.
119. **Lewis, W. K.,** personal communication, 1986.
120. **Croce, C. M.,** Chromosome translocations in human cancer, *Cancer Res.,* 46, 6019, 1986.
121. **Poustka, A., Pohl, T. M., Barlow, D. P., Frischauf, A-M., and Lehrach, H.,** Construction and use of human chromosome jumping libraries from NotI-digested DNA, *Nature,* 325, 353, 1987.
122. **Schwartz, D. C. and Cantor, C. R.,** Separation of yeast chromosome-sized DNA by pulsed field gradient gel electrophoresis, *Cell,* 37, 67, 1984.
123. **Van Ommen, G. J. B. and Verkerk, J. M. H.,** Restriction analysis of chromosomal DNA in a size range up to two million base pairs by pulsed field gradient electrophoresis, in *Human Genetic Diseases,* Davies, K. E. Ed., IRL Press, Oxford, 1986, 113.
124. **Anand, R.,** Pulse field gel electrophoresis: a technique for fractionating large DNA molecules, *Trends Genet.,* 2, 278, 1986.
125. **Carle, G. F., Frank, M., and Olson, M. V.,** Electrophoretic separations of large DNA molecules by periodic inversion of the electric field, *Science,* 232, 65, 1986.
126. **Carle, G. F. and Olson, M. V.,** Separation of chromosomal DNA molecules from yeast by orthogonal field alteration gel electrophoresis, *Nucleic Acids Res.,* 12, 5647, 1984.
127. **Brown, W. R. A. and Bird, A. P.,** Long range restriction site mapping of mammalian genomic DNA, *Nature,* 322, 477, 1986.
128. **Bird, A. P.,** CpG-rich islands and the functions of DNA methylation, *Nature,* 321, 209, 1986.
129. **Bird, A., Taggart, M., Frommer, M., Miller, O. J., and Macleod, D.,** A fraction of the mouse genome that is derived from islands of nonmethylated, CpG-rich DNA, *Cell,* 40, 91, 1985.

Chapter 9

GENE REARRANGEMENT IN LEUKEMIAS AND LYMPHOMAS

W. J. Smith

TABLE OF CONTENTS

I. INTRODUCTION: THE IMMUNOGLOBULIN GENES

The advent of recombinant DNA technology in the 1970s provided the scientific community with powerful and precise tools to examine many biological processes. The ability to generate and replicate recombinant DNA probes which encode specific genes, or portions of genes, was quickly exploited by immunologists studying the immunoglobulin (Ig) genes.[1] The availability of myelomas expressing monotypic Ig facilitated the isolation of human and murine Ig genes. Functionally similar genes in different species often show sequence homologies as a result of evolutionary relationships. Consequently, clones isolated from one species, e.g., mouse, can be used to obtain their human equivalent. (See Tables 1 and 2.)

Comparisons between human and murine Ig genes revealed that they share structural as well as functional characteristics.[1] Each Ig variable gene domain is composed of two (or, in the case of the Ig heavy chain [IgH], three) gene segments which undergo somatic recombination to generate a functional exon in a cell committed to the B cell lineage (Figure 1). The segments are the variable (V), joining (J), and, in IgH, diversity (D) regions. Each cell undergoes a specific V-(D-)J rearrangement which becomes the "hallmark" of that cell if it undergoes clonal expansion. The transcription of the V domain, in conjunction with the constant (C) region, generates a heavy or light chain Ig mRNA. The IgH locus contains several C regions which are utilized to synthesize the different heavy chain classes. The kappa (κ) locus consists of a sole C region per haploid copy of the genome. In contrast, the lambda chain (λ) C segment is encoded by a highly polymorphic locus. The segmental organization is responsible for the enormous diversity of Ig chains which can be synthesized in response to antigen. The recombination mechanism is governed by recognition sequences which consist of 2 conserved sequences, a nonamer and a heptamer, separated from each other by a nonconserved spacer region composed of either 12 or 23 nucleotides. Recombination between a V region and a D or J segment can only occur if a twelve nucleotide spacer is brought into conjunction with a 23 spacer (Figure 2).[1] This ensures that V-J joining occurs in light chain genes and V-D-J in heavy chain loci. Additional flexibility is achieved by "N" region addition in which nucleotides not encoded by the V gene are inserted by terminal deoxyribonucleotidyl transferase (Tdt) at the junction with the D segment.[2] Somatic mutation in V gene segments and flexibility at the point of V-J joining also contribute to the repetoire of the Ig molecules.[1]

The IgH locus is situated on chromosome 14 at q32, Cκ on chromosome 2p11-12, and Cλ at 22q11.[3] The correlation between cytogenetic abnormalities in these regions and certain B cell neoplasms has been studied by various groups.[3-5]

The fact that Ig rearrangement is correlated with commitment to the B cell lineage has facilitated clonal analysis of cell populations. If one considers a monoclonal population of B cells, they will all possess identical rearranged genes for both heavy and light Ig chains. This particular configuration can be identified by examining DNA extracted from the clone. However, if a heterogeneous B cell population was analyzed, one would be unable to identify any clear pattern since the signals generated by each particular B cell would be too weak to be detected on a Southern blot. In the case of a leukemia or lymphoma, the total lymphoid population would be composed of normal lymphocytes at various differentiation stages, nonlymphoid cells, and the clone of neoplastic cells. The first two groups of cells would generate a germline signal superimposed on a low level of nonclonal hybridization. Non-germline signals (i.e., rearranged) would indicate the presence of the neoplastic clone. This could be identified if it exceeded 5% of the population.[6]

The definition of a neoplastic state is that it is a clonal proliferation of cells.[7] However, the analysis of various "benign" conditions, e.g., angioimmunoblastic lymphadenopathy (AILD) and lymphomatoid papulosis, by molecular methods has revealed the presence of clonal proliferations in these apparently non-neoplastic cell populations.[8-10] Similarly, Jh

Table 1
ILLUSTRATION OF RECOMBINANT DNA PROBES UTILIZED IN GENOTYPIC ANALYSES

Probe	Code name	Ref.
Heavy chain, joining region (Jh)	C76R51A	13
κ light chain, constant region (Cκ)	pUCR17	3
λ light chain, constant region (Cλ)	pUCλ5	39
Constant region of T cell receptor (β chain)	pucCβ	56

Table 2
CD NOMENCLATURE EMPLOYED IN THIS CHAPTER

Antigen	Alternative name	M. WT. (kDa)	Cellular location	Comments
CD3	T3	19—29	T cells	Associated with T. C. R.
CD4	T4	55	Helper/inducer T cells Macrophages	Receptor for H. I. V.
CD7		40	T cells	Receptor for IgM
CD8	T8	32—33	Cytoxic/supressor T cells Splenic sinusoidal cells	
CD10	cALLA	100	Stem cells Renal epithelium, etc.	Marker for cALL
CD25	Tac	55	Activated cells Macrophages	Interleukin II receptor

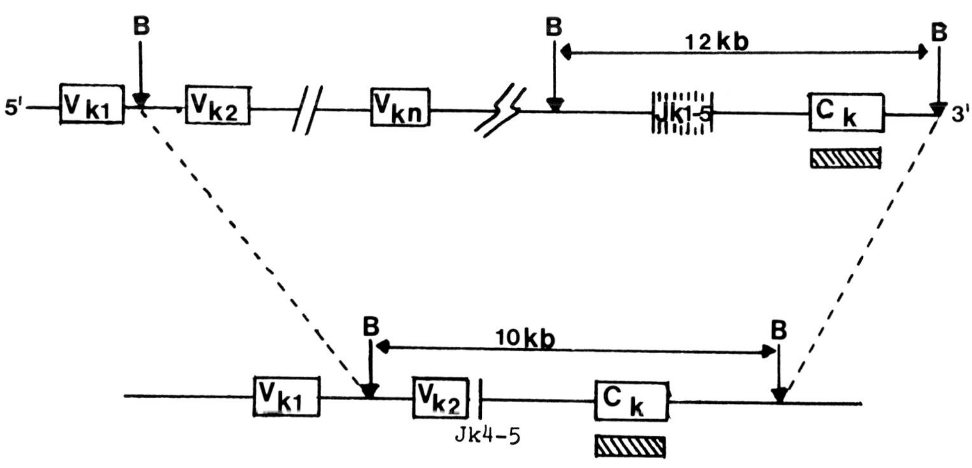

FIGURE 1. Germline organization of the κ light chain gene. The rearranged gene is formed from variable (Vκ). Joining (Jκ) and constant (Cκ) gene segments. The intervening DNA is excised before mRNA transcription. In a B cell neoplasm expressing monotypic light chain, every cell will have undergone an identical Cκ gene rearrangement. In contrast, a nonclonal B cell proliferation will give numerous gene fragments of different sizes at a level below the threshold for detection by routine hybridization studies. Kb; kilobases.

and light chain rearrangements have been detected in Stage A immunoproliferative small intestinal disease (IPSID) which are not usually classified as lymphoma.[11] It is possible that the clonal populations represent neoplastic clones of cells, the proliferation of which is controlled by the immune system in benign conditions. Another theory is that the clones are "preneoplastic" and require an additional mutational event in order to become malignant. A proportion of patients with lymphomatoid papulosis develope malignant lymphomas and

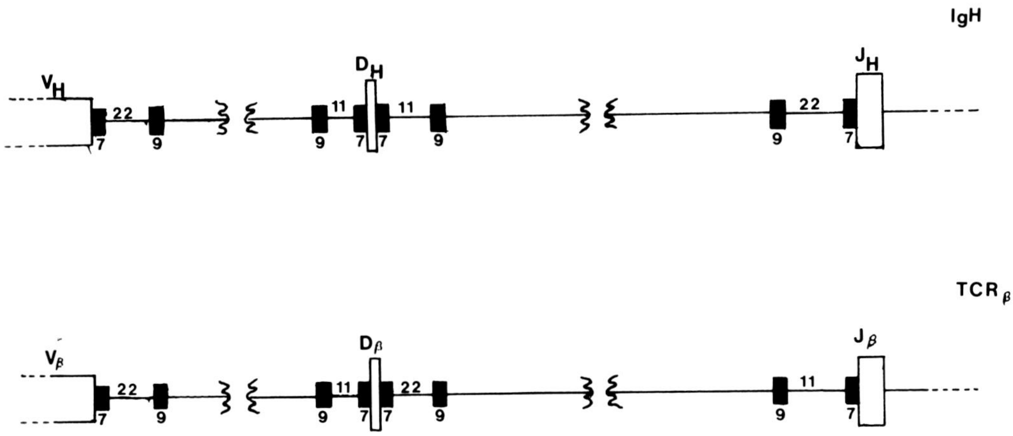

FIGURE 2. Recombination signal distribution in IgH and T cell receptor B genes. Septamer and nonamer sequences are indicated as 7 and 9, respectively. The spacing between these signals in either 11 or 22 nucleotide is indicated.

the comparison of the gene configurations in the benign and malignant conditions of the same patient would determine whether the same clone of cells was present in both states.[10]

The technique known as Southern blotting is utilized in these clonal analyses.[12] High molecular weight genomic DNA is purified from the sample and digested with restriction endonucleases, which recognize specific nucleotide sequences. This generates restriction fragments of various lengths. Separation of these fragments by electrophoresis through an agarose gel is followed by their transfer to a nitrocellulose filter, forming a replica of the gel. The identification of fragments which encode the region of interest is performed by the hybridization of a radioactive plasmic containing the appropriate cloned gene, e.g., the joining region of the IgH gene.[12] Plasmids are extra-chromosomal elements which can be replicated in host bacteria. Many plasmids have been genetically altered to provide a range of cloning sites into which restriction fragments of DNA encoding particular genes, or parts of genes, can be inserted. Selection systems based on antibiotic resistance or the ability to metabolize certain substrates facilitates the identification of plasmids containing recombinant DNA. The stringency of hybridization of the recombinant sequences to the genomic DNA can be controlled by the temperature and salt concentration of the hybridization and washing buffers: this is of particular interest in studies on gene families, e.g., those coding for the V regions of Ig molecules. After washing the filter to remove excess probe, an autoradiograph is obtained by exposing it to X-ray film which provides a permanent record of the data. Radioactive probes can be removed from the filters, allowing the same filter to be reprobed to gain information about the configuration of other genes.

The sensitivity of the technique can result in artifacts: incomplete digestion of DNA with restriction enzymes; contamination of the samples with bacterial or plasmid DNA; and inadequate transfer of the fragments to the filter may all result in misleading data. The recombinant DNA probes used must be well characterized to ensure the validity of the results obtained.

II. Ig GENE REARRANGEMENT IN HEMOPOIETIC MALIGNANCIES

A. B Cell Leukemias

One of the first applications of molecular techniques to a clinical problem was the characterization of "non-T/non-B" acute lymphocytic leukemias (ALL) by Korsymeyer et al.[14] They identified rearranged heavy, and in some cases, light chain genes in seven out of eight cases which did not synthesize detectable cytoplasmic Ig. Interpretation of these data led them to postulate a developmental hierarchy in which successful IgH rearrangement was followed by attempts to generate productive κ genes. If aberrant κ recombinations occur, the λ genes are utilized in order to obtain a viable Ig molecule. Further studies on non-T/non-B ALL cases confirmed this model.[15-17] DNA extracted from T-ALL samples only demonstrated germline configuration Ig genes.[15]

The Ig genes in DNA from the leukemic cells from 93 children with non-T ALL was examined and in all cases at least one rearranged μ allele was observed.[18] Eighteen of the samples revealed more than two DNA nongermline fragments which hybridized to the Cμ probe. In eight of these cases, the additional fragment was due to the presence of an extra chromosome 14. However, the identification of at least three hybridizing fragments in the other ten cases indicated that more than one leukemic clone was present, either as a result of clonal evolution or the occurrence of more than one transformation event. Preliminary data suggest that these cases tend to be more resistant to therapy.

The identification of Ig rearrangement in non-T ALL has been utilized in a sensitive molecular assay to identify one leukemic cell in 500 normal bone marrow cells from patients in remission.[19] This technique exceeds the sensitivity of morphological evaluation (1/20) and may be of use when the remission status is equivocal or when bone marrow transplantation is under consideration.

Although Ig rearrangement is useful in the diagnosis of non-T ALL, it must be remembered that IgH rearrangements have been identified in T cell neoplasms and cell lines.[16,20,21] Conversely, clonal rearrangements of the constant region of the β chain (Cβ) of the T cell receptor (TCR) have been detected in a small porportion of B-cell lines and leukemias.[22] However, these cases are rare and should not discourage the use of a valuable technique in conjunction with immunophenotyping.

Blast cells from children with ALL that carry the 4;11 translocation or with ANLL (acute nonlymphocytic leukemia) often express both lymphoid and myeloid antigens.[17,23-27] Analysis of the Ig genes of blast cells with the t(4;11) translocation from six children has demonstrated IgH rearrangement in 5/6 cases and light chain rearrangement in one case.[23,24] Similar studies on 63 cases of childhood ANLL revealed four examples with nongermline fragments that hybridized to the Jh probe and one with TCR Cβ rearrangement.[26,27] These results can be interpreted as indicating that cells with mixed lineage characteristics arise as a result of either aberrant gene expression in lymphoid cells or the transformation of a multipotential stem cell. Follow up studies on children with t(4;11) ALL have indicated that the rearrangement of IgH genes may continue after the initial transformation event, thus generating sublines of leukemic clones.[23] Such findings have implications for the treatment and analysis of these leukemias.

The examination of Ig gene configuration in cell samples from 46 adults with ANLL has shown four cases with Jh rearrangement.[28] In one example, the rearranged fragments detected in blast cells were not present in the polymorphonuclear leukocytes isolated during remission, indicating that there is no clonal relationship between the two populations. In another case, evidence of leukemic blast cells differentiating to mature granulocytes was provided by the demonstration of identical IgH configurations in the two cell types. The group also used a cloned X-chromosome probe which distinguishes between maternal and paternal copies of the gene HPRT (hypoxanthine phospho-ribosyl-transferase) by a restriction polymorphism to identify clonality in mature granulocytes from two patients. This analysis is only useful for female patients, but it does provide support for the hypothesis that the leukemic blast cells can differentiate to mature granulocytes in ANLL. It is not clear at present whether the leukemic transformation has taken place in a stem cell which has the ability to undergo Ig rearrangement and to differentiate along the myeloid pathway. An alternative explanation is that Ig rearrangement in myeloid cells is evidence of lineage infidelity.[28]

Controversy over the origin of hairy cell leukemia (HCL) has been resolved by the demonstration of rearranged heavy and light chain Ig genes and their corresponding mRNAs in eight cases.[29] The correlation between the molecular and immunological data, except for the presence of the IL2 receptor (CD25), indicates a B cell origin for the "hairy" cells. The extension of this study has confirmed this conclusion.[30] The occasional coexistence of HCL and diffuse histiocytic lymphoma has been interpreted as a clonal evolution of the HCL into lymphoma. However, an immunological and molecular analysis of cells from a patient with HCL and a large cell immunoblastic lymphoma revealed that the two malignant clones possessed different IgH and κ gene configurations, implying separate origins for each clone.[31] In a similar case, a patient with HCL and macroglobulinema was shown to possess two clones of malignant B cells by Southern blot analysis.[32]

Chronic lymphocytic leukemia (CLL) is a monoclonal proliferation of surface-Ig positive B cells which express monotypic light chains.[33] The clonality of the disease has been confirmed by the demonstration of IgH rearrangement.[21,33,34] However, TCR Cβ rearrangement was observed in 1/3 cases of CLL in one study.[21] A proportion of patients with CLL develop lymphoma during the course of the disease.[33] Phenotypic data indicate that the neoplastic population are transformed B cells rather than macrophages. Analysis of the Ig genes of peripheral blood lymphocytes and ascites cells from a patient with Richter's syndrome showed that the two populations possessed different IgH gene configurations.[35] Unless one postulates a transforming event prior to IgH rearrangement, these results indicate separate clonal origins for the two neoplasms.

The monoclonal nature of B-PLL (B cell prolymphocytic leukemia) has been demonstrated by immunological and molecular methods.[5,34] In 5/5 cases, both alleles of the IgH gene were rearranged. Immunological analysis of one case demonstrated that the neoplastic clone expressed both κ and λ light chains.[5] However, only κ gene rearrangement was detected by Southern blotting, probably because the proportion of the population expressing λ chains (8%) was below the threshold of sensitivity of the technique.

A consistent karyotypic abnormality known as the Philadelphia chromosome (Ph) characterizes chronic myeloid leukemia (CML). Cytogenetic and enzymatic studies have indicated the clonal nature of the disease, which is derived from the transformation of a progenitor cell.[33] The overproduction of granulocytes marks the chronic phase of the disease which usually progresses to an acute period, the blast crisis. Approximately one third of patients enter a lymphoid blast crisis in which the neoplastic cells generally express Tdt and CD10 and possess rearranged IgH genes.[34,36,37] In all cases of myeloid blast crisis examined, only germline configurations of immunoglobulin genes have been identified.[34,36,37] Two cases of "mixed" blast crises have been analyzed and the CD10-positive cells, which displayed myeloid antigens, were shown to have germline Ig genes.[37,38] The analysis of two separate episodes of blast crisis in one patient has revealed that, although both clones possessed the same IgH gene configuration, their light chain genes differed.[37] This data has been interpreted as indicating a common lymphoid progenitor cell for both clones which had not undergone light chain gene rearrangement at transformation. It is suggested that the blast crisis represent the expansion of subclones derived from the progenitor neoplastic cell which has undergone further Ig gene rearrangement. Distinguishing between patients with lymphoid rather than myeloid blast crises has obvious clinical consequences.

Molecular analysis of CML has focused on the Ph which is composed of a translocation between chromosomes 9 and 22. The translocation of the oncogene *c-abl* from chromosome 9 to the Ph chromosome (22q-) and its possible relationship to the Ig λ chain locus, which is situated on 22q11, has been investigated.[39] There is no evidence to connect the λ locus with the creation of the Ph chromosome.[39] However, the breakpoint cluster region (bcr) on chromosome 22 has been cloned and shown to be fused to *c-abl* in the progenitor cell responsible for the chronic myeloid and blastic phases of CML.[40] There is no evidence to indicate that the blast phase is preceeded by further alteration to the bcr-*c-abl* region.

However, the exact role played by transcripts of this locus in the progression of the disease is unclear at present.

B. B Cell Lymphoma

The analysis of Ig gene configurations in lymphomas was a natural extension of the studies on leukemia. The Southern blot technique facilitates the identification of a minority population of clonal B cells within a variety of normal cell types.[41] This is of particular value in cases where reactive lymphocytes, which are difficult to distinguish from neoplastic lymphoid cells, are present or when the conventional pathological data are insufficient to differentiate between lymphoma and other conditions, e.g., an undifferentiated carcinoma.

Non-Hodgkin's lymphoma (NHL) are a heterogeneous group of lymphoid neoplasms: immunological data has shown that in adults 75% of cases are B cell in origin, 20% T cell and 5% lack surface Ig or E-rosette receptors (''null'' NHLs).[42] Initial studies on unequivocal B cell lymphomas demonstrated IgH and light chain gene rearrangement in every case.[6,41] Ig rearrangement was not detected in a reactive follicular hyperplasia or a variety of non-B cell lymphomas.[6] Two cases were studied in which there was no evidence of a predominance of B or T cells or of monoclonality, based on the monotypic expression of light chains.[41] However, both samples demonstrated rearranged IgH genes, indicating a clonal expansion of B cells. It was possible to distinguish a minority monoclonal B cell population within three apparent T cell lymphomas. Since the TCR probes were not available at the time it was not possible to formally test whether the T cells were clonal.

The lineage of NHL ''null'' cells has eluded classification by immunological methods. Genetic analysis of these lymphomas by two groups has enabled them to assign a B or T cell lineage in every case. Forty-nine out of 54 cases were B cell malignancies which suggests that the majority of ''null'' lymphomas are in fact of B cell lineage.[42,43] The failure of these lymphomas to express Ig, despite the somatic recombination of their Ig genes, may be due to malfunctions at the translational or transcriptional level. These studies demonstrate that good immunophenotyping in conjunction with genetic analysis can determine the lineage of most lymphoid neoplasms.

The detection of Ig rearrangement in NHLs has resulted in attempts to identify lymphoma cells in the peripheral blood and bone marrow aspirates by Southern blotting.[44,45] B cell clones have been observed in the peripheral blood of 15/17 patients with active phase low grade B cell lymphona by this method.[44] In seven cases, the configuration of the IgH genes were identical in DNA from paired samples of peripheral blood lymphocytes and lymph node biopsies. Blood samples from 12 patients in remission were also studied and seven had indications of clonal B cells. Long term follow up of these patients will clarify the clinical significance of these findings. Bone marrow aspirates have proved to be suitable material for the characterization of B cell lymphomas.[45] Identical Ig gene configurations were identified in paired samples of bone marrow aspirates and lymph node biopsies available from seven patients. Aspirates from different sites indicated a common B cell clone throughout the marrow. The ability to identify clonal proliferation in lymphomas without the necessity to perform excisional biopsies is of value in the assessment of the disease. Possible extensions of this type of sampling include the analysis of T cell lymphomas and, with the availability of more gene probes, the identification of clones with specific chromosomal translocations.

The development of lymphoproliferative lesions in immunosuppressed patients following organ transplantation has led to controversy as to whether they are monoclonal or polyclonal.[46,47] Since polyclonal proliferations do not give rise to nongermline fragments hybridizing to the Ig probes, the genetic analysis of tissue from ten immunosuppressed cardiac transplant patients was undertaken. Despite the absence of surface Ig, monoclonal populations of B cells were detected in all samples.[47] Follow up studies on five of the patients indicated that, although monoclonal B cell populations were still present, their Ig gene configurations differed from the original biopsies in every case.[48] However, there was no evidence of more one B cell clone per biopsy site at any one time. This data is interpreted as a multisite, multiclonal proliferation, which may explain the rapid clinical course of these disorders since a fatal tumor mass can be generated at multiple sites rather than spreading from one location to another. It is possible that the multiple clones arise from a common progenitor which has retained its ability to undergo rearrangement. There is some evidence from one case which supports this hypothesis, but further markers of clonality are required to test the hypothesis rigorously.

During their studies of B cell lymphomas, Sklar et al. have identified 5 to 10% of cases which possess more than one clone of malignant cells.[48,49] Biclonal proliferations can only be identified in Southern blots by the presence of more than two nongermline fragments hybridizing to the IgH probe: a biclonal proliferation in which one allele per clone had undergone rearrangement is indistinguishable from a monoclonal population with both alleles rearranged. The preparation of anti-idiotype antibodies, which distinguishes one B cell population from another, facilitates cell sorting experiments in order to determine the genetic configurations of the Ig genes in each clone. Cell cloning experiments and the use of additional clonal markers are required to determine the relationship, if any, between the two populations. The design of treatment protocols in such neoplasms should take into account the possibility that more than one malignant clone may be present.

The Reed-Sternberg cell, the malignant cell in Hodgkin's disease, is of uncertain origin and there is conflicting evidence as to whether it is of the lymphoid or myeloid-macrophage lineage.[33] A single case has been reported in which a patient with Hodgkin's disease developed a leukemic phase.[50] The analysis of the Ig genes of the neoplastic cells in this case indicated a monoclonal B cell proliferation. A study of 35 cases of Hodgkin's disease demonstrated Ig gene rearrangement in 2/9 samples with a high Reed-Sternberg cell content; the rest had germline Ig genes.[51] There was no evidence of TCR rearrangement in any case.

The molecular analysis of the Ig genes in B cell lymphomas has been extended by studies in which the sequences of the rearranged genes have been determined.[4,52,53] Of follicular lymphomas, 60% are characterized by a t(14q32;18q21) translocation. The breakpoint on 14q32 has been cloned and shown to contain the Ig enhancer region in proximity to a previously unidentified transcriptional unit (18q21).[4] Although this unit has not yet been fully characterized, its involvement in the translocation may indicate a similar function to oncogenes which are implicated in cytogenetic abnormalities e.g., *c-myc* in a t(8;14) translocation seen in Burkitt's Lymphoma.[3] The breakpoint regions in cell lines derived from a Burkitt's lymphoma and a pre-B ALL carrying the t(8;14) translocation have been cloned and sequenced.[52] Comparisons between rearranged and normal clones have shown that at each joining site, the sequences recognized by the V-D-J recombinase are present. Since the progenitor cell of these tumors is a pre-B cell, it is capable of undergoing further Ig gene rearrangement. Errors in recombinase activity are assumed to result in the t(8;14) translocations. DNA analysis of multiple biopsies from a patient with B cell lymphoma demonstrated that, despite an alteration in idiotype, the same B cell clone was present over a 15-month period.[53] Sequencing of the IgH variable regions revealed that somatic mutation in the second complementarity determining region was responsible for the change in idiotype. Although it is likely that such detailed molecular studies would only be undertaken on a small number of cases, they may help to identify the genetic basis for B cell lymphomas.

III. THE T CELL RECEPTOR GENES

T cells recognize antigen in the context of their own major histocompatablity complex (''self'' MHC).[54] The receptor is a heterodimer, composed of an α and a β chain, which is recognized by clonotypic antibodies. The isolation of recombinant DNA clones encoding

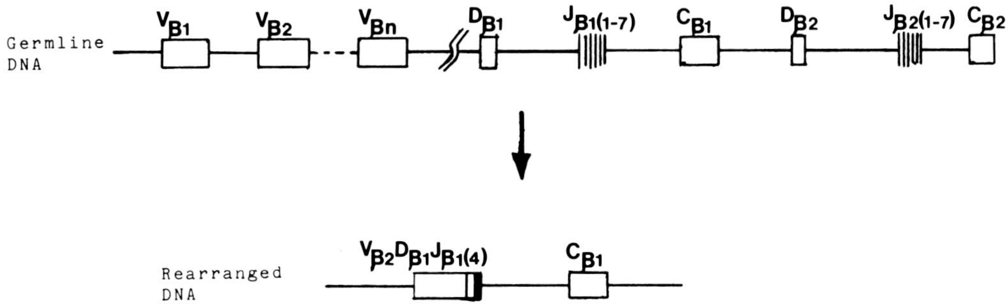

FIGURE 3. Assembly of the T-cell receptor gene from separately encoded variable (Vβ) diversity (Dβ) joining (Jβ) and constant (Cβ) gene segment.

these chains from murine and human gene libraries revealed a segmental structure similar to Ig genes (Figure 3) and led to the concept of them belonging to the immunoglobulin super-gene family.[54] The recombination mechanisms utilized in the formation of functional TCR genes resemble those seen in the Ig system (Figure 2). However, the arrangement of the recognition sequences flanking the V and J segments in the TCR β locus allow for functional V-J joining as well as the conventional V-D-J.

In humans the α locus is unusual as the Jα region, composed of numerous J regions, extends 35 to 60 kilobases upstream of a single Cα segment.[55] It has been suggested that this region is particularly prone to breakage, generating chromosomal translocations: this will be discussed in a later section.[55] Dα segment(s) have not been identified. In the haploid genome, the TCR β locus is composed of multiple Vβ regions, two Dβs, twelve functional Jβs, two Jβ pseudogenes and two Cβ segments.[54] The two Cβ regions are tandemly linked and each has its own associated cluster of joining and diversity segments: it is postulated that the clusters arose as a result of gene duplication since they show a high degree of homology.[56] A third member of the TCR gene family, the γ locus, has been identified by its ability to undergo genetic recombination in T cells.[54] The human γ genes are composed of two tandemly linked Cγ regions, each with its own Vγ and Jγ segments.[57]

The chromosomal locations of each of the TCR genes have been identified by *in situ* hybridization and Southern blotting of DNA extracted from human/murine somatic hybrids. The α chain locus is at 14q11-12 which is a region associated with translocations identified in human T cell neoplasms, e.g., the chromosomal inversion t(14q11; 14q32) in T-CLL.[59,60] Chromosome 14 abnormalities are also associated with childhood ALL, adult T cell leukemia, and T cell malignancies arising in patients with ataxia telaniectasia.[59,61,62] The genes for the β and γ chains are both on chromosome 7: the β locus is at 7q32 and γ at 7p15.[63,64]

The rearrangement of the TCR genes occurs in a hierarchical order: the somatic recombination of the γ locus occurs early in T cell differentiation and is followed by the β gene.[57,65] Rearrangement of the Cβ locus can occur in a variety of ways: one or two of the Cβ1 or Cβ2 alleles can be rearranged or one or both Cβ1 alleles may be deleted. Rearrangement of the Cβ genes occurs prior to the coordinate expression of the heterodimer TCR with CD3.[66] Consequently, clonal expansions of immature (i.e., CD3-negative) T cells can be detected by Southern blotting. The size of the Jα region complicates the analysis of gene rearrangement in the α locus, but it generally occurs after the recombination of the β gene.[65] Studies on the TCR gene configurations in T cell neoplasms have tended to concentrate on the β chain.

IV. T CELL GENE REARRANGEMENT IN HEMOPOIETIC MALIGNANCIES

A. T Cell Leukemias

The initial studies on gene rearrangement in human T cell neoplasms were undertaken by

Tak Mak's group.[67] They identified the germline pattern of the β chain genes in a variety of nonlymphoid and B cell samples and then extended the study to a range of T cell lines.[67,68] Nongermline patterns were detected in thymic leukemic cell lines, indicating that the β chain locus undergoes rearrangement at an early stage in ontogeny. Helper, killer, and suppressor T cells all possessed rearranged TCR β chain genes.

CD7-positive blast cells are identified in approximately 20% of childhood ALL cases which are, therefore, classified as T-ALLs.[33] Rearranged Cβ and germline Ig genes have been observed in the majority of cases analyzed.[15,16,22,68-72] Although it has been suggested that the patterns of Cβ rearrangement in T-ALL are nonrandom, other authors have published data which refute this hypothesis.[22,68,71,72] Two cases have been reported in which the mediastinal mass typical of T-ALL was present but the immunological profiles were inconsistent with this diagnosis.[73] Genetic analysis demonstrated IgH rearrangement: the Cβ genes were not examined. Rearranged Cβ and IgH genes have been detected in approximately 10% of T-ALLs studied.[16,20,21,68,70,71] The configurations of the TCR Cβ and Ig genes have been examined in 39 cases of childhood non-T, non-B ALL.[72] IgH rearrangement was detected in all cases but 25% of the series also exhibited nongermline Cβ gene configurations. There were no other indications that these ten patients differed from the rest of the group and only clinical follow up will reveal the significance, if any, of this finding. The reason why both gene systems undergo somatic recombination in certain cases of malignancies is unknown: it may reflect errors which occur in normal lymphocytes at a low frequency, or it may be connected with the neoplastic process.

Adult T cell leukemia/lymphoma (ATLL) is associated with the human T cell leukemia/lymphoma virus-1 (HTLV-1).[74] The malignant cells express CD3, CD4, CD8, and CD25. All cases of ATLL studied exhibited at least two rearranged Cβ alleles while the Ig genes retained a germline configuration.[16,22,69,71,74,75] Three nongermline fragments which hybridized to the Cβ probe were identified in one sample.[74] Karyotypic analysis indicated a tandem duplication of the long arm of chromosome 7 present in the malignant cells. It is likely that the chromosomal duplication had preceeded the Cβ gene rearrangement. The ability to identify the neoplastic clone enabled Waldmann's group to monitor the reemergence of the original leukemic clone during therapy utilizing an anti-CD25 antibody.[22]

The majority of CLL and prolymphocytic leukemia (PLL) cases are of B cell origin, but in approximately 5% of cases, the neoplastic proliferation is of T cells.[33] The immunological phenotype of the neoplastic cells in CLL is CD3+, CD4+, CD8−, surface Ig-negative. The PLL malignant cells are usually CD3+ but may be CD4+ or CD8+. The data from the genetic analysis of T-CLL and T-PLL confirm that they are monoclonal proliferations of T cells.[16,21,22,68-71,76,77] The monoclonality and malignancy of clinically indolent CLL has been questioned, but the genetic data confirm that the observed T cell population is clonal.[76]

Lymphocytes from patients with Sezary cell leukemia have been analyzed for T cell clonality by several groups.[22,69,71,77] In all cases, Cβ rearrangement was detected.

T cell clonality has also been detected in Ph+ve CML blast crisis and in 3/24 samples from patients with AML.[78-80] The significance of these findings is unclear: they may resemble aberrant genetic events in normal cells which are not normally detected, or they may be connected with the neoplastic process. Another hypothesis is that the neoplastic clones arise from progenitor cells which are capable of lymphoid and myeloid differentiation, presumably after the genes encoding the TCR β chain have undergone rearrangement.[79]

B. T Cell Lymphomas

The isolation and characterization of the TCR genes has facilitated the determination of clonality in T cell lymphomas.[69,70,81,82] Until these probes were available, only cytogenetic abnormalities or the production of enzymes encoded by genes located on the X-chromosome could be used to identify T cell clones. Cβ rearrangement was detected in 28/32 cases of

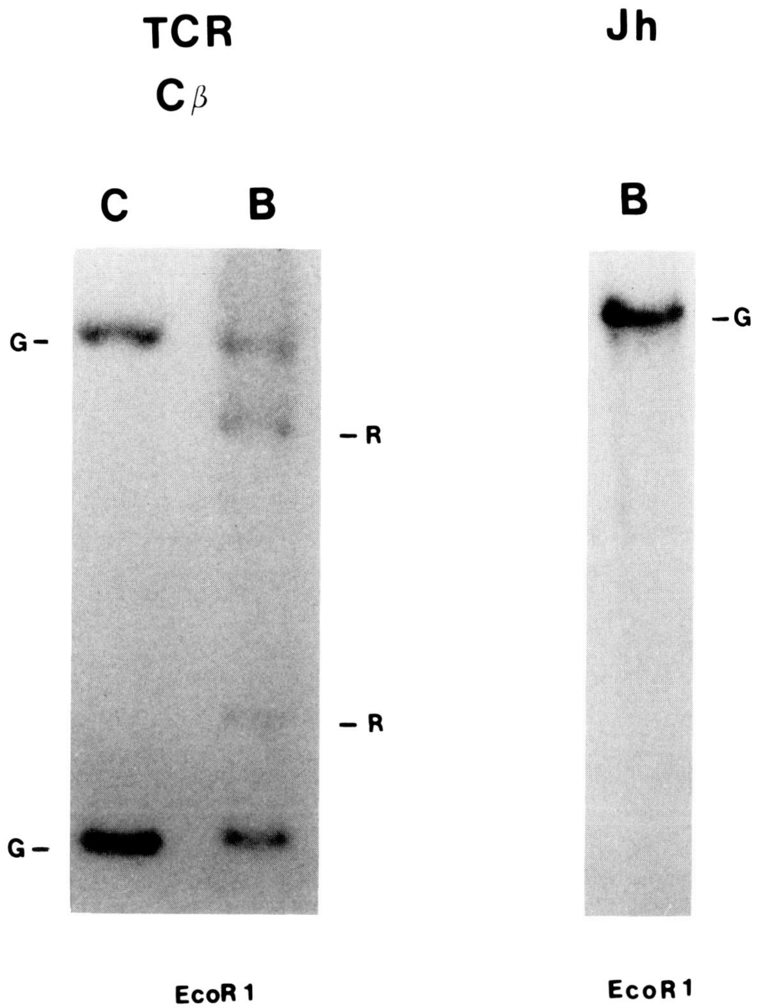

FIGURE 4. Example of a genotypic analysis of a case which exhibited a histological morphology consistent with a B cell follicular lymphoma. Immunophenotyping was inconclusive, but Southern blot analysis, utilizing several restriction enzymes to exclude polymorphisms, revealed the presence of a T cell lymphoma. T.C.R. Cβ, T cell receptor β chain; Jh, joining region of immunoglobulin heavy chain; C, control DNA; B, biopsy DNA; G, germline configuration (11.5 and 4 kb.); and R, rearranged genetic configuration. HindIII and BamH1 digests confirmed the presence of two rearranged alleles (EcoR1 nongermline fragments were 8.8 and 4 kb); EcoR1, restriction enzyme.

T-NHL examined.[70,83] Dual rearrangement of Ig and TCR genes had occurred in four samples: this is analogous to aberrant rearrangement in B cell neoplasms.[21] However, other groups have not observed Jh rearrangement in T cell lymphomas.[81,82] The lack of detectable rearrangement in some cases may be due to the clone only representing 5 to 10% of the cellular population or misdiagnosis of a reactive T cell population as a neoplastic expansion.[70] The identification of T cell clonality by molecular methods in precursor T (lymphoblastic) neoplasms is of particular use when the immature phenotype of the T cells makes a diagnosis of malignancy problematical (Figure 4).

Distinguishing between lymph node involvement in advanced mycosis fungoides (M.F.) and dermatopathic lymphadenopathy, a reactive lymphoid hyperplasia often associated with chronic skin disease, can be problematical. Studies on DNA extracted from lymph node biopsies from patients with M.F. have confirmed the T cell clonal nature of the disease.[70,81,85]

The configurations of the Cβ genes in matched biopsies from lymph nodes and histologically involved tissue, e.g., skin, were compared and in each case found to be identical.[85] This confirms that the disease is monoclonal even when several sites are involved. Clonal cells have been detected in the peripheral blood of these patients and this may provide a relatively noninvasive method of monitoring the disease during treatment.[85] However, the situation in earlier stages of the disease (stage I and II), which does not always progress to frank lymphoma, is less clear since TCR Cβ gene rearrangement has not been detected.[83] A clonal proliferation of T cells may be present but at levels indetectable by the Southern blotting technique or the initial stages of M.F. may be polyclonal. The association of M.F. with Hodgkin's disease was investigated by comparing the Cβ gene configurations in serial biopsies from a patient with M.F. who developed Hodgkin's disease.[81] The germline pattern of Cβ genes seen in the malignant lymph node, which was diagnosed as reflecting Hodgkin's disease, demonstrated that this was not a conversion of the cutaneous T cell lymphoma.

Lennert's lymphoma was initially described as a variant of Hodgkin's disease with a strong epithelioid component.[86] Cytogenetic studies indicated chromosomal abnormalities associated with T cell neoplasms. Immunophenotyping and genotyping have confirmed that Lennert's lymphoma is a CD4+ T cell lymphoma.[86,87] Serial biopsies from one patient have suggested that subclones of the lymphoma have replaced the original neoplasm.[86]

The determination of T cell clonality by immunological and genetic methods in malignant histiocytosis of the intestine (MHI) has shown that it is of T cell rather than of histiocytic origin.[88] Consequently, it has been suggested that the term "enteropathy-associated T cell lymphoma" is a more accurate description of this condition.[89] The existence of neoplasms in which the cell of origin is histiocytic has been questioned by some authors following the molecular study of MHI and "histiocytic" malignancies.[90] In one study, 5/6 cases which were judged to be histiocytic by morphological criteria were found to have either rearranged Ig or Cβ genes.[90] However, only 1/5 cases of large cell lymphoma which expressed macrophage antigens possessed nongermline configurations of TCR Cβ genes; all had germline configurations of Ig genes.[83]

The association between T cell neoplasms and cytogenetic abnormalities has already been mentioned briefly.[60-63] Detailed molecular analysis of these translocations has defined the DNA sequences of the chromosomal breakpoints in two cases of T-ALL and one case of T cell lymphoma.[91-93] The cytogenetic profile of the malignant cells in the T-ALLs investigated revealed a translocation between 11p13 and 14q13.[91] Hybridization data demonstrated that the chromosomal breakpoint at 14q13 had separated the TCR Cα region from the V segments. The breakpoint on chromosome 11 had occurred between the catalase and calcitonin genes, in a region close to the putative Wilms' tumor locus (11p13). The relationship, if any, between this alteration in genetic material and the leukemiogenesis is not clear at present (see Cowell, J., Chapter 8).

The study of a cell line, SUPT-1, derived from a patient with childhood T cell lymphoma has revealed that the DNA recombinase can function at both the Ig and TCR loci.[92,93] The tumor carried an inversion of chromosome 14 (q11.2; q32.2). Since the IgH locus is at 14q32 and the TCRα at 14q11, it was of interest to study the DNA sequences around both breakpoints. This revealed that a "fusion" gene ("IgT"), composed of an Ig V region and a TCR Jα and Cα, had been formed by a rearrangement of genetic material.[93] The role of IgT in oncogenesis is a matter of speculation until it is known whether it is present in other T cell neoplasms with an inverted chromosome 14 and whether IgT transcripts are functional in the neoplastic cell.

V. CONCLUSIONS

The isolation and characterization of the immunoglobulin and the T cell receptor recombinant DNA probes has been of value in many clinical problems studied by this methodology.

The ability to discriminate between reactive and malignant lymphoid populations, the identification of the evolution of subclones of neoplastic clones, and the facility to determine whether one tumor has evolved into another are all of benefit to the clinician.[23,31-33,94] However, the interpretation of data generated by this technology must be performed in the context of all the clinical, histological, and immunological information that is available. Sensitive assays are prone to artifacts and the neoplastic process itself may lead to malfunctions in the somatic recombination of Ig and TCR genes. If these factors are taken into consideration, the analysis of the genetic configurations of the Ig and TCR genes has a role to play in the diagnosis of lymphoproliferative disorders.

REFERENCES

1. **Honjo, T.,** Immunoglobulin Genes, *Ann. Rev. Immunol.,* 1, 499, 1983.
2. **Desiderio, S. V., Yancopulos, G. D., Paskind, M., Thomas, E., Boss, M. A., Landau, N., Alt., F. A., and Baltimore, D.,** Insertion of N regions into heavy-chain genes is correlated with expression of terminal deoxytranferase in B cells, *Nature,* 311, 752, 1984.
3. **Rabbitts, T. H.,** Cytogenetics and molecular biology combine in the investigation of chromosomal translocation and human leukaemia, *Mol. Biol. Med.,* 1, 275, 1983.
4. **Bakhshi, A., Jensen, J. P., Goldman, P., Wright, J. J., McBride, O. W., Epstein, A. L., and Korsmeyer, S. J.,** Cloning the chromosomal breakpoint of t(14;18) human lymphomas: clustering around Jh on chromosome 14 and near a transcriptional unit on 18, *Cell,* 41, 899, 1985.
5. **Brito-Babapulle, V., Melo, J. V., Foroni, L., Robinson, D., Parreira, L., Brozovic, M., and Catovsky, D.,** Neoplastic κ and λ cells in a B-PLL with chromosome translocations of both light chain regions, *Int. J. Cancer,* 34, 769, 1984.
6. **Clearly, M. L., Chao, J., Warnke, R., and Sklar, J.,** Immunoglobulin gene rearrangement as a diagnostic criterion of B cell lymphoma, *Proc. Natl. Acad. Sci. U.S.A.,* 81, 593, 1984.
7. **Davey, M. P. and Waldmann, T. A.,** Clonality and lymphoproliferative lesions, *N. Engl. J. Med.,* 315, 509, 1986.
8. **Weiss, L. M., Strickler, J. G., Dorfman, R. F., Horning, S. J., Warnke, R. A., and Sklar, J.,** Clonal T-cell populations in angioimmunoblastic lymphadenopathy and angioimmunoblastic lymphadenopathy-like lymphoma, *Am. J. Pathol.,* 122, 392, 1986.
9. **O'Connor, N. T. J., Crick, J. A., Wainscoat, J. S., Gatter, K. C., Stein, H., Falini, B., and Mason, D. Y.,** Evidence for monoclonal T lymphocyte proliferation in angioimmunoblastic lymphadenopathy, *J. Clin. Pathol.,* 39, 1229, 1986.
10. **Weiss, L. M., Wood, G. S., Trela, M., Warnke, R. A., and Sklar, J.,** Clonal T-cell populations in lymphomatoid papulosis, *N. Engl. J. Med.,* 315, 475, 1986.
11. **Smith, W. J., Price, S. K., and Isaacason, P. G.,** Immunoglobulin gene rearrangement in immunoproliferative small intestinal disease (IPSID), *J. Clin. Pathol.,* in press, 1987.
12. **Southern, E. M.,** Detection of specific sequences among DNA fragments separated by gel electrophoresis, *J. Mol. Biol.,* 98, 503, 1975.
13. **Flanagan, J. D. and Rabbitts, T. H.,** The sequence of an immunoglobulin epsilon heavy chain constant region gene and evidence for three nonallelic genes, *EMBO J.,* 1, 655, 1982.
14. **Korsmeyer, S. J., Heiter, P. A., Ravetch, J. V., Poplack, D. G., Waldmann, T. A., and Leder, P.,** Developmental hierarchy of immunoglobulin gene rearrangements in human leukaemic pre-B-cells, *Proc. Natl. Acad. Sci. U.S.A.,* 78, 7096, 1981.
15. **Korsmeyer, S. J., Arnold, A., Bakshi, A., Ravetch, J. V., Siebenlist, U., Hieter, P. A., Sharrow, S. O., Lebien, T., Kersey, J. H., Poplack, D. G., Leder, P., and Waldmann, T. A.,** Immunoglobulin gene rearrangement and cell surface antigen expression in acute lymphocytic leukemias of T and B cell precursor origins, *J. Clin. Invest.,* 71, 301, 1983.
16. **Aisenberg, A. C. and Wilkes, B. M.,** The genotype and phenotype of T cell and non-T, non-B acute lymphoblastic leukemia, *Blood,* 66, 1215, 1985.
17. **Stong, R. C., Korsmeyer, S. J., Parkin, J. L., Arthur, D. C., and Kersey, J. H.,** Human acute leukemia cell line with the t(4;11) chromosomal rearrangement exhibits B lineage and monocytic characteristics, *Blood,* 65, 21, 1985.

18. **Kitchingham, G. R., Mirro, J., Stass, S., Rovigatti, U., Melvin, S., Williams, D. L., Raimondi, S. C., and Murphy, S. B.,** Biologic and prognostic significance of the presence of more than two μ heavy chain genes in childhood acute lymphoblastic leukemia of B precursor cell origin, *Blood,* 67, 698, 1986.
19. **Zehnbauer, B. A., Pardoll, D. M., Burke, P. J., Graham, M. L., and Vogelstein, B.,** Immunoglobulin gene rearrangements in remission bone marrow specimens from patients with acute lymphoblastic leukemia, *Blood,* 67, 835, 1986.
20. **Kitchingham, G. R., Rovigatti, U., Mauer, A. M., Melvin, S., Murphy, S. B., and Stass, S.,** Rearrangement of immunoglobulin heavy chain genes in T cell acute lymphoblastic leukemia, *Blood,* 65, 725, 1985.
21. **Pelicci, P. G., Knowles, D. M., and Favera, R. D.,** Lymphoid tumours displaying rearrangements of both immunoglobulin and T cell receptor genes, *J. Exp. Med.,* 162, 1015, 1985.
22. **Waldmann, T. A., Davis, M. M., Bongiovanni, K. F., and Korsmeyer, S. J.,** Rearrangements of genes for the antigen receptor on T cells as markers for lineage and clonality in human lymphoid neoplasms, *N. Engl. J. Med.,* 313, 776, 1985.
23. **Mirro, J., Kitchingham, G. R., Williams, D., Lauzon, G. J., Lin, C. C., Calihan, T., and Zipf, T. F.,** Clinical and laboratory characteristics of acute leukaemia with the 4;11 translocation, *Blood,* 67, 689, 1986.
24. **Srivastava, B. I. S., Wright, J. J., and Bakhshi, A.,** Immunoglobulin chain gene rearrangements in a t(4;11) acute leukaemia with monocytoid blasts, *Br. J. Haematol.,* 63, 321, 1986.
25. **Rovigatti, U., Mirro, J., Kitchingham, G., Dahl, G., Ochs, J., Murphy, S., and Stass, S.,** Heavy chain immunoglobulin gene rearrangement in acute nonlymphocytic leukaemia, *Blood,* 63, 1023, 1984.
26. **Ha, K., Minden, M., Hozumi, N., and Gelfand, E. W.,** Immunoglobulin gene rearrangement in acute myelogenous leukaemia, *Cancer Res.,* 44, 4658, 1984.
27. **Mirro, J., Zipft, T. F., Pui, C. H., Kitchingham, G., Williams, D., Melvin, S., Murphy, S., and Stass, S.,** Acute mixed lineage leukaemia: clinicopathologic correlations and prognostic significance, *Blood,* 66, 1115, 1985.
28. **Fearon, E. R., Burke, P. J., Schiffer, C. A., Zehnbauer, B. A., and Vogelstein, B.,** Differentiation of leukaemia cells to polymorphonuclear leukocytes in patients with acute nonlymphocytic leukaemia, *N. Engl. J. Med.,* 315, 15, 1986.
29. **Korsmeyer, S. J., Greene, W. C., Cossman, J., Hsu, S., Jensen, J. P., Neckers, L. M., Marshall, S. L., Bakhshi, A., Depper, J. M., Leonard, W. J., Jaffe, E. S., and Waldmann, T. A.,** Rearrangement and expression of immunoglobulin genes and expression of Tac antigen in hairy cell leukemia, *Proc. Natl. Acad. Sci. U.S.A.,* 80, 4522, 1983.
30. **Cleary, M. L., Wood, G. S., Warnke, R., Chao, J., and Sklar, J.,** Immunoglobulin gene rearrangements in hairy cell leukaemia, *Blood,* 64, 99, 1984.
31. **Downing, J. R., Grossi, C. E., Smedberg, C. T., and Burrows, P. D.,** Diffuse large cell lymphoma in a patient with hairy cell leukaemia: immunoglobulin gene analysis reveals separate clonal origins, *Blood,* 67, 739, 1986.
32. **Giardina, S. L., Schroff, R. W., Woodhouse, C. S., Golde, D. W., Oldham, R. K., Cleary, M. L., Sklar, J., Pritkin, N., and Foon, K. A.,** Detection of two distinct malignant B cell clones in a single patient using anti-idiotype monoclonal antibodies and immunoglobulin gene rearrangement, *Blood,* 66, 1017, 1985.
33. **Foon, K. A. and Todd, R. F.,** Immunological classification of leukaemia and lymphoma, *Blood,* 68, 1, 1986.
34. **Foroni, L., Catovsky, D., Rabbitts, T. H., and Luzzatto, L.,** DNA rearrangements of immunoglobulin genes correlate with phenotypic markers in B cell malignancies, *Mol. Biol. Med.,* 2, 63, 1984.
35. **van Dongen, J. J. M., Hooijkaas, H., Michiels, J. J., Grosveld, G., de Klein, A., van det Kwast, Th.H., Prins, M. E. F., Abels, J., and Hagermeijer, A.,** Richter's syndrome with different immunoglobulin light chains and different heavy chain gene rearrangements, *Blood,* 64, 571, 1984.
36. **Ford, A. M., Molgaard, H. V., Greaves, M. F., and Gould, H. J.,** Immunoglobulin gene organisation and expression in haemopoietic stem cell leukaemia, *EMBO J.,* 2, 997, 1983.
37. **Bakhishi, A., Minowada, J., Arnold, A., Cossman, J., Jensen, J., Whang-Pen, J., Waldmann, T. A., and Korsmeyer, S. J.,** Lymphoid blast crises of chronic myelogenous leukaemia represent stages in the development of B cell precursors, *N. Engl. J. Med.,* 309, 826, 1983.
38. **Ha, K., Freedman, M. F., Hrincu, A., Petsche, D., Poon, A., and Gelfand, E. W.,** Separation of lymphoid and myeloid blasts in the mixed blast crisis of chronic myelogenous leukaemia: no evidence for Ig gene rearrangement in CALLA-positive blasts, *Blood,* 66, 1404, 1985.
39. **Rabbitts, T. H., Foster, A., and Matthews, J. G.,** The breakpoint of the Philadelphia chromosome 22 in chronic myeloid leukaemia is distal to the immunoglobulin lambda light chain constant region genes, *Mol. Biol. Med.,* 1, 11, 1983.
40. **Zalcberg, J. R., Friedlander, M. L., and Minden, M. D.,** Molecular evidence for the clonal origin of blast crisis in chronic myeloid leukaemia, *Br. J. Cancer,* 53, 459, 1986.

41. **Arnold, A., Cossman, J., Bakhshi, A., Jaffe, E. S., Waldmann, T. A., and Korsmeyer, S. J.**, Immunoglobulin-gene rearrangements as unique clonal markers in human lymphoid neoplasms, *N. Engl. J. Med.*, 309, 1593, 1983.
42. **Knowles, D. M., Dodson, L., Burke, J. S., Wang, J. Y., Bonetti, F., Pelicci, P. G., Flug, F., Dalla-Favera, R., and Wang, C. Y.**, SIg- E- ('Null-cell') Non-Hodgkin's lymphomas, *Am. J. Pathol.*, 120, 356, 1985.
43. **Cleary, M. L., Trela, M. J., Weiss, L. M., Warnke, R., and Sklar, J.**, Most null large cell lymphomas are B lineage neoplasms, *Lab. Invest.*, 53, 521, 1985.
44. **Hu, E., Thompson, J., Horning, S., Trela, M., Lowder, J., Levy, R., and Sklar, J.**, Detection of B-cell lymphoma in peripheral lymphoma by DNA hybridisation, *Lancet*, 2, 1092, 1985.
45. **Hu, E., Horning, S., Flynn, S., Brown, S., Warnke, R., and Sklar, J.**, Diagnosis of B cell lymphoma by analysis of immunoglobulin gene rearrangements in biopsy specimens obtained by fine needle aspiration. *J. Clin. Oncol.*, 4, 278, 1986.
46. **Cleary, M. L., Warnke, R., and Sklar, J.**, Monoclonality of lymphoproliferative lesions in cardiac-transplant recipients, *N. Engl. J. Med.*, 310, 477, 1984.
47. **Cleary, M. L. and Sklar, J.**, Lymphoproliferative disorders in cardiac transplant recipients are multiclonal lymphomas, *Lancet*, 2, 489, 1984.
48. **Sklar, J., Cleary, M. L., Thielmans, K., Gralow, J., Warnke, R., and Levy, R.**, Biclonal B-cell lymphoma, *N. Engl. J. Med.*, 311, 20, 1984.
49. **Siegelman, M. H., Cleary, M. L., Warnke, R., and Sklar, J.**, Frequent biclonality and Ig gene alterations among B cell lymphomas that show multiple histologic forms, *J. Exp. Med.*, 161, 850, 1985.
50. **Linch, D. C., Berliner, N., O'Flynn, K., Kay, L. A., Jones, H. M., Maclennan, K., Huehns, E. R., and Goff, K.**, Hodgkin-cell leukaemia of B cell origin, *Lancet*, 1, 78, 1985.
51. **O'Connor, N. T. J., Crick, J. A., Gatter, K. C., Mason, D. Y., Falini, B., and Stein, H.**, Cell lineage in Hodgkin's disease, *Lancet*, 1, 158, 1987.
52. **Haluska, F. G., Finver, S., Tsujimoto, Y., and Croce, C. M.**, The t(8;14) chromosomal translocation in B cell malignancies results from mistakes in V-D-J joining, *Nature*, 324, 158, 1986.
53. **Cleary, M. L., Meeker, T. C., Levy, S., Lee, E., Trela, M., Sklar, J., and Levy, R.**, Clustering of extensive somatic mutations in the variable region of an immunoglobulin heavy chain from a human B cell lymphoma, *Cell*, 44, 97, 1986.
54. **Hood, L., Kronenberg, M., and Hunkapiller, T.**, T cell antigen receptors and the immunoglobulin supergene family, *Cell*, 40, 225, 1985.
55. **Yoshikai, Y., Clark, C. P., Taylor, S., Sohn, U., Wilson, B. I., Minden, M. D., and Mak, T. W.**, Organisation and sequences of the variable, joining and constant region genes of the human T cell receptor α chain, *Nature*, 316, 837, 1985.
56. **Sims, J. E., Tunnacliffe, A., Smith, W. J., and Rabbitts, T. H.**, Complexity of human T-cell antigen receptor β-chain constant- and variable-region genes, *Nature*, 312, 541, 1984.
57. **Lefranc, M. P. and Rabbitts, T. H.**, Two tandemly organised human genes encoding the T-cell γ constant-region sequences show multiple rearrangement in different T cell types, *Nature*, 316, 464, 1985.
58. **Caccia, N., Bruns, G. A., Kirsch, I. R., Hollis, G. F., Bertness, V., and Mak, T. W.**, T cell receptor α chain genes are located on chromosome 14 at 14q11-12 in humans, *J. Exp. Med.*, 161, 1255, 1985.
59. **Croce, C. M., Isobe, M., Palumbo, A., Puck, J., Ming, J., Tweardy, D., Erikson, J., Davis, M., and Rovera, G.**, Gene for α-chain of human T cell receptor: location on chromosome 14 region involved in T cell neoplasms, *Science*, 227, 1044, 1985.
60. **Zech, L., Gahrton, G., Hammarstrom, L., Juliusson, G., Mellsted, H., Robert, K. H., and Smith, C. I. E.**, Inversion of chromosome 14 marks human T cell chronic lymphocytic leukaemia, *Nature*, 308, 858, 1984.
61. **Williams, D. L., Look, A. T., Melvin, S. L., Roberson, P. K., Dahl, G., Flake, T., and Stass, S.**, New chromosomal translocations correlate with specific immunophenotypes of childhood acute lymphoblastic leukaemia, *Cell*, 36, 101, 1984.
62. **Fukuhara, S., Hinuma, Y., Gotoh, Y., and Uchino, H.**, Chromosome aberrations in T lymphocytes carrying adult T cell leukaemia-associated antigens (ATLA) from healthy adults, *Blood*, 61, 205, 1983.
63. **Morton, C. C., Duby, A. D., Eddy, R. L., Shows, T. B., and Siedman, J. G.**, Location of gene for β subunit of human T cell receptor at band 7q35, a region prone to rearrangements in T cells, *Science*, 228, 580, 1985.
64. **Rabbitts, T. H., Lefranc, M. P., Stinson, M. A., Sims, J. E., Schroder, J., Steinmetz, M., Spurr, N. L., Solomon, E., and Goodfellow, P. N.**, The chromosomal location of T cell receptor genes and a T cell rearranging gene: possible correlation with specific translocations in human T cell leukaemia, *EMBO J.*, 4, 1461, 1985.
65. **Sangster, R. N. Minowada, J., Suciu-Foca, N., Minden, M., and Mak, T. W.**, Rearrangement and expression of the alpha, beta and gamma chain T cell receptor genes in human thymic leukaemia cells and functional T cells, *J. Exp. Med.*, 163, 1491, 1986.

66. **Royer, H. D., Acuto, O., Fabbi, M., Tizard, R., Ramachandran, K., Smart, J. E.,and Reinherz, E. L.,** Genes encoding the Tiβ subunit of the antigen/MHC receptor undergo rearrangement during intrathymic ontogeny to surface T3-Ti expression, *Cell,* 39, 261, 1984.
67. **Toyonaga, B., Yanagi, Y., Suciu-Foca, N., Minden, M., and Mak, T. W.,** Rearrangements of T cell receptor gene YT35 in human DNA from thymic leukaemia T cell lines and functional T cell clones, *Nature,* 311, 385, 1984.
68. **Minden, M. D., Toyonaga, B., Ha, K., Yanagi, Y., Chin, B., Gelfand, E., and Mak, T. W.,** Somatic rearrangement of T cell antigen receptor genes in human T cell malignancies, *Proc. Natl. Acad. Sci. U.S.A.,* 82, 1224, 1985.
69. **Flug, F., Pellicci, P. G., Bonetti, F., Knowles, D. M., and Dalla-Favvers, R.,** T cell receptor gene rearrangements as markers of lineage and clonality in T cell neoplasms, *Proc. Natl. Acad. Sci. U.S.A.,* 82, 3460, 1985.
70. **O'Connor, N. T. J., Weatherall, D. J., Feller, A. C., Jones, D., Pallesen, G., Stein, H., Wainscoat, J. S., Gatter, K. C., Isaacson, P., Lennert, K., Ramsay, A., Wright, D. H., and Mason, D. H.,** Rearrangement of the T cell receptor β chain gene in the diagnosis of lymphoproliferative disorders, *Lancet,* 1, 1295, 1985.
71. **Rabbitts, T. H., Stinson, A., Foster, A., Foroni, L., Luzzatto, L., Catovsky, D., Hammarstrom, L., Smith, C. I. E., Jones, D., Karpas, A., Minowada, J., and Taylor, A. M. R.,** Heterogeneity of T cell β chain gene rearrangements in human leukaemias and lymphomas, *EMBO J.,* 4, 2217, 1985.
72. **Tawa, A., Hozumi, N., Minden, M., Mak, T. W., and Gelfand, E. W.,** Rearrangement of the T cell receptor β chain gene in non-T cell, non-B cell acute lymphoblastic leukaemia of childhood, *N. Engl. J. Med.,* 313, 1033.
73. **Ha, K., Minden, M., Hozumi, N., and Gelfand, E. W.,** Phenotypic heterogeneity at the DNA level in childhood leukaemia with a mediastinal mass, *Cancer,* 56, 509, 1985.
74. **Jarrett, R. F., Mitsuya, H., Mann, D. L., Cossman, J. F., Broder, S., and Reitz, M. S.,** Configuration and expression of the T cell receptor β chain gene in human T-lymphotrophic virus-1 infected cells, *J. Exp. Med.,* 163, 383, 1986.
75. **Maeda, M., Shimizu, A., Ikuta, K., Okamoto, H., Kashihara, M., Uchiyama, T., Honjo, T., and Yodoi, J.,** Origin of human T-lymphotrophic virus 1-positive T cell lines in adult T cell leukaemia, *J. Exp. Med.,* 162, 2169, 1985.
76. **Foa, R., Pelicci, P. G., Migone, N., Lauria, F., Pizzolo, G., Flug, F., Knowles, D. M., and Dalla-Favera, R.,** Analysis of T cell receptor beta chain gene rearrangement demonstrates the monoclonal nature of T cell lymphoproliferative disorders, *Blood,* 67, 247, 1986.
77. **Aisenberg, A. C., Krontiris, T. G., Mak, T. W., and Wilkes, B. M.,** Rearrangement of the gene for the beta chain of the T cell receptor in T cell chronic lymphocytic leukaemia and related disorders, *N. Engl. J. Med.,* 313, 530, 1985.
78. **Falini, B., Tablico, A., Pelicci, P., Dalla-Favera, R., Donti, E., Rambotti, P., Grigani, F., and Martelli, M. F.,** T cell receptor beta chain gene rearrangement in a case of Ph′-positive chronic myeloid leukaemia blast crisis, *Br. J. Haematol.,* 62, 776, 1986.
79. **Chan, L. C., Furley, A. J., Ford, A. M., Yardumian, D. A., and Greaves, M. F.,** Clonal rearrangement and expression of the T cell receptor beta gene and involvement of the breakpoint cluster region in blast crisis of CGL, *Blood,* 67, 533, 1986.
80. **Cheng, G. Y., Minden, M. D., Toyonaga, B., Mak, T. W., and McCullwch, E. A.,** T cell receptor and immunoglobulin gene rearrangements in acute myeloblastic leukaemia, *J. Exp. Med.,* 163, 414, 1986.
81. **Bertness, V., Kirsch, I., Hollis, G., Johnson, B., and Bunn, P. A.,** T cell receptor gene rearrangements as clinical markers of human T cell lymphomas, *N. Engl. J. Med.,* 313, 534, 1985.
82. **Ramsay, A. D., Smith, W. J., Earl, H. M., Souhami, R. L., and Isaacson, P. G.,** T cell lymphomas in cases: a clinicopathological study of eighteen cases, *J. Pathol.,* 152, 63, 1987.
83. **O'Connor N. T. J.,** Genotypic analysis of lymph node biopsies, *J. Pathol.,* 151, 185, 1987.
84. **Pittaluga, S., Raffeld, M., Lipford, E. H., and Cossman, J.,** 3A1 (CD7) expression preceeds Tβ gene rearrangement in precursor T (lymphoblastic) neoplasms, *Blood,* 68, 134, 1986.
85. **Weiss, L. W., Hu, E., Wood, G. S., Moulds, C., Cleary, M. L., Warnke, R., and Sklar, J.,** Clonal rearrangements of T cell receptor genes in mycosis fungoides and dermatopathic lymphenadenopathy. *N. Engl. J. Med.,* 313, 539, 1985.
86. **Feller, A. C., Griesser, G. H., Mak, T. W., and Lennert, L.,** Lympoepitheliod lymphoma (Lennert's lymphoma) is a monoclonal proliferation of helper/inducer T cells, *Blood,* 68, 663, 1986.
87. **O'Connor, N. T. J., Feller, A. C., Wainscoat, J. S., Gatter, K. C., Pallesen, G., Stein, H., Lennert, L., and Mason, D. Y.,** T cell origin of Lennert's lymphoma, *Br. J. Haematol.,* 64, 521, 1986.
88. **Isaacson, P. G., Spencer, J., Connolly, C. E., Pollock, D. J., Stein, H., O'Connor, N. T. J., Bevan, D. H., Kirkham, N., Wainscoat, J. S., and Mason, D. Y.,** Malignant histiocytosis of the intestine: a T cell lymphoma, *Lancet,* 2, 688, 1985.

89. **O'Farrelly, C., Feighery, C., O'Briain, D. S., Stevens, F., Connolly, C., and McCarthy, C.,** Humoral response to wheat protein in patients with coeliac disease and enteropathy associated T cell lymphoma, *Br. Med. J.*, 293, 908, 1986.
90. **Weiss, L. W., Trela, M. J., Cleary, M. L., Turner, R. R., Warnke, R. A., and Sklar, J.,** Frequent immunoglobulin and T cell receptor gene rearrangements in 'histiocytic' neoplasms, *Amer. J. Pathol.*, 121, 369, 1985.
91. **Lewis, W. H., Michalopoulos, E. E., Williams, D. L., Minden, M. D., and Mak, T. W.,** Breakpoints in the human T cell antigen receptor α chain locus in two T cell leukaemia patients with chromosomal translocations, *Nature,* 317, 544, 1985.
92. **Denny, C. T., Yoshikai, Y., Mak, T. W., Smith, S. D., Hollis, G. F., and Kirsch, I. R.,** A chromosome 14 inversion in a T cell lymphoma is caused by site-specific recombination between immunoglobulin and T cell receptor loci, *Nature,* 320, 549, 1986.
93. **Baer, R., Chen, K., Smith, S. D., and Rabbitts, T. H.,** Fusion of an immunoglobulin variable gene and a T cell receptor constant gene in the chromosome 14 associated with T cell tumours, *Cell,* 43, 705, 1985.
94. **O'Connor, N. T. J., Gatter, K. C., Wainscoat, J. S., Crick, J., Jones, D. B., Delsol, G., Ralfkiaer, E., de Wolf-Peeters, C., Angus, B., and Mason, D. Y.,** Practical value of genotypic analysis for diagnosing lymphoproliferative disorders, *J. Clin. Pathol.*, 40, 147, 1987.

Chapter 10

THE N-MYC ONCOGENE IN PEDIATRIC TUMORS: DIAGNOSTIC, PROGNOSTIC AND BIOLOGICAL ASPECTS

J. A. Garson

TABLE OF CONTENTS

I. INTRODUCTION

The exponential growth in research on the molecular biology of cancer that has occurred over the past few years has provided us with significant new insights into the fundamental nature and complexities of the neoplastic process. The previously distinct fields of viral oncogenesis, chemical carcinogenesis, cytogenetics, and molecular genetics have converged dramatically around the central unifying concept of the oncogene. Despite this impressive step forward in understanding of basic mechanisms, clinical oncology in general has yet to benefit significantly from these advances. However, clinical correlations are now being made and in the case of neuroblastoma at least, these promise to bear directly upon the management of the cancer patient. In the discussion that follows, we shall briefly review some of the essential facts about oncogenes in general, in order to provide a suitable context for a more detailed consideration of N-myc and its role in pediatric tumors.

II. BIOLOGICAL MECHANISMS

A. Oncogenes

Oncogenes are a class of gene that, when activated by one of several possible mechanisms, are associated with the malignant transformation of cells *in vitro* or with the development of tumors *in vivo*.[1,2] They were first identified in animal tumor viruses and fall into two broad categories. In the first category, which will not be further discussed here, are genes such as E1a of adenovirus which are of truly viral origin and not homologous with any known eukaryote gene. In the second group are the oncogenes of the acutely transforming retroviruses, which are closely related to normal cellular genes of mammalian or avian origin.[3] Approximately 20 such retroviral oncogenes (v-onc) are known, each associated with a particular type of animal tumor (Table 1).

Interest in oncogenes increased when it was discovered by DNA hybridization studies (for description of Southern blot hybridization, see Chapter 9 by W. Smith) that normal cellular DNA from a wide variety of species, including man, contained sequences highly homologous with those of the v-oncs.[4] The term cellular oncogene (c-onc) or proto-oncogene is used to describe the normal cellular counterpart of a retroviral oncogene. It is now thought that v-oncs represent proto-oncogenes that have been "highjacked" from the host genome by retroviruses at some stage during their evolution.[1]

Oncogenes have also been identified in human tumor samples by DNA transfection experiments[5] in which tumor derived DNA is introduced into, and causes malignant transformation of, the mouse fibroblast cell line NIH/3T3. In the majority of cases, the gene responsible for inducing the malignant change has been shown to be the proto-oncogene c-ras which has been activated by a single point mutation.[6] Such mutations may arise "spontaneously" or be induced experimentally by a variety of chemical carcinogens.[3]

Activation of proto-oncogenes may also be caused by mechanisms such as "promoter insertion", in which viral regulatory sequences integrate into the host genome in the vicinity of c-oncs and increase their level of expression.[7] Chromosomal translocation,[8,9] a feature of many tumors, is another means by which normally innocuous proto-oncogenes may become activated and, thus, involved in the neoplastic process. In Burkitt's lymphoma[10] for example, the proto-oncogene, c-myc, becomes activated by juxtaposition to one or other of the immunoglobulin genes, during a reciprocal translocation most frequently involving chromosome 8 and chromosome 14 (see Chapter 9 by W. Smith in this volume). Finally, proto-oncogenes may be activated by gene amplification,[11,12] a process which increases the number of copies of the gene available for transcription; this mechanism will be considered in detail later in this chapter.

In view of their postulated role in tumor pathogenesis, the biochemical functions of proto-

Table 1
ORIGIN AND FUNCTION OF ONCOGENES

Oncogene	Viral origin or method of detection	Possible function
abl	Abelson murine leukaemia virus	Tyrosine kinase
erb-A	Avian erythroblastosis virus	Steroid receptor
erb-B	Avian erythroblastosis virus	Tyrosine kinase (EGF receptor)
ets	Avian leukaemia virus E26	?
fps	Fujinami sarcoma virus	Tyrosine kinase
fes	Snyder-Theilen feline sarcoma virus	Tyrosine kinase
fms	McDonough feline sarcoma virus	Tyrosine kinase (CSF-1 receptor)
fos	FBJ murine osteo-sarcoma virus	Nuclear
mil	Mill Hill 2 avian sarcoma virus	Serine kinase
raf	3611 murine sarcoma virus	Serine kinase
mos	Moloney murine sarcoma virus	Serine kinase
myb	Avian myeloblastosis virus	Nuclear, DNA binding
myc	Avian myelocytomatosis virus MC29	Nuclear, DNA binding
N-myc	Amplified in neuroblastoma	Nuclear, DNA binding
L-myc	Amplified in certain lung tumours	Nuclear
neu	Identified by DNA transfection	Tyrosine kinase
Ha-ras	Harvey murine sarcoma virus	GTP binding
Ki-ras	Kirsten murine sarcoma virus	GTP binding
N-ras	Identified by DNA transfection	GTP binding
rel	Avian reticuloendotheliosis virus	?
ros	UR2 avian sarcoma virus	Tyrosine kinase
sis	Simian sarcoma virus	Analogue of PDGF
ski	SKV770 avian virus	?
src	Rous sarcoma virus	Tyrosine kinase
yes	Y73 avian sarcoma virus	Tyrosine kinase

oncogenes in the normal cell are of considerable interest. Many findings now indicate that the protein products of c-oncs are fundamentally involved in information pathways between the surface membrane and the nucleus. These regulate the key functions of cell growth, division, and differentiation. The oncogene products so far analyzed (see Table 1) fall into five groups:[2,13] (1) proteins homologous to growth factors, e.g., c-sis, which codes for the beta chain of platelet derived growth factor;[14] (2) membrane bound proteins possessing tyrosine kinase activity and related to growth factor receptors, e.g., v-erb B, which codes for a truncated form of the epidermal growth factor receptor;[15] (3) cytoplasmic proteins with serine kinase activity, e.g., the products of c-raf and c-mos; (4) membrane bound proteins with GTPase activity, possibly mediating interactions between cell surface receptors and effector enzyme systems, e.g., the p21 c-ras protein; and (5) proteins located in the cell nucleus, e.g., the products of c-myb, c-fos, and the myc gene family[16] (c-myc, N-myc and L-myc). The biological functions of this last and most enigmatic group, the nuclear oncoproteins, will be discussed further in a later section.

B. Gene Amplification

As mentioned above, gene amplification is one of the mechanisms by which proto-oncogenes can become activated. In lower organisms, such as amphibians and Drosophila, selective increase in gene copy number (i.e., amplification) occurs normally during certain stages of development.[17] Even in mammals, the phenomenon is not exclusively associated with the neoplastic process, but may be seen when cells are placed under a variety of selective conditions.[12,18] The best known example of this is the amplification of the dihydrofolate reductase gene, leading to drug-resistance in response to methotrexate exposure.[19] At the cytological level, amplified genes are associated with characteristic karyotype abnormalities known as homogenously staining chromosomal regions (HSRs) and extrachromosomal double minute chromatin bodies (DMs). HSRs (so called because they tend to stain uniformly with Giemsa in G-band preparations) are relatively stable structures but DMs lack centromeres, are thus comparatively unstable and may disappear from cells altogether or participate in the formation of HSRs by chromosomal reintegration.[18]

HSRs and DMs have been reported in a wide variety of human tumor cell lines[20] and, in several instances, these have been shown by quantitative Southern blotting techniques to be associated with oncogene amplification. Genes of the myc family appear to be the most commonly involved, but amplifications of c-Ki-ras, c-myb, c-abl, c-erb B, and most recently the neu oncogene, have also been reported.[21] Although HSRs and DMs are particularly prevalent in human neuroblastoma,[22] the nature of the amplified gene(s) in these tumors remained unknown until 1983, when Schwab et al.[23] demonstrated their partial sequence homology to the proto-oncogene, c-myc. This c-myc related sequence, subsequently designated N-myc, is not associated with any known retrovirus, but is nevertheless regarded as a true proto-oncogene in view of its biological properties. Similarly, the proto-oncogene L-myc was discovered by virtue of its partial sequence homology with c-myc and its presence in amplified form in certain lung tumors.[24]

In situ hybridization studies using radioactive (^3H) probes have localized the normal single copy N-myc gene to the distal short arm of chromosome 2 (2p23-24) and confirmed that neuroblastoma HSRs are, indeed, the location of amplified N-myc sequences.[25] However, the HSRs are found, in the majority of cases, at apparently random sites throughout the genome, far distant from the normal single copy locus on chromosome 2, thus suggesting that amplification and translocation of N-myc may be interrelated processes. Little is known about these processes or about the structure and arrangement of the amplified DNA sequences in HSRs, although large inverted duplications are thought to be a common feature.[26] This lack of structural information may partly be due to the relatively low spacial resolution associated with silver grain scatter in autoradiographic *in situ* techniques. In order to overcome this problem and gain more information about HSR structure, we have developed a very high resolution, nonradioactive *in situ* technique using biotinylated DNA probes and a sensitive enzymatic detection system.[27] Using this technique,[28] we have been able to localize, more precisely than autoradiographic studies, the position of the normal single copy N-myc gene to 2p24. We have also demonstrated a previously unrecognized periodic microstructure within HSRs of a neuroblastoma cell line exhibiting N-myc amplification (Figure 1). Hybridization of the biotinylated N-myc probe in this cell line occurred at regular intervals, dividing the HSR into several (usually 5) alternating stained and unstained blocks. Although the nature of the nonhybridizing DNA between the blocks of N-myc bearing sequences remains unknown, recent molecular studies by Shiloh et al.[29] on the IMR-32 neuroblastoma cell line may provide a clue. They demonstrated that the IMR-32 HSR located in chromosome 1 was constructed not only of amplified DNA from the immediate region of the N-myc gene at 2p23-24, but also of distant sequences located more proximally at 2p13. A novel amplification/relocation/rejoining mechanism was postulated to account for their findings. The striated staining pattern of HSRs seen in our *in situ* hybridization studies may well represent direct morphological evidence of such a mechanism. Alternatively, the blocks of nonhybridizing sequences might represent amplified satellite DNA that has been incorporated into the HSR, as previously described in methotrexate resistant mouse cell lines.[30]

There is considerable uncertainty over the size of the N-myc amplicon, i.e., the amount of flanking DNA that is coamplified with the N-myc gene. Estimates vary from as little as 2.9×10^2 kb,[31] to as much as 2.4×10^3 kb.[32] From our high resolution *in situ* studies, assuming a figure of 3×10^6 kb for the size of the total human haploid genome, we estimate that the amplicon of the neuroblastoma cell line Kelly contains approximately 1.5×10^3

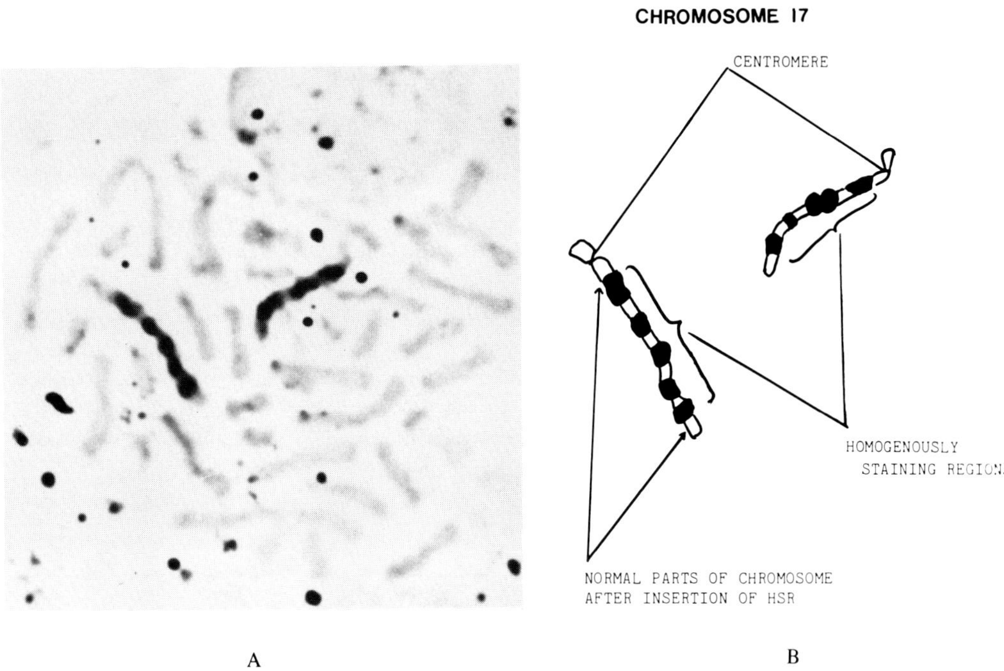

FIGURE 1. Metaphase from human neuroblastoma cell line showing striated HSRs after *in situ* hybridization with biotinylated N-myc probe. The HSRs have inserted into chromosome 17 in this particular cell line — phase contrast illumination.

kb of DNA. These discrepancies may simply be due to differences in experimental methods, but more probably reflect genuine differences in the size and structure of the amplicon between different cell lines, as has been noted previously in the methotrexate resistant mouse cell system.[33] The function, if any, of the large amount of DNA that is coamplified with N-myc is entirely unknown at present.

C. N-myc: Structure and Biological Properties

As mentioned above, N-myc was originally discovered during low stringency hybridization studies by virtue of its partial sequence homology with the nuclear proto-oncogene c-myc.[23] Subsequent sequencing of the entire N-myc gene[34] has defined the extent of this homology and revealed striking similarities with c-myc in its overall topography. Both genes contain three exons of similar length with coding elements being located in the second and third exons only and both genes have unusually long 5′ untranslated regions in their mRNAs. These long noncoding mRNA regions contain imperfect, inverted repeats (dyad symmetries) which by forming stable stem and loop structures,[5] are thought to be involved in translational control of gene expression.[35] Although the exact mechanism is uncertain, the proposed stem and loop structures are assumed to interfere with the interaction between the myc mRNA and its ribosomes.

Comparison of the proteins encoded by N-myc and c-myc also reveals remarkable similarities, with many short stretches of identical amino acids. These similarities are most marked in the carboxyl-terminal portions of the proteins which are characterized by the presence of numerous basic amino acids.[34] The resulting histone-like quality of these regions is thought to underlie the DNA-binding capabilities of both c-myc and N-myc proteins.[36,37] Other biochemical/physical similarities between the myc proteins include their predicted molecular weights (48 Kda, c-myc and 49 Kda, N-myc), their anomalous positions on SDS-polyacrylamide gels (62/66 Kda doublet, c-myc; 65/67 Kda doublet, N-myc), their phosphorylated state, and their extremely short half lives of approximately 30 min. Marked instability (i.e., short $t^{1}/_{2}$) is also a feature of other nuclear proteins, such as the products of the fos and myb proto-oncogenes.[38] This property suggests that the myc proteins are designed to undergo rapid changes in abundance and are, therefore, more likely to serve regulatory than structural purposes within the cell. Direct evidence of such a regulatory role has recently been provided by Bernards et al.[39] who demonstrated N-myc mediated down modulation of MHC class 1 antigens in rat neuroblastoma cells.

In addition to the structural and functional similarities that have been outlined above, both c-myc and N-myc possess the ability to transform embryonic fibroblasts in culture when cotransfected with the activated ras oncogene.[40] It is thought that the two cooperating oncogenes provide distinct transforming functions, the myc gene conferring "immortality" while the ras gene confers the properties of anchorage independence and loss of contact inhibition.[16]

Several observations suggest that N-myc may be involved in regulating cellular differentiation. Firstly, Thiele et al. have demonstrated that retinoic acid induced morphological differentiation of human neuroblastoma cells is preceded by a dramatic fall in N-myc mRNA expression.[41] Secondly, it has been shown by *in situ* hybridization studies on neuroblastoma tissue sections, that primitive undifferentiated neuroblasts express higher levels of N-myc mRNA than the more differentiated cells of the tumor.[42] Thirdly, analysis of mRNA extracted from developing mouse embryos has demonstrated that while c-myc expression is relatively generalized, expression of N-myc is restricted with respect to both tissue and embryonic stage.[43] Finally, there is a highly significant correlation between the extent of N-myc amplification in human neuroblastoma and the stage of the disease; the highest levels of amplification being associated with the least differentiated and most advanced tumors.[44,45] The clinical implications of this correlation will be considered further in the following section.

III. CLINICAL ROLE

A. Prognostic Implications of N-myc Amplification

Neuroblastomas are usually classified into four stages[46] (Evans classification) according to standard clinical and pathological criteria. Stage I defines a tumor confined to the organ or structure of origin. Stage II indicates that the tumor extends in continuity beyond the organ or structure of origin but does not cross the midline; regional ipsilateral lymph nodes may be involved. Stage III tumors extend beyond the midline and may involve regional lymph nodes bilaterally. Stage IV refers to large primary tumors with distant metastases involving bone, bone marrow, organs, soft tissues, or remote lymph nodes. Stage IV-s defines a group of patients (usually less than 1 year of age) with small primaries similar to stage I or II tumors, but with remote tumor in liver, skin, or bone marrow. This clinical staging system correlates well with prognosis so that patients with stage I or II disease have a 75 to 90% chance of disease-free survival at 2 years, whereas stage III and IV patients have only a 10 to 30% chance.[44] Paradoxically, stage IV-s neuroblastomas have a favorable outcome in approximately 80% of cases.[47]

Brodeur et al. were the first to report by quantitative Southern blotting analysis, a correlation between N-myc amplification in neuroblastoma and advanced clinical stage.[44] They detected between 3- and 300-fold amplification of the N-myc gene in 38% (24 of 63) of untreated tumors. Amplification was found in 0 of 15 patients with stage I or II disease but in 24 of 48 cases with stage III or IV disease. These findings were later corroborated and extended in a large study[45] by Seeger et al. who also detected N-myc amplification in 38% of untreated neuroblastomas (34 of 89). They reported amplification in 2 of 16 tumors in stage II, 13 of 20 in stage III, and 19 of 40 in stage IV. In contrast, 8 stage I and 5 stage IV-s tumors had only 1 copy of N-myc per haploid genome. Correlation of N-myc amplification with progression-free survival revealed that patients with amplification had the worst prognosis ($p<0.0001$) and that the degree of amplification was also significant. Thus at 18 months after diagnosis, patients whose tumors had 1, 3 to 10, or greater than 10 copies of N-myc per haploid genome, had a 70%, 30% or 5% chance of progression-free survival, respectively. Even within individual stages, the presence of N-myc amplification correlated with rapid disease progression, so that of 16 stage II tumors, 2 of 2 with N-myc amplification metastasized, whereas only 1 of 14 without amplification did so.

These results suggest that N-myc amplification is a useful predictor of biological behavior in neuroblastoma and indeed, that it represents a new and clinically important independent prognostic variable in this disease. However, the correlation with prognosis is by no means perfect since some patients with advanced stage disease do badly despite having only a single copy of N-myc per haploid genome. Several possible explanations have been put forward to account for this anomalous situation. For example, a small subset of neoplastic cells with N-myc amplification may be present in the tumor but at too low a level to be detectable by Southern blotting. It is also possible that overexpression may be due to faulty transcriptional regulation of a single copy N-myc gene rather than due to genomic amplification, as has been demonstrated in certain cases of retinoblastoma.[48] Alternatively, an as yet unidentified mutation may activate the N-myc gene in these cases, or N-myc may be superseded by the action of other oncogenes. Despite this reservation, it is clear that irrespective of clinical stage, patients whose tumors exhibit N-myc amplification have a high probability of early disease progression and a poor outcome with conventional cytotoxic therapy regimes. It is for this group of patients that potentially more effective, but as yet unproven modes of treatment, such as monoclonal antibody targeting[49] and autologous bone marrow transplantation[50] seem most appropriate at present.

Until early 1987, amplification of N-myc in neuroblastoma was virtually the only example of a direct association between a proto-oncogene abnormality and the clinical behavior of a human tumor. Very recently, however, Slamon et al.[21] have provided another example of such an association by demonstrating a very strong correlation between amplification of the neu oncogene and both survival and time to relapse, in patients with breast cancer. Indeed neu amplification in this disease was found to be of greater prognostic value than that of any other known prognostic variable, including clinical stage at diagnosis, patient age, lymph node involvement, and hormone-receptor status. In view of the very high incidence of the disease, approximately 119,000 new cases per year in the U.S., and the range of possible treatment options, the overall clinical impact of this finding is likely to be considerably greater than in a relatively rare disease such as neuroblastoma. Furthermore, since the neu oncogene product probably functions as a growth factor receptor (EGF receptor related) involved in the pathogenesis of the tumor, the identification of its ligand and development of specific antagonists or toxin conjugated antibodies could provide new therapeutic opportunities. In neuroblastoma, where the amplified oncogene product is located in the nucleus rather than on the cell membrane, such an approach would not be feasible although some alternative form of molecular targeting might, nevertheless, be envisaged.[1]

B. N-myc Specificity — A New Tool in Differential Diagnosis?

N-myc amplification was originally described in human neuroblastoma cell lines[23] and later reported in both retinoblastoma[48] and in small cell carcinoma of the lung with neuroendocrine properties.[51] The apparent restriction of the phenomenon to tumors of this type gave rise to the assumption that N-myc amplification was exclusively a property of tumors of neuroectodermal origin.[44,52] This in turn led to the suggestion[42,53] that the presence of N-myc amplification/overexpression might be useful as a marker in the differential diagnosis of the often morphologically indistinguishable, small round cell tumors of childhood (e.g., neuroblastoma, rhabdomyosarcoma, Ewing's sarcoma, and lymphoblastic leukemia/lymphoma).

In order to further test these claims of neural specificity, we looked for evidence of N-myc amplification in a wide variety of pediatric tumors, tissues, and cell lines. As expected, we detected amplification of N-myc in approximately 44% (n = 9) of stage IV tumors but in none of the stage I and II cases. N-myc amplification was seen in 83% (n = 6) of neuroblastoma cell lines and 80% (n = 5) of human neuroblastoma xenografts grown in nude mice. A wide range of other tumor types, including 14 Ewing's sarcomas, 11 medulloblastomas, 4 Schwannomas, 3 leukemic cell lines, and other miscellaneous non-neuroectodermal tumors showed no evidence of N-myc amplification. In addition to these findings, which were entirely compatible with the concept of neural specificity, we unexpectedly detected N-myc amplification and rearrangement in a grade III astrocytoma taken from a child with a frontal intracerebral mass.[54] This demonstrated that amplification of N-myc could occur in tumors of glial as well as of neural origin, a not entirely surprising finding since both are derived from the neuroectoderm. Much more disturbing was the discovery of ten-fold N-myc amplification in a recurrent embryonal rhabdomyosarcoma.[55] Since rhabdomyosarcoma is a tumor of mesodermal origin, this observation seriously challenges the concept of absolute neuroectodermal specificity for N-myc amplification. The possibility that this tumor was a misdiagnosed neuroblastoma was excluded by demonstration of desmin expression and the presence of characteristic cytoplasmic cross-striations.[56] N-myc amplification in another embryonal rhabdomyosarcoma was subsequently reported independently in a Japanese study.[57] In view of these findings, we would advocate extreme caution in using N-myc amplification as a differential diagnostic marker for pediatric tumors. As more extensive screening of tumor biopsy material is carried out, further apparently paradoxical examples of N-myc amplification may well emerge.

As mentioned above, amplification of the N-myc gene in the original rhabdomyosarcoma case[55] was observed in the recurrent tumor, the initial biopsy taken 18 months earlier from the same site having had only a single copy of N-myc per haploid genome. Such an increase in N-myc copy number during the course of the disease in an individual patient has not previously been reported, but represents an important observation because it lends direct support to the hypothesis[42,44,45] that N-myc amplification is primarily concerned with progression of the malignant phenotype rather than with the initiation of neoplasia per se. Further compelling evidence in support of this hypothesis has recently been provided by Bernards et al. who demonstrated that experimentally induced (by gene transfer) overexpression of the N-myc gene in a rat neuroblastoma cell line resulted in increased metastatic ability and accelerated *in vivo* growth rate.[39] It is tempting to speculate that the N-myc mediated down modulation of MHC class 1 antigen expression reported in the same study, might contribute to such neoplastic progression by allowing MHC supressed tumor cell subpopulations to evade cytotoxic T cell mediated immune surveillance.

When N-myc mRNA expression rather than DNA amplification is considered, the concept of neuroectodermal specificity as originally formulated is further weakened. Thus, Nisen et al., employing quantitative Northern blotting analysis, have reported greatly enhanced levels of N-myc expression in 12 of 13 Wilms' tumors in the absence of genomic amplification.[58] Since Wilms' tumor is derived from primitive renal cells, it is of interest to note that both human and murine fetal kidney also express significant levels of N-myc mRNA. In addition, Nisen et al. detected N-myc expression in a hepatoblastoma. They conclude that, "N-myc expression is not limited to neuroectodermal tumours as previously thought, but is a marker for several neoplasms that derive from primitive cell precursors". It is thus becoming apparent that with regard to N-myc expression, the original concept of neuroectodermal specificity will have to be drastically revised, if not altogether abandoned; clearly much work remains to be done in defining the full extent of N-myc expression in both normal and neoplastic tissues.

C. The Role of *In Situ* Hybridization and Immunohistology

N-myc mRNA expression has also been examined by *in situ* hybridization using radioiodinated DNA probes on tissue sections.[42,47] Unlike Northern blotting of tissue extracts, this technique has the potential advantage of being able to detect small numbers of cells with increased expression in a largely negative population. On the other hand, the possibility of sampling errors is considerably greater with the *in situ* technique. Despite these differences, the two approaches have produced remarkably concordant results when compared directly on the same clinical samples. Furthermore, N-myc expression analyzed *in situ* has been shown,[47] like genomic amplification, to correlate well with clinical outcome, although the number of patients so far analyzed by *in situ* methods has been low. If *in situ* analysis is eventually to find a place in routine diagnostic laboratories, replacement of ^{125}I labeled probes by nonisotopic reagents will be desirable. Kabisch et al. have made a start in this direction by using biotin labeled DNA probes to detect N-myc mRNA expression in metastatic neuroblastoma cells in bone marrow aspirates.[59] Whether such techniques will prove to be of value clinically remains to be established.

An alternative, and technically much simpler approach to the study of N-myc expression in tissue sections, would be to use antibodies specific for the N-myc gene product for immunohistochemical staining. Such antibodies have recently been described, several of which appear to be suitable for immunohistology. Ikegaki et al., using monoclonal antibodies raised against an N-myc fusion protein made in *E. coli,* detected nuclear staining in the neuroblastoma cell line IMR5 by indirect immunofluorescence.[60] Similarly, Slamon et al. reported nuclear staining in the LA-N-5 neuroblastoma cell line with rabbit antisera raised against portions of the N-myc protein produced by a bacterial expression vector.[53] These authors also described intense staining of malignant neuroblasts in clinical biopsy material from two neuroblastoma patients. One of these tumors had no evidence of genomic amplification, thus demonstrating again that as in retinoblastoma, amplification is not the only mechanism involved in determining the level of N-myc expression in human tumors.

Preliminary experiments in this laboratory have also indicated that N-myc antisera may be useful in immunohistochemistry. Using sheep antisera raised against synthetic peptides (peptide sequence deduced from the known nucleotide sequence of the N-myc gene) we have observed nuclear staining in a variety of neuroblastoma cell lines, xenografts, and primary tumors (Figure 2). Despite considerable heterogeneity in the staining intensity of individual cells, the overall staining levels we observe correlate well with Southern and Northern blotting analyses of the same samples. However, there are indications that the extremely labile nature of the N-myc protein is likely to cause problems in quantitative studies of N-myc expression in clinical samples. The same proviso applies to *in situ* hybridization studies on clinical material because of the very unstable nature of N-myc mRNA. In spite of these reservations, we feel that much information of biological and, hopefully, also of direct clinical value will be obtained in the near future by the use of these newly available immunological reagents.

IV. CONCLUSION

In summary, despite considerable doubts about the neuroectodermal specificity of the phenomenon, N-myc amplification represents a valuable new clinical tool for assessing the prognosis and, thus, optimizing the management of children with neuroblastoma. At the same time, it promises to provide important insights into the fundamental molecular mechanisms involved in the complex processes of both cellular differentiation and neoplastic progression.

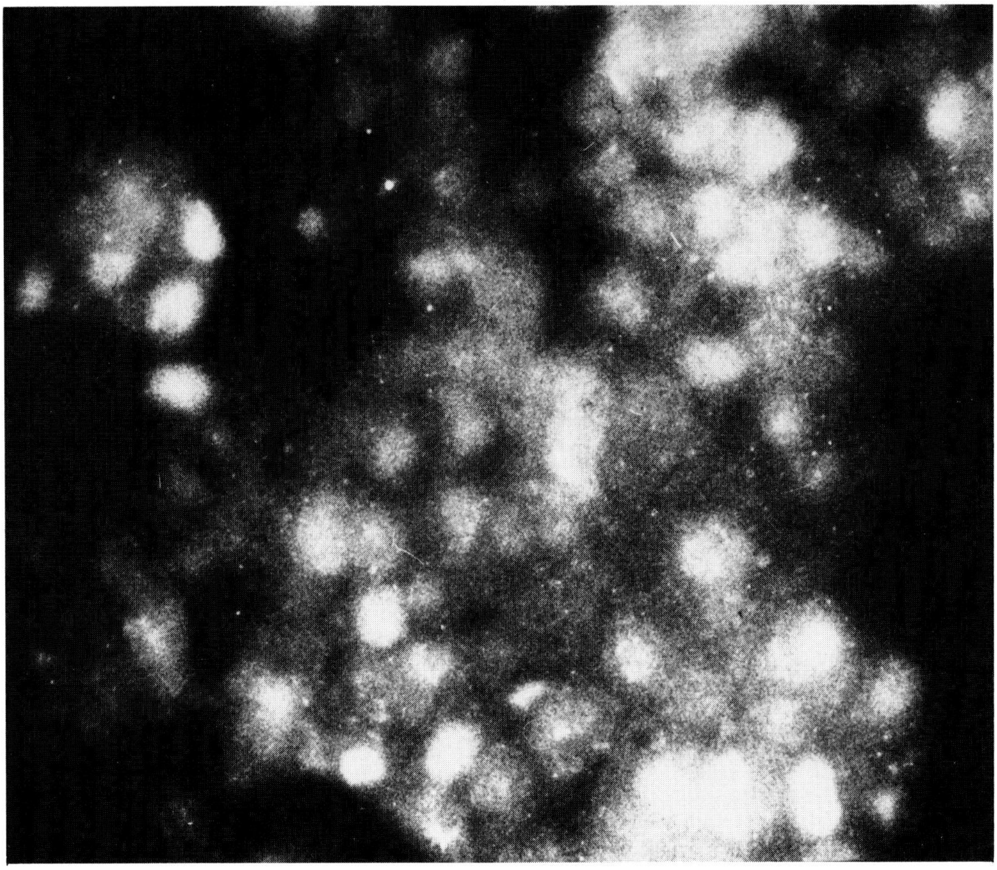

FIGURE 2A. Frozen section of N-myc amplified human neuroblastoma xenograft, stained by indirect immunofluorescence, with sheep antiserum raised against synthetic N-myc peptide. Note that the intensity of nuclear staining varies considerably from cell to cell.

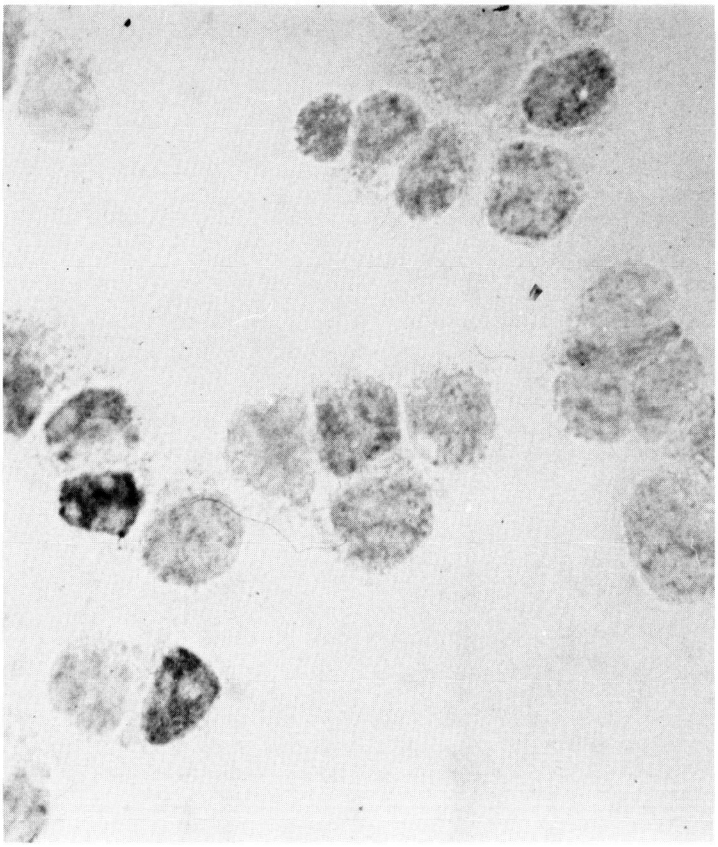

FIGURE 2B. Cytocentrifuge preparation of human neuroblastoma cell line showing N-myc amplification, stained by the ABC peroxidase technique using sheep antiserum raised against synthetic N-myc peptide. Note that the staining is nuclear and varies in intensity from cell to cell.

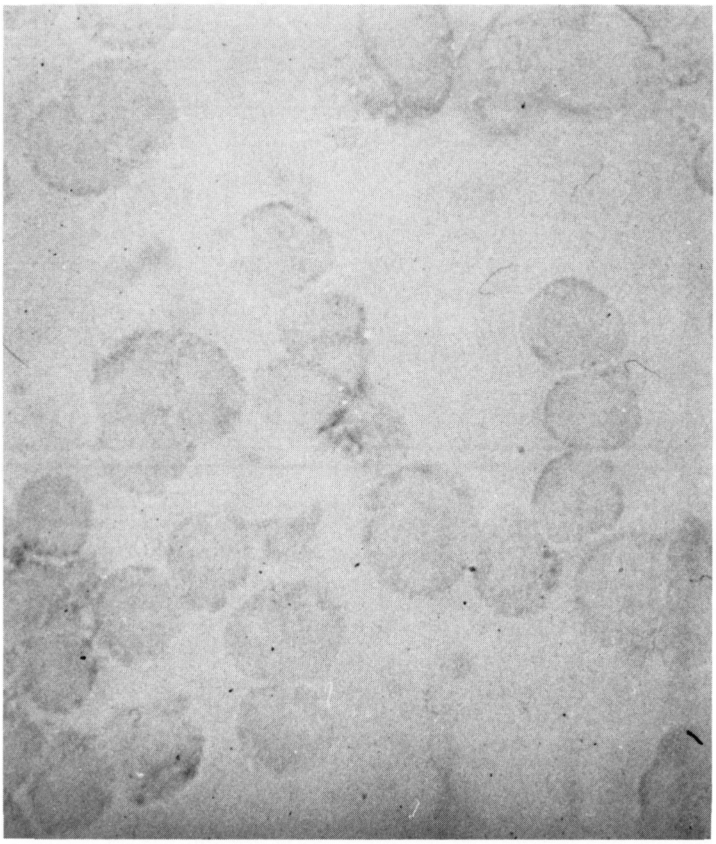

FIGURE 2C. Negative control for Figure 2B, stained with peptide absorbed antiserum.

REFERENCES

1. **Weiss, R.,** The oncogene concept, *Cancer Rev.,* 2, 1, 1986.
2. **Garrett, C.,** Critical review: oncogenes, *Clin. Chim. Acta,* 156, 1, 1986.
3. **Bishop, J.,** Trends in oncogenes, *Trends Genet.,* 1(9), 245, 1985.
4. **Stehelin, D., Varmus, H., Bishop, J., and Vogt, P.,** DNA related to the transforming gene(s) of avian sarcoma viruses is present in normal avian DNA, *Nature,* 260, 170, 1976.
5. **Paul, J.,** Oncogenes, *J. Pathol.,* 143, 1, 1984.
6. **Capon, D., Seeburg, P., McGrath, J., Hayflick, J., Edman, U., Levinson, A., and Goeddel, D.,** Activation of Ki-ras2 gene in human colon and lung carcinomas by two different point mutations, *Nature,* 304, 507, 1983.
7. **Neel, B., Hayward, W., Robinson, H., Fang, J., and Astrin, S.,** Avian leukosis virus-induced tumours have common proviral integration sites and synthesise discrete new RNAs: oncogenesis by promotor insertion, *Cell,* 23, 323, 1981.
8. **Pedersen-Bjergaard, J., Andersson, P., and Philip, P.,** Possible pathogenetic significance of specific chromosome abnormalities and activated proto-oncogenes in malignant diseases of man, *Scand. J. Haematol.,* 36, 127, 1986.
9. **Heim, S. and Mitelman, F.,** Proliferation-specific and differentiation-associated chromosomal break points in human neoplasia — a unifying model, *Hereditas,* 104, 307, 1986.
10. **Taub, R., Kirsch, I., Morton, C., Lenoir, G., Swan, D., Tronick, S., Aaronson, S., and Leder, P.,** Translocation of the c-myc gene into the immunoglobulin heavy chain locus in human Burkitts lymphoma and murine plasmacytoma cells, *Proc. Nat. Acad. Sci. U.S.A.,* 79, 7837, 1982.

11. **Schimke, R.**, Gene amplification in cultured animal cells, *Cell,* 37, 705, 1984.
12. **Stark, G.**, DNA amplification in drug resistant cells and in tumours, *Cancer Surv.*, 5(1), 1, 1986.
13. **Marshall, C.**, Oncogenes, *J. Cell Sci.*, Suppl. 4, 417, 1986.
14. **Waterfield, M., Scrace, G., Whittle, N., Stroobant, P., Johnsson, A., Wasteson, A., Westermark, B., Heldin, C., Huang, J., and Deuel, T.**, Platelet derived growth factor is structurally related to the putative transforming protein p28 sis of simian sarcoma virus, *Nature,* 304, 35, 1983.
15. **Downward, J., Yarden, Y., Mayes, E., Scrace, G., Totty, N., Stockwell, P., Ullrich, A., Schlessinger, J., and Waterfield, M.**, Close similarity of epidermal growth factor receptor and v-erb-B oncogene protein sequences, *Nature,* 307, 521, 1984.
16. **Weinberg, R.**, The action of oncogenes in the cytoplasm and nucleus, *Science,* 230, 770, 1985.
17. **Kafatos, F., Orr, W., and Delidakis, C.**, Developmentally regulated gene amplification, *Trends Genet.*, 1(11), 301, 1985.
18. **Cowell, J.**, Double minutes and homogenously staining regions: gene amplification in mammalian cells, *Ann. Rev. Genet.*, 16, 21, 1982.
19. **Alt, F., Kellems, R., Bertino, J., and Schimke, R.**, Selective multiplication of dihydrofolate reductase genes in methotrexate-resistant variants of cultured murine cells, *J. Biol. Chem.*, 253, 1357, 1978.
20. **Alitalo, K.**, Amplification of cellular oncogenes in cancer cells, *Trends Biochem. Sci.*, 10, 194, 1985.
21. **Slamon, D., Clark, G., Wong, S., Levin, W., Ullrich, A., and McGuire, W.**, Human breast cancer: correlation of relapse and survival with amplification of the HER-2/ neu oncogene, *Science,* 235, 177, 1987.
22. **Gilbert, F., Feder, M., Balaban, G., Brangman, D., Lurie, D., Podolsky, R., Rinaldt, V., Vinikoor, N., and Weisband, J.**, Human neuroblastomas and abnormalities of chromosomes 1 and 17, *Cancer Res.*, 44, 5444, 1984.
23. **Schwab, M., Alitalo, K., Klempnauer, K., Varmus, H., Bishop, J., Gilbert, F., Brodeur, G., Goldstein, M., and Trent, J.**, Amplified DNA with limited homology to myc cellular oncogene is shared by human neuroblastoma cell lines and a neuroblastoma tumour, *Nature,* 305, 245, 1983.
24. **Nau, M., Burke, J., Brooks, J., Battey, J., Sausville, E., Gazdar, A., Kirsch, I., McBride, O., Bertness, V., Hollis, G., and Minna, J.**, L-myc, a new myc-related gene amplified and expressed in human small cell lung cancer, *Nature,* 318, 69, 1985.
25. **Schwab, M., Varmus, H., Bishop, J., Grezschik, K., Naylor, S., Sakaguchi, A., Brodeur, G., and Trent, J.**, Chromosome localisation in normal human cells and neuroblastomas of a gene related to c-myc, *Nature,* 308, 288, 1984.
26. **Ford, M. and Fried, M.**, Large inverted duplications are associated with gene amplification, *Cell,* 45, 425, 1986.
27. **Garson, J., Van-den-Berghe, J., and Kemshead, J.**, High resolution *in situ* hybridisation technique using biotinylated N-myc oncogene probe reveals periodic structure of HSRs in human neuroblastoma. *Cytogenet. Cell Genet.*, 45, 10, 1987.
28. **Garson, J., Van-den-Berghe, J., and Kemshead, J.**, Novel non-isotopic *in situ* hybridisation technique detects small (1Kb) unique sequences in routinely G-banded human chromosomes: fine mapping of N-myc and B-NGF genes, *Nucleic Acids Res.*, 15(12), 4761, 1987.
29. **Shiloh, Y., Shipley, J., Brodeur, G., Bruns, G., Korf, B., Donton, T., Schreck, R., Seeger, R., Sakai, K., and Latt, S.**, Differential amplification, assembly and relocation of multiple DNA sequences in human neuroblastomas and neuroblastoma cell lines, *Proc. Natl. Acad. Sci. U.S.A.*, 82, 3761, 1985.
30. **Bostock, C. and Clark, E.**, Satellite DNA in large marker chromosomes of methotrexate-resistant mouse cells, *Cell,* 19, 709, 1980.
31. **Kinzler, K., Zehnbauer, B., Brodeur, G., Seeger, R., Trent, J., Meltzer, P., and Vogelstein, B.**, Amplification units containing human N-myc and c-myc genes, *Proc. Natl. Acad. Sci. U.S.A.*, 83, 1031, 1986.
32. **Brodeur, G. and Seeger, R.**, Gene amplification in human neuroblastomas:basic mechanisms and clinical implications, *Cancer Genet. Cytogenet.*, 19, 101, 1986.
33. **Caizzi, R. and Bostock, C.**, Gene amplification in methotrexate-resistant mouse cell lines. IV. Different DNA sequences are amplified in different resistant lines, *Nucleic Acids Res.*, 10(21), 6597, 1982.
34. **Stanton, L., Schwab, M., and Bishop, J.**, Nucleotide sequence of the human N-myc gene, *Proc. Natl. Acad. Sci. U.S.A.*, 83, 1772, 1986.
35. **Saito, H., Hayday, A., Wiman, K., Hayward, W., and Tonegawa, S.**, Activation of the c-myc gene by translocation: a model for translational control, *Proc. Natl. Acad. Sci. U.S.A.*, 80, 7476, 1983.
36. **Donner, P., Greiser-Wilke, I., and Moelling, K.**, Nuclear localisation and DNA binding of the transforming gene product of avian myelocytomatosis virus, *Nature,* 296, 262, 1982.
37. **Ramsay, G., Stanton, L., Schwab, M., and Bishop, J.**, Human proto-oncogene N-myc encodes nuclear proteins that bind DNA, *Mol. Cell. Biol.*, 6(12), 4450, 1986.
38. **Rogers, S., Wells, R., and Rechsteiner, M.**, Amino-acid sequences common to rapidly degraded proteins: The PEST hypothesis, *Science,* 234, 364, 1986.

39. **Bernards, R., Dessain, S., and Weinberg, R.,** N-myc amplification causes down modulation of MHC class 1 antigen expression in neuroblastoma, *Cell,* 47, 667, 1986.
40. **Schwab, M., Varmus, H., and Bishop, J.,** Human N-myc gene contributes to neoplastic transformation of mammalian cells in culture, *Nature,* 316, 160, 1985.
41. **Thiele, C., Reynolds, C., and Israel, M.,** Decreased expression of N-myc precedes retinoic acid-induced morphological differentiation of human neuroblastoma, *Nature,* 313, 404, 1985.
42. **Schwab, M., Ellison, J., Busch, M., Rosenau, W., Varmus, H., and Bishop, J.,** Enhanced expression of the human gene N-myc consequent to amplification of DNA may contribute to malignant progression of neuroblastoma, *Proc. Natl. Acad. Sci. U.S.A.,* 81, 4940, 1984.
43. **Zimmerman, K., Yankopoulos, G., Collum, R., Smith, R., Kohl, N., Denis, K., Nau, M., Witte, O., Allerand, D., Gee, C., Minna, J., and Alt, F.,** Differential expression of myc family genes during murine development, *Nature,* 319, 780, 1986.
44. **Brodeur, G., Seeger, R., Schwab, M., Varmus, H., and Bishop, J.,** Amplification of N-myc in untreated human neuroblastomas correlates with advanced disease stage, *Science,* 224, 1121, 1984.
45. **Seeger, R., Brodeur, G., Sather, H., Dalton, A., Siegel, S., Wong, K., and Hammond, D.,** Association of multiple copies of the N-myc oncogene with rapid progression of neuroblastomas, *N. Engl. J. Med.,* 313(18), 1111, 1985.
46. **Evans, A., D'Angio, G., and Koop, C.,** Diagnosis and treatment of neuroblastoma, *Pediatr. Clin. North Am.,* 23, 161, 1976.
47. **Grady-Leopardi, E., Schwab, M., Ablin, A., and Roseman, W.,** Detection of N-myc oncogene expression in human neuroblastoma by *in situ* hybridisation and blot analysis: relationship to clinical outcome, *Cancer Res.,* 46, 3196, 1986.
48. **Lee, W., Murphree, A., and Benedict, W.,** Expression and amplification of the N-myc gene in primary retinoblastoma, *Nature,* 309, 458, 1984.
49. **Kemshead, J., Jones, D., Lashford, L., Pritchard, J., Gordon, I., Breatnach, F., and Coakham, H.,** ^{131}-I coupled to monoclonal antibodies as therapeutic agents for neuroectodermally derived tumours: fact or fiction?, *Cancer Drug Deliv.,* 3, 25, 1986.
50. **Kemshead, J., Heath, L., Gibson, F., Katz, F., Richmond, F., Treleaven, J., and Ugelstad, J.,** Magnetic microspheres and monoclonal antibodies for the depletion of neuroblastoma cells from bone marrow. Experiences, improvements and observations, *Br. J. Cancer,* 54, 771, 1986.
51. **Nau, M., Carney, D., Battey, J., Johnson, B., Little, C., Gazdar, A., and Minna, J.,** Amplification, expression and rearrangement of c-myc and N-myc oncogenes in human lung cancer, *Curr. Top. Microbiol. Immunol.,* 113, 172, 1984.
52. **Schwab, M.,** Amplification of N-myc in human neuroblastomas, *Trends Genet.,* 1(10), 271, 1985.
53. **Slamon, D., Boone, T., Seeger, R., Kieth, D., Chazin, V., Lee, H., and Souza, L.,** Identification and characterisation of the protein encoded by the human N-myc oncogene, *Science,* 232, 768, 1986.
54. **Garson, J., McIntyre, P., and Kemshead, J.,** N-myc amplification in malignant astrocytoma, *Lancet,* 2, 718, 1985.
55. **Garson, J., Clayton, J., McIntyrre, P., and Kemshead, J.,** N-myc oncogene amplification in rhabdomyosarcoma at relapse, *Lancet,* 1, 1496, 1986.
56. **Altmannsberger, M., Weber, K., Droste, R., and Osborne, M.,** Desmin is a specific marker for rhabdomyosarcoma of human and rat origin, *Am. J. Pathol.,* 118, 85, 1985.
57. **Mitani, K., Kurosawa, H., Suzuki, A., Hayashi, Y., Hanada, R., Yamanoto, K., Komatsu, A., Kobayashi, N., Nakagome, Y., and Yamada, M.,** Amplification of N-myc in rhabdomyosarcoma, *Jpn. J. Cancer Res.,* (Gann), 77, 1062, 1986.
58. **Nisen, P., Zimmerman, K., Cotter, S., Gilbert, F., and Alt, F.,** Enhanced expression of the N-myc gene in Wilms' tumours, *Cancer Res.,* 46, 6217, 1986.
59. **Kabisch, H., Heinsolm, S., Milde, K., Loning, T., Barth, S., and Erthmann, R.,** Detection of neuroblastoma cells in bone marrow by *in situ* hybridisation, *Eur. J. Paediatr.,* 145, 323, 1986.
60. **Ikegaki, N., Bukovsky, J., and Kennett, R.,** Identification and characterisation of the N-myc gene product in human neuroblastoma cells by monoclonal antibodies with defined specificities, *Proc. Natl. Acad. Sci. U.S.A.,* 83, 5929, 1986.

INDEX

A

B

C

D

E

F

G

H

M

N

O

P

Q

R

S